Joint Mobilization/ Manipulation

EXTREMITY AND SPINAL TECHNIQUES

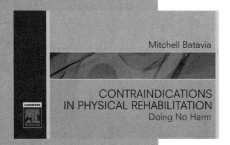
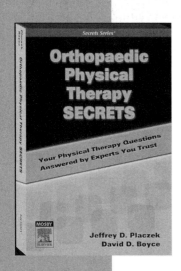
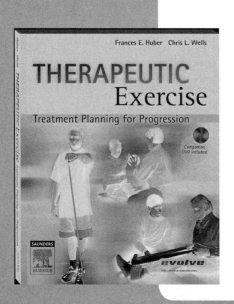

Joint Mobilization/ Manipulation

EXTREMITY AND SPINAL TECHNIQUES

SUSAN L. EDMOND, P.T., D.Sc., O.C.S.
Associate Professor
Doctor of Physical Therapy
University of Medicine and Dentistry of New Jersey

SECOND EDITION

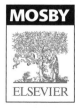
MOSBY

ELSEVIER

MOSBY
ELSEVIER

11830 Westline Industrial Drive
St. Louis, Missouri 63146

JOINT MOBILIZATION/MANIPULATION: ISBN-13: 978-0-323-02726-7
EXTREMITY AND SPINAL TECHNIQUES ISBN-10: 0-323-02726-1

Notice

Neither the Publisher nor the Author assume any responsibility for any loss or injury and/or damage to persons or property arising out of or related to any use of the material contained in this book. It is the responsibility of the treating practitioner, relying on independent expertise and knowledge of the patient, to determine the best treatment and method of application for the patient.

The Publisher

Previous editions copyrighted 1993 by Mosby, Inc.

Library of Congress Cataloging-in-Publication Data

Edmond, Susan L.
    Joint mobilization/manipulation: extremity and spinal techniques/Susan L. Edmond. – 2nd ed.
        p. ; cm.
    Rev. ed. of: Manipulation and mobilization/Susan L. Edmond. c1993.
    Includes bibliographical references and index.
    ISBN-13: 978-0-323-02726-7 (alk. paper)
    ISBN-10: 0-323-02726-1 (alk. paper)
    1. Manipulation (Therapeutics) 2. Extremities (Anatomy)—Diseases—Physical therapy. 3. Spine—Diseases—Physical therapy. I. Edmond, Susan L. Manipulation and mobilization. II. Title. III. Title: Joint mobilization manipulation.
    [DNLM: 1. Manipulation, Orthopedic. 2. Manipulation, Spinal. WB 535 E24j 2006]
RD736.M25E35 2006
615.8′2—dc22

2006044895

ISBN-13: 978-0-323-02726-7
ISBN-10: 0-323-02726-1

Acquisitions Editor: Kathy Falk
Developmental Editor: Patricia Gillivan
Publishing Services Manager: Pat Joiner
Project Manager: Jennifer Clark
Designer: Andrea Lutes

Printed in the United States of America.

Last digit is the print number: 9 8 7 6 5 4 3

To
Derek,
my son,
for being in my life.

Reviewers

Katherine L. Beissner, Ph.D., P.T.
Ithaca College
Ithaca, New York

Lee C. Grinonneau, M.S., P.T.
Owens State Community College
Toledo, Ohio

Peter M. Leininger, M.S., P.T., O.C.S., C.S.C.S.
The University of Scranton
Scranton, Pennsylvania

L. Vince Lepak III, P.T., M.P.H., C.W.S.
University of Oklahoma Health Sciences Center
Tulsa, Oklahoma

Becky J. Rodda, P.T., M.H.S., O.C.S., O.M.P.T.
University of Michigan–Flint
Flint, Michigan

Richard Biff Williams, Ph.D., A.T.C., L.A.T.
University of Northern Iowa
Cedar Falls, Iowa

Preface

The motivation for writing the first edition of this book was to provide entry-level students and practicing clinicians with a practical guide for learning the art and science of joint mobilization/manipulation. Since the publication of the first edition in 1993, much has changed in the discipline of manual therapeutic techniques. One notable change is the increased emphasis on evidence-based practice. Implicit in the use of evidence-based practice is the critical appraisal of theories and techniques that are commonly used to evaluate and treat patients using the best available research.

I firmly believe that we serve our patients most effectively when we consistently apply results from clinical research to our decisions regarding patient care. In this edition, I have incorporated information from available research regarding evaluation and intervention techniques associated with joint mobilization/manipulation. There is much we have yet to learn about this discipline, and I have identified some of the areas in which additional research is needed. I trust that with the changes and additions to this second edition, I have provided the reader with an important resource for advancing the understanding and implementation of effective evaluation and treatment procedures involving mobilization/manipulation of the extremities and spine.

Susan L. Edmond, P.T., D.Sc., O.C.S.

Acknowledgments

To my colleague, Robyn Lieberman, whose editing, advice, and support made this book happen, and who contributed her time to model for videos and stills.

To my students and colleagues, who continually educate and inspire me.

To the folks at Elsevier, especially Marion, Pat, and Bruce, for their patience and guidance, and to Jill and Fred for their video and photo expertise.

Susan L. Edmond, P.T., D.Sc., O.C.S.

How to Use This Manual

This book was designed to provide the student of manual therapy with a text to accompany formal coursework as well as a resource for self-teaching joint mobilization/manipulation techniques. Suggestions for how this book can further assist in the learning of these manual techniques come in the following paragraphs.

If the student is practicing these techniques with another student, then one student can act as the patient, while the other student can act as the therapist. The 'patient' should read the description of the technique while the 'therapist' performs the technique on the 'patient.' Both clinicians should examine the description of the technique, comparing it with the manner in which the technique is being performed, and provide feedback regarding whether the technique is being executed correctly. The 'patient' then changes roles to 'teacher', and directs the 'therapist' to carry out additional tasks related to clinical situations, such as performing a specific grade of mobilization/manipulation, or performing the technique in the restricted range for a specific direction. Again, both clinicians critique the manner in which the procedure is executed.

Also, the student might find it helpful to mark the photographs in the book with a symbol designating the stabilizing hand (such as an X) and the mobilizing/manipulating hand (such as an □ or an O). This should be done *after* the student has read the description of the technique, so that the specific information (regarding which bone to stabilize and which bone to mobilize/manipulate when performing a specific technique) is reinforced during the process of marking the photographs.

Contents

Section I

Introduction

CHAPTER 1

General Concepts

DEFINITION

Joint mobilization has been defined by Maitland[1] as an externally imposed, small-amplitude passive motion that is intended to produce gliding or traction at a joint. Joint manipulation traditionally has been defined as a specific technique in which the articular capsule is passively stretched by delivering a quick thrust maneuver to the joint, and has been considered by many clinicians to be a particular type of joint mobilization technique. In an attempt to consolidate these definitions, the American Physical Therapy Association[2] presented the following definition of *mobilization/manipulation*: a manual therapy technique comprising a continuum of skilled passive movements to the joints or related soft tissues (or both) that are applied at varying speeds and amplitudes, including a small-amplitude/high-velocity therapeutic movement. This definition encompasses multiple techniques, including those referred to by Maitland[1] in the aforementioned definition (called *passive accessory mobilization/manipulation*), passive joint movement techniques induced by active contraction of the patient's own muscles (called *muscle energy*), and passive joint movements that occur simultaneously with active range of motion (called *mobilization with movement*) or passive range of motion (called *passive physiological mobilization/manipulation*). As a general rule, passive accessory joint mobilization/manipulation and passive physiological joint mobilization/manipulation can be performed using either quick thrust or slower amplitude maneuvers, whereas muscle energy and mobilization with movement are performed using slower maneuvers.

HISTORY

Joint mobilization/manipulation has been a part of medicine since recorded history. There is some evidence that manual techniques were used in Thailand around 2000 B.C. as well as in ancient Egypt. Hippocrates used manual traction in the treatment of spinal deformities. In Europe during the 1600s, bonesetters developed an entire practice consisting of joint mobilization/manipulation techniques. This discipline persisted throughout the 1800s. Although ignorant of much of the anatomical and physiological basis for mobilization/manipulation, bonesetters used a series of techniques that were often successful in reducing pain and deformity.

The practices of osteopathic and chiropractic medicine were conceived of in the late 19th to early 20th century. Osteopathic and chiropractic medicine are based on the theory that diseases, including spinal conditions, are due to vertebral joint impairment. Some of the techniques practiced by osteopaths and chiropractors resemble those of bonesetters.

Osteopathy is based on the premise that disease processes frequently manifest themselves in the neuromusculoskeletal system, resulting in *somatic dysfunction*. Somatic dysfunction is defined as impairment in the skeletal, arthrodial, and myofascial systems with resultant alteration in vascular, lymphatic, and neural tissue. Manipulative therapy is believed to normalize the somatic system.

The osteopathic neuromusculoskeletal examination includes a determination of the presence of joint asymmetry, joint movement restrictions, and soft tissue texture changes. Treatment includes manipulation, mobilization, and muscle energy, among other techniques.

Chiropractors also believe that disease processes can manifest themselves in the neuromusculoskeletal system, causing somatic dysfunction, although they place greater emphasis on the role of the spinal nerves. The chiropractic examination also focuses primarily on joint asymmetry and restrictions, and treatment most often consists of thrust joint manipulation.

Osteopaths continue to use mobilization/manipulation as an adjunct to medical intervention, but have expanded their education to a level comparable to that of medical physicians, with additional training in mobilization/manipulation. Most chiropractors now believe that most diseases cannot be cured by spinal manipulation and focus their treatments to address specifically spinal impairments. Both of these disciplines have contributed to the knowledge base of manual therapy as currently practiced by physical therapists.

PRACTITIONERS CONTRIBUTING TO THE KNOWLEDGE BASE OF JOINT MOBILIZATION AND MANIPULATION

Numerous practitioners, including medical physicians and physical therapists, have contributed to the current knowledge base of joint mobilization/manipulation evaluation and intervention techniques.

Mennell

Mennell developed the concept that joint adhesions are a common cause of joint impairments, as they alter movement between two joint surfaces. He advocated that clinicians evaluate patients for loss of joint motion. He also promoted the concept that this loss of joint motion could be treated effectively with mobilization techniques.

Cyriax

Cyriax was an orthopedic physician who contributed to the development of a system of examination of patients with musculoskeletal impairments commonly used by physical therapists. This system focuses on using different tests to selectively isolate one soft tissue from another to determine which soft tissue is responsible for the patient's symptoms. He advocated including mobilization as part of this examination. Cyriax also brought into common use some of the thrust joint manipulation techniques practiced today, many of which were developed to treat spinal disc conditions.

Kaltenborn

Kaltenborn proposed that the clinician should evaluate patients for joint mobility restrictions and soft tissue changes, and treat with glide and traction mobilizations. Glide mobilization interventions should be performed in a specific direction, based on the evaluation of the restriction in range of motion and the shape of the articular surface. He also developed the concepts of close-packed and loose-packed joint positions; testing with compression, distraction, and gliding; and a three-grade (I, II, III) categorization system for describing joint mobilization techniques.

Maitland

Maitland is a strong advocate of performing a thorough examination on each patient to determine the position, movement, or test that reproduces the patient's symptoms. This examination includes testing osteokinematic (physiological range of motion) and accessory (joint) movements. Maitland also developed a system of determining the "irritability," or acuity of a patient's symptoms, based on the intensity of symptoms as they relate to the physical examination and to functional activities, and an intervention strategy in which the aggressiveness of treatment is based on this determination. Intervention often includes joint mobilization/manipulation. The direction of the intervention mobilization/manipulation is determined primarily by the direction of the examination technique that reproduced symptoms. Maitland also developed the four-grade (I, II, III, IV) categorization system of mobilization intervention techniques that is in common use today and extended this system to include grade V thrust manipulations.

Mulligan

Mulligan built on the approach established by Maitland. He advocates combining joint mobilization/manipulation techniques with active range of motion, a technique he calls *mobilization with movement*. This technique entails applying a mobilization force to a joint while the patient performs a specific movement. Mulligan believes this method of joint mobilization/manipulation is effective in correcting mechanical impairments such as positional faults and increasing joint range of motion.

Paris and Grimsby

Also worthy of mention for their roles in the development of manipulative therapy are Paris and Grimsby, who helped to systematize and disseminate information regarding mobilization/manipulation to clinicians.

Paris proposed that intervention should focus on correcting joint mobility impairments, thus minimizing the role of pain.

Summary

The role of joint mobilization/manipulation in the evaluation and intervention of movement impairments is strongly influenced by the experiences, insight, and charisma of numerous clinicians. In some cases, these different philosophies and strategies of mobilization/manipulation evaluation and intervention conflict with one another. Little, if any, research has compared the specific tenets of these various philosophies with one another. At this time, it is unclear whether or under what circumstances choosing one discipline or practitioner's approach over another would result in better outcomes and, if so, which approach is optimal.

EVIDENCE-BASED PRACTICE

Traditionally, much of the practice of physical therapy, and specifically joint mobilization/manipulation, has evolved because of the influence of practitioners who were able to organize their clinical experience into a cohesive entity and disseminate this information to other clinicians. These clinicians are to be commended for their insight and effort. Nevertheless, as Rothstein[3] eloquently stated, "we do a disservice to the pioneers of manual therapy when we worship their words and fail to advance the scientific basis on which they first developed."

Evidence-based practice is a process of health care decision making that has evolved since the 1970s and is increasingly influencing physical therapy practice. One consequence of the movement toward evidence-based practice is the critical evaluation of health care theories and techniques using the best available research.

Adhering to evidence-based practice principles involves not only applying the *best research evidence* to a patient scenario, but also integrating *clinical expertise* and *patient values* into the decision-making process.[4] Using the "best research evidence" entails the conscientious, explicit, and judicious use of clinically relevant research in making decisions about the care of individual patients.[4,5] The integration of clinical expertise involves the ability to use clinical skills and past experience to identify a patient's unique health status and the risks and benefits of potential interventions. Finally, each patient has unique preferences, concerns, and expectations that have an impact on the outcome of the therapeutic intervention. Patient care decisions should entail the identification and consideration of patient values.[4]

Take the example of a patient who reports experiencing a recent exacerbation of low back pain accompanied by radicular symptoms of numbness and weakness in the L4 nerve root distribution that had been treated successfully in the past with spinal thrust joint manipulation. A review of the literature on the efficacy of spinal manipulation for acute lumbar radiculopathy suggests that spinal manipulation might not be effective for these patients. The decision whether to intervene with spinal manipulation would involve a process of weighing the evidence, which does not strongly support the intervention, with the patient's expectations, which do support the intervention, and the clinician's own experience with using spinal manipulation on patients with similar signs and symptoms. One of several solutions to this clinical dilemma might be to use the least aggressive manipulation procedure known to the clinician, perform it only once during that treatment session, and monitor the result of that intervention carefully for the purpose of determining future actions. By adhering to the tenets of evidence-based practice, we are recognizing the importance of all three of the aforementioned components, and not just information gleaned from research studies.

The objective of this book is to describe the strategies and techniques commonly used by physical therapists to examine, evaluate, and treat musculoskeletal impairments with joint mobilization/manipulation and to evaluate them in relation to the current best evidence. The specific articles referenced in this book were chosen based on best research evidence principles, relative to the specific issue being addressed.

There are numerous concerns with determining the validity of studies addressing the efficacy of manual techniques in the treatment of patients with musculoskeletal conditions. Foremost is the issue with the strong placebo effects that accompany interventions involving the laying on of hands, especially the placebo effects associated with thrust joint manipulations accompanied by an audible crack. One additional concern is that many musculoskeletal conditions are self-limiting: many patients improve with time regardless of the intervention. For these reasons, in this book, priority was given to reporting efficacy studies that used a placebo or comparison group.

One other major concern with study validity involves the difficulty in blinding clinicians and subjects to the intervention the subjects are receiving. Especially in relation to clinician blinding, most intervention studies investigating mobilization/manipulation techniques were unsuccessful in avoiding this pitfall, adversely affecting the validity of these study results.

One issue related to spine research, but applicable to all musculoskeletal impairments, is the manner in which impairments are classified. If joint mobilization/manipulation is extremely effective with one type of back pain, but relatively ineffective with other types, studies that do not correctly classify patients in such a way as to identify this trend would not be likely to show positive effects from the mobilization/manipulation intervention. Many studies do not make any attempt to classify subjects beyond identifying them as having pain in a particular location. At best, subjects also are classified based on symptom acuity. An alternative explanation for results of studies indicating that joint mobilization/manipulation is not efficacious would be that the inclusion criteria was not suitable for finding an effect.

INDICATIONS FOR JOINT MOBILIZATION AND MANIPULATION

Numerous rationales for performing joint mobilization/manipulation have been advanced. The major indications recognized by physical therapists and the evidence supporting or refuting these indications are discussed in this section. Many of these indications most likely operate in conjunction with one another. For example, it is possible that, in addition to the reasons outlined under "pain reduction," pain also might be reduced through other mechanisms, such as muscle relaxation, an increase in the range of motion of periarticular muscles, or an increase in nutrition to the joint.

Increasing Joint Extensibility and Joint Range of Motion

Theory

All joints are capable of physiological movement. Physiological movement occurs when muscles contract concentrically or eccentrically, or when gravity causes the position of one bone of a joint to change in relation to the other bone. This type of movement is categorized as *osteokinematic motion*. The different directions of movement that each joint is capable of are called its *osteokinematic degrees of freedom,* defined as the number of components within a movement system that specify position in space. A maximum of 6 different degrees of freedom are possible in each joint: 4 degrees of freedom occur as the bone moves in both directions in two planes of motion perpendicular to one another, and 2 degrees of freedom occur as the bone rotates around an axis perpendicular to the joint surfaces. In most cases, the joint motion accompanying functional activities is the result of a combination of more than one osteokinematic motion.

Joints also undergo *arthrokinematic motion,* which is defined as movement between two articulating surfaces without reference to any of the external forces being applied to that joint. The number of arthrokinematic movements that occurs at each joint is determined by the number of accessory motions. *Accessory motion* has been defined as movement occurring between two joint surfaces that is produced by forces applied by the examiner[6] and, as with osteokinematic motion, usually refers only to movement in cardinal planes.

Normal accessory motion is believed to be necessary for full, pain-free osteokinematic movement to occur. Joint mobilization/manipulation entails moving a joint through its accessory motion, thereby maintaining or increasing the extensibility of articular structures. Joint mobilization/manipulation is therefore the recommended treatment for restoring normal accessory motion, which is one criterion for the restoration of normal osteokinematic motion. Although theoretically the joint capsule is the structure affected by joint mobilization/manipulation intervention techniques, most likely other periarticular tissues, such as tendons, muscles, and fascia, also are targeted when joint mobilization/manipulation is performed.

Some clinicians believe that accessory motion can be decreased even when joint range of motion is normal, and that this impairment can lead to limitations in function. For example, full shoulder elevation can occur despite the inability of the humeral head to glide fully in an inferior direction in the glenoid cavity. This limitation in accessory motion is believed to be one cause of pain from glenohumeral joint impingement syndrome.

Articular and periarticular restrictions have been shown to result from immobilization of joints. Early studies have identified many of the biomechanical and biochemical effects of immobilization on joint capsules. With immobilization, there is a decrease in water content, resulting in a reduction in the distance between the fibers constituting the joint capsule. This causes an increase in fiber cross-link formation, which produces adhesions. In the absence of movement, as new collagen tissue is produced, additional cross-linking occurs. Immobilization also produces adhesions between synovial folds. Additionally, fibrofatty connective tissue proliferates within the joint and adheres to cartilaginous structures. Finally, the strength of collagen tissue decreases, resulting in a decrease in the load-to-failure rate.[7-9]

Joint mobilization/manipulation is thought to reverse these changes by promoting movement between capsular fibers. This movement is believed to result in an increase in interstitial water content and interfiber distance. It also is believed that when joints are mobilized/manipulated, synovial tissue stretches in a selective manner, causing a gradual rearrangement of collagen tissue with a reduction of cross-link formation and the development of parallel fiber configuration in newly forming collagen tissue. More aggressive manipulation techniques are thought to break adhesion in the joint capsule and synovial folds and increase the length of capsular fibers. These responses to mobilization/manipulation are believed to have the mechanical effect of increasing the amount of arthrokinematic motion and consequently osteokinematic motion at a joint.

Studies of continuous passive motion machines have shown that movement does decrease the formation of capsular adhesions. Still, there are no studies that identify histological joint changes resulting from joint mobilization/manipulation techniques. There also is no conclusive research providing information regarding the optimal type of mobilization/manipulation intervention, the amount of time a joint should be mobilized/manipulated, or the optimal amount of force required to treat any of the many joint impairments, despite the fact that these parameters are likely to have an impact on the efficacy of joint mobilization/manipulation interventions. Nevertheless, increasing joint mobility is the most common rationale given by clinicians for performing joint mobilization/manipulation interventions.

Evidence

Numerous studies have addressed the effect of joint mobilization/manipulation on joint range of motion in several peripheral joints: the shoulder, wrist, metacarpophalangeal joints, and ankle. The earliest study was performed on mongrel dogs. The right carpal joint of 12 dogs was immobilized for 6 weeks. The dogs were randomly assigned to receive either passive range of motion or passive range of motion with the addition of joint mobilization. Outcomes were measured weekly for 4 weeks and consisted of functional range of motion and the amount of time to reach maximum range of motion during gait. The investigator concluded that although range of motion improvements were greater in the group receiving joint mobilization, the study results should be interpreted cautiously. Evidently there was a great amount of variability among study animals, including differences in the extent to which the immobilization process affected joint range of motion.[10]

A study of mobilization of hand joints was performed on 18 human subjects who were immobilized after a fracture of the metacarpophalangeal joint. Subjects were randomly assigned to receive either a home exercise program or a home exercise program with the addition of joint mobilization. Outcome measures included active and passive range of motion, evaluated three times over one week of treatment. Increases in range of motion were significantly greater in the treatment group compared with the control group. This study provides evidence to support the premise that joint mobilization, combined with exercise, improves joint range of motion.[11]

A second study addressing the effect of joint mobilization/manipulation on the metacarpophalangeal joint was performed. In this study, 33 asymptomatic subjects were randomly assigned to receive mobilization to either the left or right third metacarpophalangeal joint. The contralateral third metacarpophalangeal joint received a thrust joint manipulation. In both groups, there was an increase in range of motion, although the increase was significantly greater in the group that received manipulation.[12]

Several studies have documented increases in shoulder joint range of motion after glenohumeral joint mobilization/manipulation. In each of these studies, one objective was to determine whether gliding the glenohumeral joint in a particular direction was associated with increases in range of motion in a particular direction. Gliding techniques, performed in several different directions with sufficient force to take the joint through tissue resistance, increased motion in shoulder flexion, abduction, and rotation.[13-17] These studies are described in greater detail in Chapter 2.

In relation to the ankle joint, study results are equivocal. When 20 asymptomatic subjects received a single talocrural distraction thrust joint manipulation, there was no significant increase in dorsiflexion range of motion compared with the untreated ankle.[18] In a similar study, 41 asymptomatic subjects were randomly assigned to receive either a single talocrural distraction thrust joint manipulation or no intervention. In this study, there also was no significant increase in dorsiflexion range of motion compared with the untreated ankle.[19]

Conversely, 10 subjects whose ankles had been immobilized in a cast for 6 weeks due to a fracture were randomly assigned to receive either exercise or exercise and joint mobilization to the joints of the leg and foot, based on an accessory motion examination. Subjects who received joint mobilization in addition to exercise had a significant increase in range of motion compared with the control group.[20]

In a similar study, 22 subjects presenting to a podiatry clinic with decreased range of motion into dorsiflexion who received thrust joint manipulation were compared with subjects in a prior study who had received stretching exercises. Manipulation consisted of anterior glide of the proximal tibiofibular joint and distraction and posterior glide of the talocrural joint. The increase in dorsiflexion range of motion was significantly greater in the group receiving manipulation.[21]

In a more recent study involving ankle joint mobilizations performed on 14 subjects with lateral ankle sprains, subjects were assigned to receive mobilization with movement to the ankle, a placebo treatment, and no treatment in random order. The intervention in this study consisted of a posterior glide of the distal fibula on the tibia with repeated active ankle inversion movements. There was a significant increase in dorsiflexion range of motion after the mobilization with movement technique was performed compared with the other two conditions.[22]

Several studies addressed the effects of mobilization/manipulation on range of motion of spinal joints. In one study of 24 asymptomatic subjects with asymmetrical neck motion into side bending, the investigator concluded that there was a significant increase in cervical range of motion after thrust joint manipulation to the lower cervical spine compared with subjects assigned to receive a placebo manipulation.[23] In a second study, performed on 16 subjects with chronic neck pain, subjects showed an improvement in cervical range of motion after a thrust joint manipulation to restricted C5-6 and C6-7 segments.[24]

The relative effect of cervical spine mobilization was compared with that of thrust joint manipulation in a randomized trial of 100 subjects with neck pain. In this study, both groups experienced a similar increase in range of motion, suggesting that mobilization and manipulation are equally effective in increasing range of motion.[25]

The effect of a single thoracic spine thrust joint manipulation was studied in 78 asymptomatic subjects. Subjects were randomly assigned to receive a thoracic spine thrust manipulation to a restricted joint segment, mobility testing only, or no intervention. Thoracic spine manipulation was associated with an increase in active range of motion into left side bending, but not into right side bending or forward bending, compared with the other two groups.[26]

Several studies addressed range of motion changes after lumbar spine mobilization/manipulation. Two early studies showed improvements in range of motion after lumbar spine mobilization/manipulation. In the first study, 94 subjects were randomly assigned to receive Maitland mobilization/manipulation or a placebo treatment. Subjects receiving mobilization/manipulation experienced a significant improvement in lumbar range of motion after treatment, but no difference by 1-year follow-up, compared with the placebo group.[27] In the second study, subjects consisted of 51 women with a confirmed disc prolapse. Subjects were alternatively assigned to receive lumbar spine rotation mobilization/manipulation or diathermy, gentle flexion exercises, and patient education. The group receiving mobilization/manipulation obtained a significant increase in lumbar range of motion compared with the comparison group.[28]

A more recent study compared the relative effects of five approaches on range of motion: two different exercise programs, Maitland mobilization, an intervention consisting of physical agents, and a placebo group. A total of 250 subjects with chronic low back pain after L5 laminectomy were randomly assigned to one of the five groups. There was a significant improvement in lumbar extension range of motion in the mobilization and in the exercise groups compared with the groups receiving physical agents and no intervention, but lumbar flexion range of motion increased only in the exercise groups.[29]

In conclusion, studies addressing the effect of mobilization/manipulation on range of motion provide evidence of this association. Qualitative differences in results among studies might be due in part to differences in the type, frequency, or intensity of the mobilization/manipulation technique or to idiosyncratic differences among specific joints, subjects, or clinicians. One explanation for the result of the two studies that failed to show an association between mobilization/manipulation and range of motion is that the effect of joint mobilization/manipulation might be related to the pretreatment condition of the joint: Range of motion increases are likely to be greater in joints with signs and symptoms of impairment.

Decreasing Pain

Theory

Numerous neurological mechanisms have been proposed to explain the purported effect of pain reduction secondary to mobilization/manipulation techniques. Included are theories that propose that pain reduction occurs via activation of pain inhibitory mechanisms or pain control centers in the central or in the peripheral nervous system, or via chemical changes in peripheral nociceptors. Controversy currently exists over the validity of these theories, and to date, no single theory has emerged as being more widely accepted than others. Possibly, pain reduction from joint mobilization/manipulation is a multifaceted phenomenon.

Evidence

Several studies have shown that hypoalgesia occurs as a result of mobilization/manipulation techniques. Four of these studies addressed this effect in relation to mobilization/manipulation of peripheral joints.

In one study, 24 subjects with chronic lateral epicondylalgia were assigned to receive mobilization with movement to the elbow, a placebo treatment, and no treatment in random order. Outcome measures included pain-free grip force and pressure pain threshold, measured in the affected and unaffected arms. Results showed an increase in pain-free grip force and pressure pain threshold in the affected arm after mobilization compared with the other two conditions. There were no significant changes in the unaffected arm.[30]

The same mobilization intervention was investigated in a follow-up study of 24 subjects, also with chronic lateral epicondylalgia. The design of this study was similar to that of the first study, although in this study, outcomes were measured only on the affected limb, and thermal pain threshold was also measured. Results showed an increase in pain-free grip force and pressure pain threshold, but no change in thermal pain threshold with mobilization, compared with the other two conditions.[31]

A third study, performed by many of the same researchers and using the same study design as in the last two studies, investigated the effects of mobilization on pain in 14 subjects with lateral ankle sprains. The intervention was a mobilization with movement posterior glide of the distal fibula on the tibia with repeated active ankle inversion movements. There were no changes in pressure or thermal pain threshold after any of the three conditions.[22]

A different group of investigators studied the effects of knee mobilization on 31 rats. These animals were injected with capsaicin, a drug that causes hyperalgesia. The rats were randomly assigned to receive no contact; manual contact; or 3, 9, or 15 minutes of knee mobilization. Hyperalgesia, determined by withdrawal threshold, was decreased for 30 minutes in the group that received 9 and 15 minutes of mobilization, but not in either of the control groups or the group that received treatment for 3 minutes.[32]

Several studies addressing mobilization/manipulation and pain assessed this association in relation to the spine. In one study, 30 subjects with mid to lower cervical pain of insidious onset were studied. These subjects received an anterior glide mobilization procedure that involves taking the articular tissue through tissue resistance (grade III) to the C5 facet on the painful side, a placebo condition consisting of manual contacts, and a control condition consisting of no physical contact between subject and clinician in random order. After the mobilization technique, subjects experienced a significant increase in pressure pain thresholds and a decrease in visual analogue scores compared with the other two conditions.[33]

Pain from lateral epicondylalgia also was shown to decrease as a result of C5 side glide mobilizations in two studies. In the first study, 15 subjects received mobilization while positioned in a predetermined upper limb tension test position, placebo treatment, and no treatment in random order. Pressure pain threshold, pain-free grip strength, and pain scores improved after treatment compared with the placebo and control group conditions.[34] The second study was performed on 24 subjects with chronic lateral epicondylalgia, using the same study design. In this study, there also was evidence of greater hypoalgesia after mobilization compared with the other two conditions.[35]

The hypoalgesic effect of thoracic spine mobilization versus thrust manipulation also was studied. In this study, in which 50 asymptomatic subjects were randomly assigned to receive either mobilization or manipulation, there was a statistically significant elevation in pain tolerance to an experimentally induced electrical pain stimulus after manipulation compared with the group that received mobilization.[36]

In a randomized controlled trial involving the lumbar spine, the hypoalgesic effect of mobilization was compared with that of thrust manipulation in 30 subjects with chronic mechanical low back pain. The outcome was pain/pressure threshold of selected myofascial points at three times up to 30 minutes after treatment. There were no differences in pain/pressure threshold between the two groups.[37]

A different study of the hypoalgesic effects of lumbar spine mobilization was performed on 30 subjects with rheumatoid arthritis. These subjects were randomly assigned to receive 12 minutes of mobilization or rest. Mobilization consisted of manual oscillations that did not take the joint to tissue resistance (grades I and II) to T12 and L4 for a total of 12 minutes. Subjects receiving this intervention experienced an increase in pain threshold in their spine, knees, and ankles compared with the group receiving rest.[38]

In conclusion, there is evidence of a hypoalgesic effect after joint mobilization/manipulation. This effect seems to occur regardless of the technique being used, the joint being treated, or the impairment being addressed.

Promoting Muscle Relaxation

Theory

As with pain reduction, relaxation of periarticular muscles is believed to occur with mobilization/manipulation by means of neurological mechanisms: mobilization/manipulation stimulates joint receptors, which is thought to reflexively relax periarticular musculature.

Evidence

The effect of spinal thrust joint manipulation on muscle activity was studied in 34 subjects with joint hypomobility, with and without musculoskeletal pain. Subjects were assigned to receive thrust manipulation to hypomobile thoracic and lumbar segments or no intervention. Subjects receiving manipulation had on average a 20% reduction in paraspinal muscle activity compared with controls, determined by electromyogram activity.[39] In a different study involving subjects with unilateral low back pain, similar results were reported in relation to hamstring muscle activity measured before and after spinal manipulation.[40]

These studies suggest that spinal manipulation reduces muscle activity in muscles associated with spinal impairment. The specific mechanism of this association is unknown.

Increasing Muscle Strength

Theory

Swelling secondary to joint impairments has been shown to be a cause of inhibition of muscles that act on that joint. Some clinicians believe that this inhibition is decreased when normal joint mechanics are restored using joint mobilization/manipulation techniques.

Evidence

The effect of joint mobilization on muscle inhibition has been studied in relation to the hip. Forty asymptomatic subjects with normal hip range of motion were randomly assigned to receive an anterior glide mobilization that does not take the joint to tissue resistance (grade I) or one that does take the joint through resistance (grade IV). Gluteus maximus isometric strength at end range was measured before and immediately after the mobilization procedure was performed. Subjects receiving grade IV mobilization had a significant increase in strength compared with subjects receiving grade I mobilization. This increase in strength occurred despite the exclusion of subjects with hip joint hypomobility from the study.[41]

Most of the studies addressing the effect of mobilization/manipulation on strength were performed using spinal mobilization/manipulation interventions. In one study performed on 16 subjects with chronic neck pain, biceps muscle strength improved after a thrust joint manipulation to restricted C5-6 and C6-7 segments.[24]

An increase in lower trapezius strength occurred after a thoracic spine mobilization intervention in a study of 40 asymptomatic subjects. These subjects were randomly assigned to receive either grade IV (through tissue resistance) or grade I (not up to tissue resistance) anterior glide mobilizations to T6-12. Subjects receiving grade IV mobilization experienced a significant increase in lower trapezius muscle strength compared with subjects receiving grade I mobilizations.[42]

In another study investigating the strength effects of mobilization/manipulation, 18 subjects with anterior knee pain and sacroiliac joint dysfunction were treated with a thrust joint manipulation to correct the sacroiliac joint dysfunction on the side of the more painful knee. After correcting the sacroiliac joint dysfunction, a significant increase in knee extension torque occurred on the symptomatic side.[43]

Joint mobilization/manipulation performed through tissue resistance seems to have the effect of increasing muscle strength in the short term, regardless of whether or not the joints receiving the intervention are impaired. This finding is puzzling, given that two other studies showed an inhibitive effect on specific muscles. In the two studies showing muscle inhibition, subjects had impairments in the joints receiving the intervention, and the muscles that showed inhibition are recognized as those that often guard the impaired joints that were treated. It is therefore possible that these muscles were in spasm. The evidence suggests that joint mobilization improves muscle performance, regardless of the presence or nature of the muscle impairment.

Improving Joint Nutrition

Theory

Articular surfaces are avascular and receive their nutrition from synovial fluid. For diffusion of nutrients to occur, the synovial fluid must circulate within the capsule to allow nutrients to contact the articular surface. In normal joints, joint movement through functional activities provides a mechanism for the circulation of synovial fluid. Joints that are restricted often cannot obtain adequate nutrition because insufficient range of motion reduces movement of synovial fluid within the synovium. Joint mobilization/manipulation is believed to improve nutrition to synovial tissue by promoting the circulation of synovial fluid within the capsule.

Evidence

There are no published research studies that address this theory.

Correcting Positional Faults

Theory

Joint surfaces can alter their position in relation to one another. If this alteration in position is severe, it is called a *dislocation*; however, if minimal, it is considered a *positional fault*. Even minimal displacement is believed to place abnormal stress on periarticular structures and can be a source of pain and neuromuscular dysfunction.

Mobilization/manipulation of one of the joint surfaces in the direction consistent with realigning it into its correct position is thought by some clinicians to normalize the static positioning of one joint surface in relation to the other, thereby reducing pain. For example, if the lunate was positioned in a posterior direction in relation to the radius, treatment would be directed toward mobilizing/manipulating the lunate in an anterior direction in relation to the radius; this could result in the restoration of normal alignment of the two articular surfaces. Other clinicians believe that the positional fault can be eliminated if the joint is mobilized/manipulated in the direction of greatest restriction. Positional faults are believed to be more common in the spine than in the extremities.

Evidence

Debate currently exists regarding even the most basic concepts related to the existence of positional faults. This is due in part to the fact that positional faults are recognized by many chiropractors as being a common source of back pain, although in the chiropractic literature, they are referred to as "subluxations."

A 1988 review of the medical and chiropractic literature concluded that there is no valid research showing that subluxations/positional faults correlate with pain or are a cause of hypomobility in the spine. The authors also concluded that spinal facet subluxations (positional faults) of less than 4.5 mm are not detectable by radiography. Furthermore, when comparing pre-manipulation and post-manipulation radiographs, clinicians were not capable of detecting a change in vertebral position after a chiropractic spinal thrust joint manipulation.[44] These findings are consistent with a more recent research study involving the sacroiliac joint, in which joint manipulation did not cause a detectable change in the relative position of the ilium on the sacrum, when measured by roentgen stereophotogrammetric analysis.[45] Even if spinal positional faults are a cause of back pain, given that these changes are not detectable using radiography, any changes in spinal alignment are not likely to be detectable using manual palpation techniques, which is the most common method used by physical therapists to identify these impairments.

Eliminating Meniscoid Impingement

Theory

Intracapsular meniscoid structures are present in some joints, most notably tibiofemoral and spinal facet articulations. Facet menisci are believed to be capable of becoming entrapped, or impinged, between the two facet joint surfaces, causing the joint surfaces to lock. This impingement is thought to occur most often with movement into spinal flexion and rotation and is accompanied by pain. Spinal manipulation techniques that allow the facet joint surfaces to gap are thought to release the entrapped meniscoid tissue and restore normal joint motion.

Evidence

No studies have specifically addressed the effect of spinal mobilization/manipulation on meniscoid impingement; however, investigators have addressed the anatomical plausibility of this theory. In one study and in a follow-up review of the literature, the investigators concluded that the morphology of the lumbar zygapophyseal menisci is incompatible with the meniscal entrapment theory.[46,47]

Reducing Spinal Joint Disc Herniation

Theory

During spinal manipulation, some clinicians believe that sufficient negative pressure is created between the vertebral bodies to draw the herniated disc material back into the intervertebral space.

Evidence

An early study addressing the effect of spinal manipulation on disc herniation reported that there was no reduction in the protruded disc or change in the nerve root in subjects undergoing manipulation under anesthesia.

Furthermore, the clinical results of manipulation intervention were superior among subjects with negative myelograms compared with subjects with myelographic evidence of disc herniation.[48]

In a 1986 review of the literature addressing this issue, Crock[49] supported these findings. He concluded that there is no evidence to justify the use of spinal manipulation to reduce disc herniations. There was, however, a reduction in pain and disability with spinal manipulation in a more recent clinical trial of 40 subjects with disc herniation in which manipulation was compared with chemonucleolysis. More studies are needed before drawing firm conclusions regarding the use of spinal mobilization/manipulation techniques for disc herniations.[50]

Systemic Physiological Effects

Theory

Many clinicians adhere to the premise that mobilization/manipulation can cause measurable changes in the physiology of numerous remote tissues. This theory ostensibly has been presented to justify the use of mobilization/manipulation for the treatment of both musculoskeletal and non-musculoskeletal disease processes.

A number of studies have shown physiological changes resulting from joint mobilization/manipulation interventions. Studies that are most commonly described in the physical therapy literature address sympathetic nervous system changes, and they are discussed below.

Evidence

Several sympathetic nervous system changes have been shown to occur as a result of peripheral joint mobilization. In one study, 19 subjects without upper quarter joint impairment received grade III (through tissue resistance) glenohumeral joint anterior glide mobilizations, a placebo treatment, and no treatment in random order. After mobilization, there was a significant increase in skin conductance and temperature of the distal fingertip on the side that was treated compared with the placebo and control conditions.[51]

A mobilization with movement technique was studied on a sample of 24 subjects with chronic lateral epicondylalgia. Subjects were assigned to receive treatment with mobilization with movement, a placebo treatment, and no treatment in random order. Several measures of sympathetic nervous system function were obtained, including cutaneous blood flow, skin conductance, skin temperature, blood pressure, and heart rate. Heart rate and blood pressure increased, and all measures of cutaneous sympathetic nervous system function were activated after the mobilization with movement technique, but were unchanged after the placebo and control conditions.[31]

Most of the studies addressing sympathetic nervous system changes resulting from joint mobilization/manipulation techniques were performed on the cervical spine. Many of the same researchers who performed the aforementioned studies of the sympathetic nervous system effects on peripheral joints performed six of these studies. Similar to the peripheral joint studies, in these studies a measure of sympathetic nervous system activity was compared under three different conditions. Subjects received a grade III (through tissue resistance) mobilization to the mid cervical spine, a sham intervention consisting of manual contact, and a control condition consisting of no manual contact in random order. In each case, the grade III mobilization resulted in the measure of increased sympathetic nervous system activity compared with the other two conditions. The first study was performed on 16 asymptomatic men. The mobilization consisted of an anterior glide to the spinous process of C5, and the outcome was skin conductance and skin temperature.[52] In the second study, a left side glide mobilization was administered to the C5 vertebra of 34 asymptomatic subjects, while also positioning the right upper extremity in one of two upper limb tension tests. These interventions resulted in an increase in skin conductance, but no change in skin temperature, compared with the other two conditions.[53] The third study was performed on 23 asymptomatic subjects using an anterior glide to the spinous process of C5. The sympathetic nervous system activities measured were respiratory rate, heart rate, and blood pressure.[54] The fourth study was performed on 24 asymptomatic subjects, in which a side glide technique resulted in an increase in systolic and diastolic blood pressure, heart rate, and respiratory rate.[55] In the fifth study, 24 subjects with lateral epicondylalgia were studied. A cervical side glide mobilization resulted in changes in skin conductance, skin temperature, and blood flow.[35] In the sixth study, 30 subjects with mid to lower cervical spine pain received an anterior glide to the C5 facet joint on the painful side. The outcome measure for this study consisted of skin conductance and temperature.[33]

A study by a different investigator of 24 asymptomatic subjects with asymmetrical neck motion into side bending reported different results. The investigator found that although there were significant changes in cervical range of motion after thrust manipulation to the lower cervical spine compared with sham manipulated subjects, there were negligible changes in heart rate, blood pressure, or blood plasma indicators of sympathetic nervous system activity.[23]

Disparity in study results might be due to differences in technique or the manner in which the technique was administered. In a separate study, investigators reported that sympathetic nervous system effects differed when the technique varied. There was a significant increase in skin conductance after a grade III (through tissue resistance) anterior glide mobilization to the spinous process of C5 performed at the rate of two oscillations per second, but no change after an intervention consisting of oscillations at the rate of one every two seconds or a baseline condition consisting of no manual contact. There were no changes in skin temperature after any of these three conditions.[56]

These studies indicate that some mobilization/manipulation techniques produce a generalized sympathoexcitatory response. Nevertheless, the relevance of an increase in sympathetic nervous system activity in the treatment of joint impairments is unclear, other than its potential indirect effect on pain reduction.

Placebo and Psychological Effects

Theory

Clinicians should not discount the psychological benefit of a treatment comprising techniques requiring touch. This is especially true in our current medical system, in which there are only a few remaining practitioners who heal by the laying on of hands.

Evidence

One common concern of researchers with any intervention study is the potential threat to validity caused by a placebo effect. This is especially the case in research involving the effect of manual techniques on pain because these techniques have been shown in numerous studies to be powerful placebos. Although clinicians are eager for patients to improve regardless of the reason for the improvement, it is important to recognize that when treating patients with pain, it is estimated that 30% of the effect is attributable to providing attention and hands-on care to patients. Patients are better served if we choose techniques that have an effect on outcomes beyond the effect of placebo. The effects of placebo are likely to have less of an influence on other outcomes, such as range of motion.

Summary

The evidence supports the use of joint mobilization/manipulation interventions to address specific impairments in patients with musculoskeletal conditions: decreased joint range of motion, pain, and impaired muscle performance. In doing so, the clinician assumes that the patient's level of functioning also will improve.

PRECAUTIONS AND CONTRAINDICATIONS

In the case of joint mobilization/manipulation intervention, it is arguably reasonable to adopt a strategy of "never saying never." There are, however, numerous conditions in which a clinician should weigh the risks and benefits carefully before choosing whether or not to administer a particular joint mobilization/manipulation intervention. Many of the precautions listed subsequently have been identified as such because they appeal to common sense: They are not evidence based.

When considering whether to perform a particular technique, it is important to take into account the amount of force produced and the duration of treatment. In general, it is a good strategy to use the least aggressive technique that would accomplish the goal of treatment. In the case of determining whether to intervene with mobilization/manipulation for all patients, especially patients with the following precautions, it is important to consider whether less aggressive techniques (joint mobilization/manipulation or some other intervention) would produce the desired outcome with less risk of an adverse reaction than more aggressive techniques, or if the best course of action is no intervention whatsoever.

Numerous precautions and contraindications relate specifically to the spine mobilization/manipulation. These are described in Chapter 9. Precautions and contraindications relating to all joints are as follows:

1. Any condition that has not been fully evaluated
2. Joint ankylosis
3. Joint hypermobility, if techniques that take the joint through its end range are being considered, unless a positional fault is being treated
4. An infection in the area being treated
5. A malignancy in the area being treated
6. An unhealed fracture in the area being treated
7. Inflammatory arthritis in the area being treated, especially if it is in a state of an exacerbation
8. Metabolic bone diseases, such as osteoporosis, Paget's disease, and tuberculosis
9. Any debilitating disease that compromises the integrity of periarticular tissue (e.g., advanced diabetes)

10. Long-term use of corticosteroids
11. When there is considerable joint effusion in the area being treated (because it is difficult to evaluate joint mobility accurately, as swelling takes up some of the slack in the joint capsule)
12. Considerable joint irritability or pain in the area being treated
13. Protective muscle spasm to the extent that the clinician is unable to evaluate mobility in the area being treated
14. Pain in adjacent segments that is aggravated by the placement of the clinician's hands when attempting to perform mobilization/manipulation techniques
15. Coagulation impairments
16. Skin rashes or open or healing skin lesions in the area being treated

REFERENCES

1. Maitland GD: Vertebral Manipulation, 5th ed. London, Butterworth, 1986.
2. American Physical Therapy Association: Guide to physical therapist practice, 2nd ed. Phys Ther 2001;81:9-746.
3. Rothstein JM: Editor's note: manual therapy—a special issue and a special topic. Phys Ther 1992;72:839-842.
4. Sackett DL, Straus SE, Richardson WS, et al: Evidence-Based Medicine: How to Practice and Teach EBM, 2nd ed. Philadelphia, Churchill Livingstone, 2000.
5. Sackett DL, Haynes RB, Guyatt GH, et al: Evidence based medicine: what it is and what it isn't. BMJ 1996;312:71-72.
6. Riddle DL: Measurement of accessory motion: critical issues and related concepts. Phys Ther 1992;72:865-874.
7. Woo SL-Y, Matthews JV, Akeson WH, et al: Connective tissue response to immobility: correlative study of biomechanical and biochemical measurements of normal and immobilized rabbit knees. Arthritis Rheum 1975;18:257-264.
8. Akeson WH: Immobilization effects on synovial joints. Biorheology 1980;17:95-110.
9. Akeson WH, Amiel D, Abel JF, et al: Effects of immobilization on joints. Clin Orthop 1987;219:28-37.
10. Olson VL: Evaluation of joint mobilization: a method. Phys Ther 1987;67:351-356.
11. Randall T, Portney L, Harris BA: Effects of joint mobilization on joint stiffness and active motion of the metacarpophalangeal joint. J Orthop Sports Phys Ther 1992;16:30-36.
12. Mierau D, Cassidy JD, Bowen V, et al: Manipulation and mobilization of the third metacarpophalangeal joint: a quantitative radiographic and range of motion study. Manual Med 1988;3:135-140.
13. Hjelm R, Draper C, Spencer S: Anterior-inferior capsular length insufficiency in the painful shoulder. J Orthop Sports Phys Ther 1996;23:216-222.
14. Roubal PJ, Dobritt D, Placzek JD: Glenohumeral gliding manipulation following interscalene brachial plexus block in patients with adhesive capsulitis. J Orthop Sports Phys Ther 1996;24:66-77.
15. Hsu AT, Ho L, Ho S, et al: Joint position during anterior-posterior glide mobilization: its effect on glenohumeral abduction range of motion. Arch Phys Med Rehab 2000;81:210-214.
16. Hsu A-T, Ho L, Ho S, et al: Immediate response of glenohumeral abduction range of motion to a caudally directed translational mobilization: a fresh cadaver simulation. Arch Phys Med Rehab 2000;81:1511-1516.
17. Hsu A-T, Headman T, Chang JH, et al: Changes in abduction and rotation range of motion in response to simulated dorsal and anterior translational mobilization of the glenohumeral joint. Phys Ther 2002;82:544-556.
18. Nield S, Davis K, Latimer J, et al: The effect of manipulation on range of movement at the ankle joint. Scand J Rehab Med 1993;25:161-166.
19. Fryer GA, Mudge JM, McLaughlin PA: The effect of talocrural joint manipulation on range of motion at the ankle. J Manip Physiol Therap 2002;25:384-390.
20. Wilson F: Manual therapy versus traditional exercises in mobilization of the ankle post-ankle fracture: a pilot study. N Z J Physiother 1991;19:11-16.
21. Dananberg HJ, Shearstone J, Guiliano M: Manipulation method for the treatment of ankle equinus. J Am Podiatr Med Assoc 2000;90:385-389.
22. Collins N, Teys P, Vicenzino B: The initial effects of a Mulligan's mobilization with movement technique on dorsiflexion and pain in subacute ankle sprains. Manual Ther 2004;9:77-82.
23. Nansel D: Effects of cervical adjustments on lateral-flexion passive end-range asymmetry and on blood pressure, heart rate and plasma catecholamine levels. J Manip Physiol Therap 1991;14:450-456.
24. Suter E, McMorland G: Decrease in elbow flexor inhibition after cervical spine manipulation in patients with chronic neck pain. Clin Biomech 2002;17:541-544.
25. Cassidy JD, Lopes AA, Yong-Hing K: The immediate effect of manipulation versus mobilization on pain and range of motion in the cervical spine: a randomized controlled trial. J Manip Physiol Therap 1992;15:570-575.
26. Gavin D: The effect of joint manipulation techniques on active range of motion in the mid-thoracic spine of asymptomatic subjects. J Manual Manip Ther 1999;7:114-122.
27. Sims-Williams H, Jayson MIV, Young SMS, et al: Controlled trial of mobilization and manipulation for patients with low back pain in general practice. BMJ 1978;11:1338-1340.
28. Nwuga VCB: Relative therapeutic efficacy of vertebral manipulation and conventional treatment in back pain management.

Am J Phys Med 1982;61:273-278.

29. Timm KE: A randomized-control study of active and passive treatments for chronic low back pain following L5 laminectomy. J Orthop Sports Phys Ther 1994;20:276-286.

30. Vicenzino B, Paungmali A, Buratowski S, et al: Specific manipulative therapy treatment for chronic lateral epicondylalgia produces uniquely characteristic hypoalgesia. Manual Ther 2001;6:205-212.

31. Paungmali A, O'Leary S, Souvlis T, et al: Hypoalgesic and sympathoexcitatory effects of mobilization with movement for lateral epicondylalgia. Phys Ther 2003;83:374-383.

32. Sluka KA, Wright A: Knee joint mobilization reduces secondary mechanical hyperalgesia induced by capsaicin injection into the ankle joint. Eur J Pain 2001;5:81-87.

33. Sterling M, Jull G, Wright A: Cervical mobilization: concurrent effects on pain, sympathetic nervous system activity and motor activity. Manual Ther 2001;6:72-81.

34. Vicenzino B, Collins D, Wright A: The initial effects of a cervical spine manipulative physiotherapy treatment on the pain and dysfunction of lateral epicondylalgia. Pain 1996;68:69-74.

35. Vicenzino B, Collins D, Benson H, et al: An investigation of the interrelationship between manipulative therapy induces hypoalgesia and sympathetoexcitation. J Manip Physiol Therap 1998;21:448-453.

36. Terrett ACJ, Vernon H: Manipulation and pain tolerance. Am J Phys Med 1984;63:217-225.

37. Cote P, Mior SA, Vernon H: The short-term effect of a spinal manipulation on pain/pressure threshold in patients with chronic mechanical low back pain. J Manip Physiol Therap 1994;17:364-368.

38. Dhoudt W, Willaeys T, Verbruggen LA, et al: Pain threshold in patients with rheumatoid arthritis and effect of manual oscillations. Scan J Rheumatol 1999;28:88-93.

39. Shambaugh P: Changes in electrical activity in muscles resulting from chiropractic adjustment: a pilot study. J Manip Physiol Therap 1987;10:300-304.

40. Fisk JW: A controlled trial of manipulation in a selected group of patients with low back pain favouring one side. N Z Med J 1979;90:228-291.

41. Yerys S, Makofsky H, Byrd C, et al: Effect of mobilization of the anterior hip capsule on gluteus maximus strength. J Manual Manip Ther 2002;10:218-224.

42. Liebler EJ, Tufano-Coors L, Douris P, et al: The effect of thoracic spine mobilization on lower trapezius strength testing. J Manual Manip Ther 2001;9:207-212.

43. Suter E, McMorland G, Herzog W, et al: Decrease in quadriceps inhibition after sacroiliac joint manipulation in patients with anterior knee pain. J Manip Physiol Therap 1999;22:149-153.

44. Brantingham JW: A critical look at the subluxation hypothesis. J Manip Physiol Therap 1988;11:130-132.

45. Tullberg T, Blomberg S, Branth B, et al: Manipulation does not alter the position of the sacroiliac joint: a roentgen stereophotogrammetric analysis. Spine 1998;23:1124-1128.

46. Engel R, Bogduk N: The menisci of the lumbar zygapophyseal joints. J Anat 1982;135:795-809.

47. Bogduk N, Engel R: The menisci of the lumbar zygapophyseal joints: a review of their anatomy and clinical significance. Spine 1984;9:454-459.

48. Chrisman D, Mittnacht A, Snook G: A study of the results following rotary manipulation in the lumbar intervertebral-disc syndrome. J Bone Joint Surg Am 1964;46:517-524.

49. Crock HV: Internal disc disruption: a challenge to disc prolapse fifty years on. Spine 1986;11:650-653.

50. Burton AK, Tillotson KM, Cleary J: Single-blind randomized controlled trial of chemonucleolysis and manipulation in the treatment of symptomatic lumbar disc herniation. Eur Spine J 2000, 9:202-207.

51. Simon R, Vicenzino B, Wright A: The influence of an anteroposterior accessory glide of the glenohumeral joint on measures of peripheral sympathetic nervous system function in the upper limb. Manual Ther 1997;2:18-23.

52. Petersen NP, Vicenzino GT, Wright A: The effects of a cervical mobilisation technique on sympathetic outflow to the upper limb in normal subjects. Physiother Theory Pract 1993;9:149-156.

53. Vicenzino B, Collins D, Wright A: Sudomotor changes induced by neural mobilisation techniques in asymptomatic subjects. J Manual Manip Ther 1994;2:66-74.

54. McGuiness J, Vicenzino B, Wright A: Influence of a cervical mobilization technique on respiratory and cardiovascular function. Manual Ther 1997;2:216-220.

55. Vicenzino B, Cartwright T, Collins D, et al: Cardiovascular and respiratory changes produced by lateral glide mobilization of the cervical spine. Manual Ther 1998;3:67-71.

56. Chiu TW, Wright A: To compare the effects of different rates of application of a cervical mobilization technique on sympathetic outflow to the upper limb in normal subjects. Manual Ther 1996;1:198-203.

Principles of Examination, Evaluation, and Intervention

EXAMINATION AND EVALUATION

All patients should undergo a full evaluation before any physical therapy intervention is performed, including treatment with joint mobilization/manipulation. The evaluation should consist of a complete history and a thorough physical examination, which includes an inspection of posture, positioning, gait, and body type; palpation of relevant soft and bony tissue; assessment of range of motion; examination of accessory movements; muscle strength testing; neurological testing; and special tests designed to rule in or out specific conditions. Radiographs should be examined whenever possible. Signs and symptoms should be consistent with the diagnosis, and a complete plan of care should be generated from the diagnosis, taking into consideration the acuity of the injury and any medical, surgical, psychosocial, or financial concerns.

Examination of accessory movements is crucial to the performance of any joint mobilization/manipulation technique. Testing is initiated by placing the joint to be examined in the *resting,* or *loose-packed* position. Kaltenborn[1] defined the resting position as the joint position in which the periarticular tissues are most lax. The resting position also is often the position that is most comfortable for patients with joint pain. Joints are tested in the resting position because this is the position with the greatest amount of accessory movement. If limitations in range of motion or pain prevent the clinician from placing the joint in the resting position, the position that is most comfortable for the patient and in which there is the least amount of soft tissue tension should be used to examine accessory movements. Kaltenborn[1] used the term *actual resting position* to describe this position.

In a study addressing hip biomechanics, hip joint separation was greater when the joint was placed in the resting position compared with the position believed to have the least joint laxity.[2] For most other joints, the resting position has not been determined using research methodology. Nevertheless, several clinicians have described resting positions for most of the joints that are treated with mobilization/manipulation techniques, presumably based on clinical experience. Resting positions are listed in the introductory section for each joint in its respective chapter. In cases in which there is evidence of a resting position, the research was cited. Otherwise, the resting position listed corresponds to the position described by Kaltenborn,[1] who developed this concept.

Accessory motions are examined by moving one of the articular surfaces of the joint in a direction that is perpendicular or parallel to the joint. These directions are determined by identifying the concave joint surface and visualizing the plane in which that joint surface would lie in if it were flattened out. This plane is called the *treatment plane.*

Passively moving either bone in a direction *perpendicular* to the treatment plane such that the bones *separate* constitutes a *traction* or a *distraction* technique, and moving either bone in a direction *perpendicular* to the treatment plane such that the two bones *approximate* one another constitutes a *compression* technique (Fig. 2-1). If the bones are moved in a direction *parallel* to the treatment plane, a *glide* accessory motion is being performed (Fig. 2-2). In many joints, glides can be performed in several directions. An *oscillation* motion often accompanies the glide mobilization. Less often, but occasionally, tractions are accompanied by this oscillation movement.

Since the treatment plane is identified in reference to the concave joint surface, it moves if the concave joint surface is part of the moving bone and remains stationary if the convex joint surface moves. A mobilization/manipulation administered to a long bone is not always performed parallel or perpendicular to the long axis of that bone. For example, because of the anteriorly directed angulation of the forearm in relation to the treatment plane of the ulna, humeroulnar traction mobilizations/manipulations are performed in a direction of 45 degrees less flexion than the angle of the forearm (Fig. 2-3) because this is the direction perpendicular to the

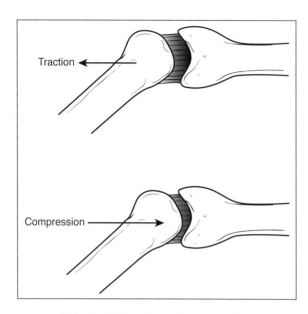

FIG. 2-1. Traction and compression.

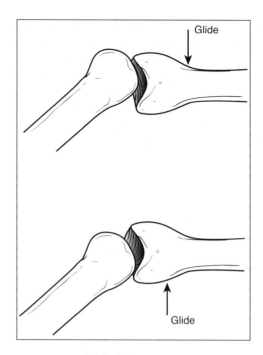

FIG. 2-2. Glides.

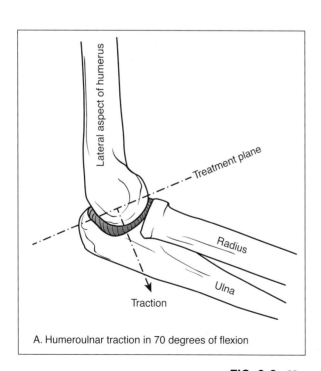

FIG. 2-3. Humeroulnar traction.

treatment plane. Based on the definition of a traction mobilization/manipulation, techniques that are directed along the axis of the long bone are not always true traction techniques. These techniques are called *long axis tractions* to distinguish them from tractions administered perpendicular to the treatment plane.

The examination procedure is performed such that the motion is taken up to and slightly through tissue resistance, and is usually performed in the same direction as the intended treatment mobilization/manipulation technique. Since it is difficult to examine accessory motion using muscle energy techniques, the indications for techniques involving muscle energy are determined by examining the corresponding accessory motion using passive accessory motion examination procedures. In the spine, because of the complexity of some techniques, in some cases, the examination technique differs from the corresponding treatment technique. In these situations, the corresponding examination technique is described along with the description of the intervention mobilization/manipulation.

As a rule, the clinician evaluates all possible accessory motions for each joint being evaluated. An accessory motion examination entails an evaluation of the *amount of excursion* or mobility present in a particular joint when moved in a particular direction, an evaluation of the *presence of pain,* and a determination of the *type of tissue resistance* felt at the end of the range for each accessory motion. The clinician evaluating the patient also should consider whether, and if so, how these accessory motion findings corroborate with other components of the physical examination.

Excursion

To understand more clearly the nature of soft tissue extensibility and its relationship to joint mobilization/manipulation, it is important to become familiar with the characteristics of the stress-strain curve (Fig. 2-4). Rules of stress-strain, or load deformation, are applicable to all solid tissue. As an external tensile force is applied to a tissue (stress or, in this case, a mobilization/manipulation force), the tissue undergoes several transitions (strain). The first stage is the elastic phase, in which the stretched tissue returns to its original configuration when the external force is removed. The second stage is the plastic phase, in which permanent elongation of the stretched tissue occurs when the external force is removed. The third stage is the failure or breaking point, in which separation of the elongated tissue occurs. Within the plastic phase, there is a point at which a decrease in load is accompanied by an increase in deformation. This is called the necking point and is an indication that the breaking point is about to be reached.

Joint mobility is evaluated by performing either a glide or a traction mobilization and by moving the bone up to and slightly through the limit of the available motion into tissue resistance. The clinician is evaluating the amount of motion that occurs up to the point where an increase in tissue resistance is felt. This point theoretically corresponds to the end of the elastic phase and the beginning of the plastic phase on the stress-strain curve.

The amount of motion from the starting position for the two joint surfaces to the point where tissue resistance is felt is graded according to the amount of excursion the bone undergoes. Most clinicians grade excursion, or

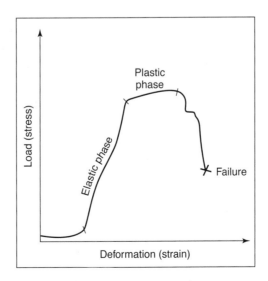

FIG. 2-4. Stress-strain curve.

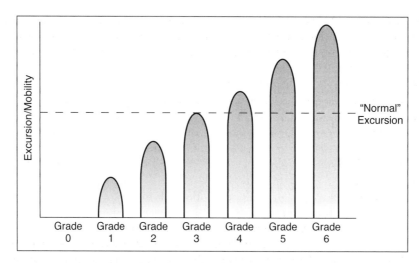

FIG. 2-5. Grades of joint excursion.

mobility, by comparing the joint being tested with the same joint on the opposite side, assuming the joint being used for comparison is not impaired. Despite this recommendation, evidence suggests that excursion at one joint is poorly correlated with excursion into the same direction at the same joint on the opposite side.[3] One alternative to this approach is to compare the perceived joint excursion with the clinician's experience with evaluating the same joint on other patients of similar age, sex, and body type, although this approach is not likely to be highly reliable.

The amount of joint excursion can be graded according to the scale shown in Figure 2-5, with the following implications for determining a plan of care:

Grade 0: There is no motion between the two articulating surfaces. Mobilization/manipulation is not indicated because the joint is ankylosed.

Grade 1: There is considerable limitation in the excursion between the two joint surfaces. Mobilization/manipulation into this accessory motion is indicated to increase joint mobility.

Grade 2: There is a slight limitation in the excursion between the two joint surfaces. Mobilization/manipulation into this accessory motion is indicated to increase joint mobility.

Grade 3: The amount of movement between the joint surfaces is normal. Mobilization/manipulation into this accessory motion is not indicated to increase joint mobility.

Grade 4: There is a slight increase in the excursion between the two joint surfaces. Mobilization/manipulation into this accessory motion is not indicated to increase joint mobility. The patient should be treated with stabilization exercises and should be educated regarding correct posture and positions to avoid. Taping and/or bracing are also treatment options.

Grade 5: There is a considerable increase in the excursion between the two joint surfaces. Mobilization/manipulation into this accessory motion is not indicated to increase joint mobility. The patient should be treated with stabilization exercises and should be educated regarding correct posture and positions to avoid. Taping and/or bracing are also treatment options.

Grade 6: The joint is unstable. Mobilization/manipulation into this accessory motion is not indicated to increase joint mobility. The patient can be treated with stabilization exercises, patient education, and taping/bracing, but this intervention is less likely to be successful than if the joint were less hypermobile.

An alternative grading scale consists of three categories: *hypomobile, normal,* and *hypermobile,* with the same plan-of-care implications as the aforementioned seven-category scale. This alternative scale is likely to be more reliable because there are fewer categories.

Pain

It is important to examine whether pain is produced or increased when evaluating accessory motion and to interpret this finding in conjunction with the results of the accessory motion examination. Pain in conjunction with hypomobility usually indicates a need for joint mobilization/manipulation intervention because treating the hypomobility would eliminate the joint impairment that might be causing the pain. Conversely, it might be a sign that there is an acute sprain with guarding or an inflamed joint. In these latter circumstances, it is important to consider whether what appears to be hypomobility is in fact muscle guarding, and if the muscle guarding is masking a hypermobile condition. If so, joint mobilization/manipulation might be detrimental. This condition can be determined by evaluating for periarticular muscle spasm and, if present, ensuring that these muscles are relaxed when evaluating joint accessory motion.

In the absence of these concerns, the examination of joint excursion, combined with a determination of the presence or absence of pain, has the following implications for determining a plan of care:

- *Hypomobility without pain* is believed to indicate a chronic adhesion or contracture. Mobilization/manipulation techniques that bring the joint through tissue resistance might be indicated in this situation, although in the absence of pain the possibility that hypomobility is a normal state for that patient also should be considered.
- *Normal mobility with pain* indicates a mild sprain without disruption of capsular fibers. Joint mobilization/manipulation for stretching of periarticular structures is not indicated in the presence of normal mobility, but the patient might benefit from more gentle mobilization techniques to decrease pain and promote normal alignment of newly forming collagen fibers.
- *Normal mobility without pain* indicates an absence of joint capsular impairment.
- *Excessive mobility with pain* indicates a partial sprain of capsular tissue, whereas excess mobility without pain indicates a complete sprain of capsular tissue. In both of these instances, stabilization techniques are indicated. When pain accompanies hypermobility, gentle mobilizations carefully administered so as not to take the joint up to tissue resistance can be used to decrease pain and promote normal alignment of newly forming collagen tissue.

Compression and distraction of the two articular surfaces of a joint are also commonly examined in relation to one another for response to pain. If pain increases with compression and is relieved with distraction, this indicates possible involvement of the articular surface. If pain is relieved with compression and increased with traction, the pain might be arising from ligamentous or other capsular structures.

If the goal of the mobilization/manipulation intervention is to decrease pain, several approaches can be considered. Maitland recommended mobilizing/manipulating into the direction of pain, with the caveat that the amount of force should be determined based on the severity of the condition. Other authors advocate always mobilizing/manipulating in a pain-free direction.

End Feel

End feels also are examined during the evaluation of accessory motion. Accessory motion end feels are either bony or firm. With bony end feels, the joint tissue resistance is felt as an abrupt change in joint extensibility, whereas firm end feels are less abrupt. A bony end feel indicates that either there is bony hypertrophy in the joint blocking additional motion, or the restrictions in the joint capsule are causing the two joint surfaces to jam together. If bony hypertrophy is blocking joint motion, performing joint mobilization/manipulation techniques might be harmful to the patient. A firm end feel indicates that capsular tissue is limiting further motion. If the firm end feel is accompanied by no pain and normal excursion, there is no joint capsular impairment involving that particular accessory motion. A firm end feel accompanied by an abnormal amount of excursion is considered an abnormal end feel. If the firm end feel is accompanied by hypomobility, joint mobilization/manipulation interventions should be considered, especially if the accessory motion is hypomobile and painful. Kaltenborn[1] stated that hypomobile joints with a firm end feel and no pain should not be treated because the hypomobility likely is not associated with the patient's symptoms. A hypermobile joint should be treated with some form of stabilization intervention, regardless of end feel.

In the situation in which a firm end feel is present, most experienced clinicians make an additional determination regarding the quality of the firm end feel, based on the relative "give" or "play" in the tissue. Firm end feels that have relatively more play are more likely to be judged hypermobile, even if the amount of joint excursion is not excessive.

INTEGRATING ACCESSORY MOTION FINDINGS WITH OTHER EXAMINATION FINDINGS

Positional Faults

The clinician might choose to identify positional faults as part of the examination procedure. If this is the case, the clinician should determine during the palpation component of the evaluation process whether the joint surfaces appear to be aligned correctly in relation to one another by comparing the position of bony landmarks with the same landmarks on the opposite side. When a suspected positional fault is identified, the clinician should examine whether the perceived alignment impairment is a positional fault or simply a bony abnormality by palpating adjacent bony landmarks. For example, if a clinician suspects, by palpating the position of a spinous process, that a thoracic vertebra has a rotational positional fault, the transverse processes corresponding to that vertebra should be asymmetrical consistent with the direction of rotation. A T5 vertebral body that is rotated right should be accompanied by a spinous process that is positioned left of midline and a right T5 transverse process that is positioned more posterior than the left T5 transverse process. If the transverse processes are aligned symmetrically, any alignment asymmetry of the spinous process is more likely to be due to a bony anomaly. There is an additional criterion for identifying the presence of a symptomatic positional fault: The joint should be hypomobile and painful with accessory motion testing.

Convex-Concave Rules

Joints are capable of several types of joint motion. Spinning is one type of joint motion (Fig. 2-6) and consists of movement of one bone on the other such that one point on both bones remains in contact with the other, and the rest of the articular surface of one bone rotates in relation to the other. The radius spins on the humerus during forearm pronation and supination. Rolling is another type of motion (Fig. 2-7) that occurs when one point on one bone comes into contact with a point on the other bone that is equidistant from the original contact point. Much of the motion associated with knee flexion and extension occurs by way of rolling motion. Gliding is the third type of motion (Fig. 2-8) and occurs when one point on one bone stays in contact with the articulating surface of the other bone, but at a new point. In relation to the spine, with forward bending movement, one facet joint glides on the other.

Kaltenborn[1] proposed that restricted range of motion is associated most often with a decrease in the gliding component. He further stated that the direction of the glide corresponds to a specific osteokinematic movement, which depends on the shape of the articular surface.

Most joints are composed of a convex surface articulating with a reciprocally shaped concave surface. If the concave surface is the moving surface, the direction of the glide is the same as the osteokinematic movement. If the convex surface is the moving surface, the direction of the glide is opposite that of the osteokinematic movement (Fig. 2-9). The direction of force imparted with an examination glide corresponds to a specific osteokinematic

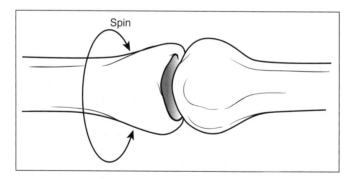

FIG. 2-6. Spin.

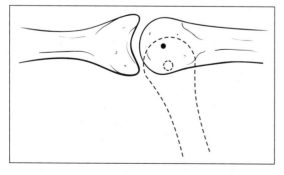

FIG. 2-7. Roll.

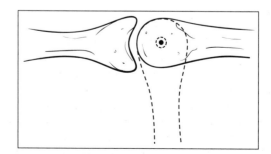

FIG. 2-8. Glide.

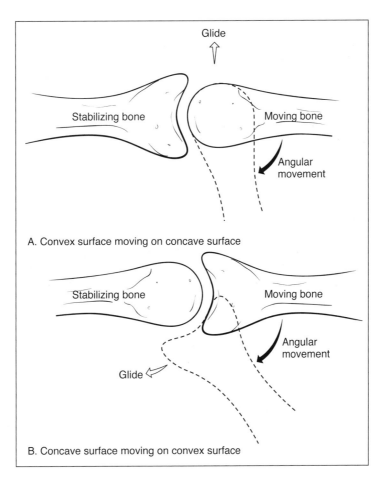

FIG. 2-9. Convex-concave rules.

movement based on the convex-concave relationship of the joint surfaces, and the grade of joint mobility (grade 1-6) given to that examination glide should correlate with the corresponding range of motion examination results.[1] If a concave tibia moves on a convex femur, as in open kinematic chain knee flexion activities, the tibia glides in the same direction as the osteokinematic motion. If knee flexion occurs in a closed kinematic chain situation, the femur moves on the tibia, and the femur glides in a direction opposite that of the osteokinematic motion. Assuming range of motion limitations correspond to the limitation in accessory motion based on these concave-convex rules, a decrease in accessory motion of the tibia gliding in a posterior direction on the femur or of the femur gliding in an anterior direction on the tibia should be present when there is a decrease in knee flexion range of motion (Fig. 2-10).

Ovoid joints are shaped such that one joint surface is concave in its entirety. This joint surface articulates with a joint surface that is convex in its entirety (Fig. 2-11). Sellar joints are shaped such that one joint surface is concave in one direction and convex in the direction perpendicular to the concave surface, similar to the shape of a saddle. The articulating joint surface is reciprocally convex to match the concave surface of its adjoining articulation and concave in the direction perpendicular to the convex surface (Fig. 2-12). The two articulating surfaces are congruent. The moving bone glides in the same direction as the osteokinematic movement in one plane of motion and opposite the direction of the osteokinematic movement occurring in the perpendicular plane.

Convex-concave rules are applied more easily when the moving joint surface is perpendicular to the axis of a long bone, as is the case with the tibia and the femur. The patellofemoral joint is an example of a joint for which the convex-concave rules are less easily conceptualized. Kaltenborn's theory of convex-concave rules, if applicable at all, most likely is less relevant to joints that move almost entirely by gliding, such as with anterior translation of the temporomandibular joint and movement at the spinal facet joints.

The validity of this strategy for determining the direction of the glide intervention to treat a range of motion restriction in a particular direction has been researched in relation to the glenohumeral joint. In each of these

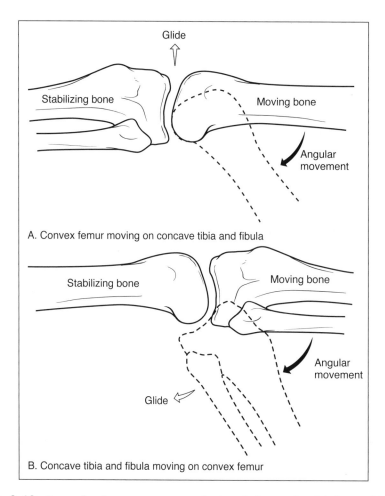

Glide

Stabilizing bone

Moving bone

Angular movement

A. Convex femur moving on concave tibia and fibula

Stabilizing bone

Moving bone

Angular movement

Glide

B. Concave tibia and fibula moving on convex femur

FIG. 2-10. Example of convex-concave rules in relation to the tibiofemoral joint.

studies, one objective was to determine whether gliding the glenohumeral joint in a particular direction was associated with increases in range of motion in a particular direction. Based on convex-concave rules, Kaltenborn[1] stated that restrictions in glenohumeral joint flexion and medial rotation should be treated with a posterior glide, restrictions in extension and lateral rotation should be treated with an anterior glide, and restrictions in abduction should be treated with an inferior glide. Some of the studies supported Kaltenborn's assertion that inferior gliding increases abduction,[4,5] anterior gliding increases lateral rotation,[6] and posterior gliding increases medial rotation.[4,6] However there is also evidence suggesting that joint mobilization/manipulation increases motion in directions that are inconsistent with Kaltenborn's assertions. In these studies, there was an increase in lateral rotation after inferior glides[7] and a combination of posterior and inferior glides[4] and an increase in abduction as a result of anterior glides[6] and posterior glides.[8]

There is insufficient evidence to support the use of Kaltenborn's convex-concave rules when treating patients with glenohumeral joint mobilization/manipulation for the purpose of increasing range of motion. Referencing some of the aforementioned studies performed on the glenohumeral joint, one investigator suggested that glenohumeral arthrokinematics are far more complicated than Kaltenborn's convex-concave rules would imply.[9] There also is insufficient evidence to support or refute the validity of these convex-concave rules in relation to other joints. Further research might find other joints to be equally complicated.

It is likely that mobilizing/manipulating a joint in multiple directions would increase osteokinematic motion in one specific direction, and that mobilizing/manipulating a joint in one direction would increase osteokinematic motion in more than one direction. Nevertheless, it is possible that the clinician would be relatively more effective with mobilization/manipulation interventions for the purpose of increasing motion in a particular direction if he or she adhered to Kaltenborn's convex-concave rules. The information that is required to apply these convex-concave rules is therefore provided in Table 2-1 and in the description of the relevant joint mobilization/manipulation procedures in subsequent chapters.

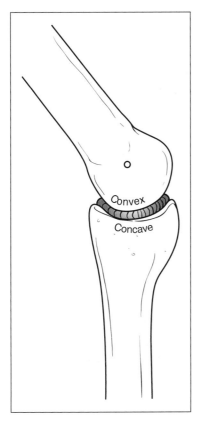

FIG. 2-11. Ovoid joint.

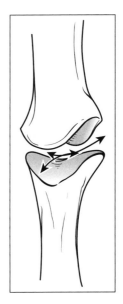

FIG. 2-12. Sellar joint.

TABLE 2-1 Articular Anatomy as per Kaltenborn and Interpretation Based on Kaltenborn's Concave-Convex Rules

Name of Joint	Articulation Anatomy	Arthrokinematic/Osteokinematic Motion
Sternoclavicular joint	*For elevation/depression:* The sternum is concave; the clavicle is convex	Osteokinematic motion and arthrokinematic glide are in the opposite direction
	For protraction/retraction: The sternum is convex; the clavicle is concave	Osteokinematic motion and arthrokinematic glide are in the same direction
Acromioclavicular joint	The acromion is concave; the clavicle is convex	Osteokinematic motion and arthrokinematic glide are in the opposite direction
Glenohumeral joint	The glenoid is concave; the humerus is convex	Osteokinematic motion and arthrokinematic glide are in the opposite direction
Humeroulnar joint	The humerus is convex; the ulna is concave	Osteokinematic motion and arthrokinematic glide are in the same direction
Humeroradial joint	The humerus is convex; the radius is concave	Osteokinematic motion and arthrokinematic glide are in the same direction
Proximal radioulnar joint	The ulna is concave; the radius is convex	Osteokinematic motion and arthrokinematic glide are in the opposite direction
Distal radioulnar joint	The ulna is convex; the radius is concave	Osteokinematic motion and arthrokinematic glide are in the same direction
Radiocarpal joints	The radius is concave; the carpals are convex	Osteokinematic motion and arthrokinematic glide are in the opposite direction
Intercarpal joints	The scaphoid is convex; the trapezium and trapezoid are concave	Osteokinematic motion and arthrokinematic glide are in the same direction
	Otherwise: The proximal bones are concave; the distal bones are convex	Osteokinematic motion and arthrokinematic glide are in the opposite direction

Continued

TABLE 2-1 Articular Anatomy as per Kaltenborn and Interpretation Based on Kaltenborn's Concave-Convex Rules—cont'd

Name of Joint	Articulation Anatomy	Arthrokinematic/Osteokinematic Motion
Carpometacarpal joint of the thumb	*For flexion/extension:* The carpal is convex; the metacarpal is concave	Osteokinematic motion and arthrokinematic glide are in the same direction
	For abduction/adduction: The carpal is concave; the metacarpal is convex	Osteokinematic motion and arthrokinematic glide are in the opposite direction
Intermetacarpal joints	*In relation to metacarpal III:* The more medial metacarpals are convex; the more lateral metacarpals are concave	Osteokinematic motion and arthrokinematic glide are in the same direction
Metacarpophalangeal joint of the thumb	The metacarpal is convex; the phalanx is concave	Osteokinematic motion and arthrokinematic glide are in the same direction
Metacarpophalangeal joints of digits 2-5	The metacarpals are convex; the phalanges are concave	Osteokinematic motion and arthrokinematic glide are in the same direction
Proximal and distal interphalangeal joints of the hand	The proximal phalanges are convex; the distal phalanges are concave	Osteokinematic motion and arthrokinematic glide are in the same direction
Hip joint	The acetabulum is concave; the femur is convex	Osteokinematic motion and arthrokinematic glide are in the opposite direction
Tibiofemoral joint	The femur is convex; the tibia is concave	Osteokinematic motion and arthrokinematic glide are in the same direction
Patellofemoral joint	The femur is concave; the patella is convex	Osteokinematic motion and arthrokinematic glide are in the opposite direction
Proximal tibiofibular joint	The tibia is convex; the fibula is concave	Osteokinematic motion and arthrokinematic glide motion are in the same direction
Distal tibiofibular joint	The tibia is concave; the fibula is convex	Osteokinematic motion and arthrokinematic glide are in the opposite direction
Talocrural joint	The tibia and fibula are concave; the talus is convex	Osteokinematic motion and arthrokinematic glide are in the opposite direction
Subtalar joint	The anterior and middle talus is convex; the anterior and middle calcaneus is concave	Osteokinematic motion and arthrokinematic glide are in the same direction
	The posterior talus is concave; the posterior calcaneus is convex	Osteokinematic motion and arthrokinematic glide are in the opposite direction
Talonavicular joint	The talus is convex; the navicular is concave	Osteokinematic motion and arthrokinematic glide are in the same direction
Calcaneocuboid joint	*For flexion/extension:* The calcaneus is convex; the cuboid is concave	Osteokinematic motion and arthrokinematic glide are in the same direction
	For abduction/adduction: The calcaneus is concave; the cuboid is convex	Osteokinematic motion and arthrokinematic glide are in the opposite direction
Intermetatarsal joints	*In relation to metatarsal II:* The more medial metatarsals are convex; the more lateral metatarsals are concave	Osteokinematic motion and arthrokinematic glide are in the same direction
Metatarsophalangeal joints	The metatarsals are convex; the phalanges are concave	Osteokinematic motion and arthrokinematic glide are in the same direction
Interphalangeal joints of the toes	The proximal phalanges are convex; the distal phalanges are concave	Osteokinematic motion and arthrokinematic glide are in the same direction
Temporomandibular joint	The temporalis is concave; the mandible is convex	Osteokinematic motion and arthrokinematic glide are in the opposite direction

Adapted from Kaltenborn FM: Manual Mobilization of the Joints: The Kaltenborn Method of Joint Examination and Treatment, Vol I: The Extremities, 6th ed. OPTP, Oslo, Norway, Norli, 2002.

Capsular Patterns

Numerous components of the physical examination, used in conjunction with the results of an accessory motion examination, can aid in determining the patient's diagnosis. One of these components entails an evaluation of the presence of a capsular pattern. According to Cyriax,[10] when the joint impairment affects the entire joint, the capsule of each joint undergoes a characteristic pattern of restriction in passive range of motion. This pattern of restriction is called the *capsular pattern*. Cyriax[10] proposed that there is a specific pattern of restriction for each joint, in which the proportional limitation in one motion is greater than one or more other motions. For example, the capsular pattern for the shoulder joint is described as lateral rotation being proportionally more limited than abduction, which is proportionally more limited than medial rotation. If a capsular pattern is present, there is a limitation in lateral rotation that is, in relation to the normal range of motion for lateral rotation, more limited than abduction, which is more limited than medial rotation. Movements not listed are irrelevant to the identification of the capsular pattern. A patient with 10 degrees of shoulder lateral rotation (10 degrees out of a possible 90 degrees of motion), 90 degrees of abduction (90 degrees out of a possible 180 degrees of motion), and 60 degrees of medial rotation (60 degrees out of a possible 90 degrees) would have a capsular pattern.

According to Cyriax,[10] if passive range of motion of a joint is limited in this characteristic pattern of restriction, this indicates that the impairment involves the entire joint capsule. Determining the presence of capsular patterns is helpful in diagnosing articular lesions because the presence of a capsular pattern would indicate that the diagnosis is therefore one in which the entire joint capsule is involved.[10] Examples of impairments involving the entire joint capsule are osteoarthritis and conditions involving trauma to the entire joint capsule. Joint conditions that do not cause a capsular pattern of restriction include knee meniscus tears, ligamentous injuries, and extra-articular lesions. Capsular patterns of restriction for all of the joints are listed in the introduction section of the respective chapter for each joint. The determination of the motion limitations that constitute a capsular pattern is not evidence-based, but rather is based on Cyriax's descriptions.

Several studies have been performed that address the validity of the concept of a capsular pattern. Some evidence suggests that subjects with knee osteoarthritis have more limitations in knee flexion than extension, as Cyriax suggested, although not in the specific proportions described by Cyriax.[11,12] In relation to subjects with hip osteoarthritis, however, no consistent pattern of restriction was found.[13]

Pain with Range of Motion

Cyriax[10] stated that a patient who has a reproduction of symptoms with active range of motion that also is reproduced with passive range of motion in the same direction is likely to have a condition involving the joint. Pain that occurs with active range of motion or with resisted isometric testing into one direction and with passive range of motion into the opposite direction is likely to be due to contractile tissue.

RELIABILITY ISSUES

Accessory motion testing is a complex task to perform. Maitland[14] provided the following description of the skills required to evaluate accessory motion: The clinician must "… apply a force to a joint and … evaluate the joint's response to that force. The student (clinician) is supposed to appreciate the amount of force applied to the joint, the speed and direction at which it is applied, the amount of movement produced at the joint, the way in which the joint moves or resists movement in response to that force, the pain produced by that movement, the presence of muscle activity evoked during the movement, and the comparison of this reaction to the expected normal response and to that of adjacent joints when palpated in a presumably similar way." For most joints, these components of accessory motion examination have not been clearly defined or studied.

The results of research on the reliability of mobilization/manipulation examination procedures are similar to those results involving other techniques commonly used by therapists to evaluate patients with musculoskeletal conditions. As a general rule, testing procedures involving the palpation of landmark position and mobility (and by implication treatment involving these skills) is associated with poor reliability,[15-17] but can be improved with training and feedback.[18,19] Pain provocation tests show greater reliability than mobility tests.[15] The results of pain provocation tests should therefore be weighted more heavily than the results involving the determination of joint position and motion. Intratester reliability almost always is higher than intertester reliability.[16,20] The implication of this latter finding for clinical practice is that measurements (and interventions) are more consistent if performed by one clinician than by two or more clinicians.

Reasons cited for poor reliability are numerous and include variability in the experience of the tester, nuances among the subjects being tested, variations in the technique itself and in the performance of the technique being performed, and asymmetrical joint anatomy. Methodological issues related to observer bias, lack of variability in the response being determined, and a low number of testers also have been cited as possible causes of poor reliability coefficients.

VALIDITY ISSUES

The determination of whether what is actually being measured reflects what the clinician intends to measure (internal validity) when he or she performs a joint mobilization/manipulation technique has not been well studied. One study evaluated this issue in relation to the cervical spine. This study addressed whether clinicians could identify the joint level responsible for symptoms in 20 subjects with chronic neck pain. Of these 20 subjects, 15 had symptomatic zygapophyseal joints determined by nerve blocks. A clinician evaluated each subject using passive accessory motions. A joint was considered to be symptomatic if it exhibited an abnormal end feel, an abnormal amount of resistance through range of motion, and pain. In all cases, the clinician was able to identify the subjects with symptomatic zygapophyseal joints and the joint level producing the pain.[21] This study exemplifies the use of one effective strategy to increase the validity of tests to identify joint impairments: using multiple tests designed to identify a specific diagnosis and arriving at that diagnosis only when the findings from these several tests corroborate with one another.

INTERVENTION

Numerous treatment parameters must be determined when designing an intervention that includes joint mobilization/manipulation. Most important are the *joint position, direction of force, amount and speed of force,* and *timing of the intervention.*

Joint Position

Treatment should be initiated with the joint in the resting position. This is the safest position in which to treat because compressive forces are minimal, and the patient's response can be observed before proceeding to more aggressive positions. Most of the techniques discussed in this book are described in the resting position for these reasons. Nevertheless, research suggests that if the goal is to increase joint mobility, positions approximating the restricted range of motion yield greater increases in joint range of motion.[5,8]

Mobilizations/manipulations should not be performed in the close-packed position. Kaltenborn[1] described the *close-packed position* as the position in which the joint capsule and ligaments are maximally tensed, and there is maximal contact between the two articular surfaces. It is believed that mobilization/manipulation in the close-packed position produces too much compressive force on the articulating surfaces.[1] As is the case with the resting position, few studies have been performed to determine the close-packed position for specific joints. To complicate this issue further, in one study investigating glenohumeral joint stiffness, the investigators concluded that close-packed positioning is most likely different for different mobilization/manipulation glides.[22] The close-packed positions are listed in the introductory section of each chapter and represent Kaltenborn's view regarding this issue, as Kaltenborn was the first clinician to address this concept in relation to joint mobilization/manipulation.

Direction of Force

If the goal of the mobilization/manipulation technique is to increase joint mobility, the direction of the mobilization/manipulation force should be the same as the hypomobile accessory motion. In most cases, the actual technique used to identify a decrease in accessory motion is also the technique used to treat this impairment. An exception to this statement involves performing some of the spinal techniques, in which case the examination technique can differ from the treatment technique.

Positional faults are treated with traction or with glide mobilization/manipulation, including muscle energy techniques. If a glide technique is chosen, most clinicians glide in the direction that would realign the two bones into the correct position, although some clinicians advocate gliding in the direction of the greatest hypomobility. The direction of the intervention mobilization/manipulation is less relevant when considering the other indications for treatment, such as pain reduction and improvement in muscle performance.

Amount and Speed of Force

Intervention mobilizations/manipulations are graded according to the amount and speed of motion imparted to the joint. Two methods of describing the grade of intervention mobilization/manipulation are in common use. The first method described, proposed by Kaltenborn,[1] involves three different grades of mobilization and is commonly used to describe traction interventions. The second method described, proposed by Maitland,[23] involves five different grades of mobilization/manipulation and is used most often to describe glide interventions. Nevertheless, both methods are appropriate for both types of mobilization/manipulation.

The Kaltenborn method[1] (Fig. 2-13) is as follows:

Grade I: A slow, small-amplitude movement that does not take the joint capsule to the limit of available joint motion

Grade II: A slow, larger amplitude movement that takes the joint capsule to the limit of available joint motion

Grade III: A slow, even larger amplitude movement that takes the joint through the limit of available joint motion and into tissue resistance

The Maitland method[23] (Fig. 2-14) is as follows:

Grade I: A slow, small-amplitude movement that does not take the joint capsule to the limit of available joint motion

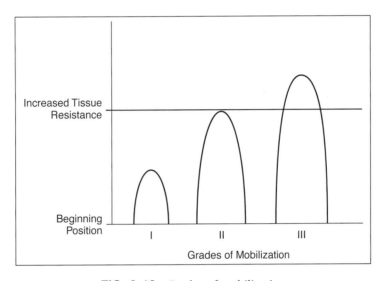

FIG. 2-13. Grades of mobilization.

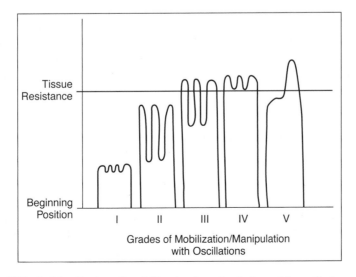

FIG. 2-14. Grades of mobilization/manipulation with oscillations.

Grade II: A slow, larger amplitude movement that does not take the joint capsule to the limit of available joint motion

Grade III: A slow, large-amplitude movement that takes the joint up to and slightly through the limit of available joint motion and into tissue resistance

Grade IV: A slow, small-amplitude movement that is performed through the limit of available joint motion and into tissue resistance

Grade V movements are used to describe thrust joint manipulations and can be defined as follows:

Grade V/thrust joint manipulation: A high-velocity, small-amplitude, nonoscillatory movement that begins at the limit of available joint motion and takes the joint into tissue resistance

The grade of movement used to evaluate joint motion corresponds to between a grade II and III using the grade I to III (Kaltenborn) scale and a grade III mobilization using the grade I to IV or V (Maitland) scale. The Maitland grading system is preferable because it includes a description of thrust joint manipulation, and it is used from this point forward in this book.

Joint mobilization/manipulation treatment techniques used to increase the mobility of joint and periarticular tissue should be forceful enough to bring the tissue into the plastic phase of the stress-strain curve (grade III or higher), but not so forceful as to reach the failure point, unless the goal is to break adhesions. The research suggests that, mobilizations/manipulations also should be at least a grade III to optimally decrease pain, improve muscle performance, promote physiological changes, and correct positional faults. In two different studies of glenohumeral joint stiffness, the authors concluded that most clinicians do not take the joint to the plastic phase of the stress-strain curve, even though their intention is to perform a mobilization that takes the joint slightly through its tissue resistance.[22,24] This finding suggests that although most clinicians performing mobilization techniques are not placing their patients at risk of joint injury, they also are not being optimally effective in treating impairments.

Maitland[23] described one method of determining how aggressively a patient can be safely treated with mobilization/manipulation techniques. This method involves examining the pattern of pain to tissue resistance with the passive range of motion corresponding to the particular mobilization/manipulation technique being considered and determining the severity of the patient's condition through history taking. If pain occurs before the end range is met with passive range of motion, and if the patient has symptoms that are easily provoked and persist for a long time, grade I and II techniques are indicated to treat the pain. If pain occurs after the end range is met with passive range of motion or if passive range of motion is pain-free, and if symptoms increase only after a moderate amount of activity and last for a short time, the patient should be able to tolerate grade III or higher mobilizations/manipulations.

Timing of Mobilization and Manipulation Intervention

Recommendations for the length of time a single mobilization maneuver should last range from two to three maneuvers a second to one maneuver every 10 seconds. There is also wide variability in the recommended total amount of time to spend mobilizing/manipulating a patient with a musculoskeletal impairment, ranging from treatments lasting seconds to treatments lasting up to 60 minutes. Other treatment parameters likely to influence outcomes from the application of a mobilization/manipulation technique include whether the technique is accompanied by an oscillatory movement and the number of technique repetitions.

Mobilization/manipulation interventions that take the joint through tissue resistance could cause irritation to stretched periarticular structures. The patient might experience soreness after treatment. If the patient experiences an increase in symptoms for more than 12 hours after treatment or experiences swelling or muscle guarding in the area of the joint being treated, either the wrong technique was performed or the treatment was too aggressive. In such cases, a re-evaluation is indicated. Finally, treatment sessions should be spaced at least 48 hours apart to allow the patient to recover from any joint irritation from the previous treatment.

TECHNIQUE

Passive Accessory and Passive Physiological Motions and Mobilization with Movement

When performing any of these techniques, either as examination or as treatment procedures, the clinician should keep the following principles in mind:

1. The patient should exhibit no muscle guarding and should be as relaxed as possible.
2. The clinician should be efficient with body mechanics and should stand with a wide base of support. The mobilizing/manipulating force should be as close to the clinician's center of gravity as possible. The force ideally

should be directed downward. If a downward force is not feasible, a horizontally directed force can be performed. This is especially important when evaluating and treating larger joints. When performing joint mobilization/manipulation techniques on the smaller joints of the hand and the foot, the role of gravity in executing the technique is relatively unimportant.

3. The joint should be tested in the resting position if the patient is capable of attaining that position. If not, the joint should be tested in the actual resting position.
4. One bone should be stabilized with the clinician's hand or other body part, a belt, a wedge, or the treatment table.
5. The other bone should be mobilized/manipulated with the clinician's hand, using body weight to provide force to the mobilization/manipulation technique when feasible.
6. The stabilizing force and the mobilizing/manipulating force should be as close to the joint surfaces as possible.
7. When performing glides on long bones, the clinician should move the distal aspect of the bone at the same time, in the same direction, and through the same distance as the mobilizing force on the proximal aspect of the bone, so that the resulting joint movement is a gliding motion and not a rotary motion.
8. The mobilization/manipulation technique should be timed with the patient's breathing such that the patient exhales while the mobilization/manipulation is being performed.
9. The patient's pain should be monitored during the mobilization/manipulation procedure, and appropriate modifications to the technique being performed should be made to minimize patient discomfort.
10. Only one movement should be performed at a time. For example, the clinician should not mobilize/manipulate a bone into posterior glide from a position of end range anterior glide because it is more difficult to determine movement in this manner.
11. Only one joint should be mobilized/manipulated at a time.
12. Each technique is an evaluative technique and an intervention technique; the clinician continually evaluates during treatment. Formal examination of accessory motion also should be made before and after the intervention.

For reasons related to patient safety and comfort, glides usually are performed with a grade I traction when feasible to decrease compression forces on the joint surfaces. Nevertheless, some clinicians advocate performing glides with compression[23] because this might aid in reducing motion at adjacent joints.

If the clinician, while mobilizing/manipulating a joint, perceives that a decrease in force is associated with a relatively large amount of deformation, this is a sign that the tissue being stretched has reached the necking point and is about to reach the breaking point in the stress-strain curve. When the clinician feels this change in tissue resistance, the technique should be terminated immediately. The exception to this assertion is when the goal is to break adhesions, in which case the force should be maintained until the breaking point has been reached.

Muscle Energy

Muscle energy is a specific type of mobilization intervention that uses a voluntary contraction of the patient's muscles to move one bone on another. To perform this technique, the joint first is placed in a specific position that facilitates optimal contraction of a particular muscle or muscle group. The patient is asked to contract that muscle or muscle group isometrically against the clinician's counter pressure. This contraction causes the muscle to pull on the bony attachment of one of the bones that compose the joint to be mobilized, moving one bone in relation to its articulating counterpart. The articulating counterpart must be stabilized for this accessory movement to occur. The contraction occurs in a precisely controlled direction with a precisely controlled joint position in all three planes and requires a distinctly executed counterforce. After holding the contraction for 3 to 7 seconds, the patient is instructed to relax, and the muscle is passively stretched. The clinician repeats the sequence from this new position. The technique is commonly performed three times before re-examination.

Muscle energy techniques have the advantage of allowing the patient to control the mobilization; if too much pain is reproduced during the maneuver, the patient can terminate the procedure. In some situations, muscle energy techniques can also alleviate joint impairment by stretching and/or strengthening muscles that influence joint mechanics.

PLAN OF CARE

Joint mobilization/manipulation should be used in conjunction with other physical therapy interventions. If pain is a component of the patient's condition, other techniques could include exercise therapeutic agents, bracing, and patient education. If improving joint mobility is the primary goal of treatment, additional techniques could include soft tissue mobilization and exercise. In this case, the goals of exercise would be to maintain the range gained from the mobilization/ manipulation techniques and to provide the patient with the strength required to perform functional activities in the newly gained range of motion.

In relation to specific conditions, there is some evidence to support the premise that combining joint mobilization/manipulation with other interventions enhances outcomes.[25-38] These studies provide only limited information, however, on the efficacy of using other interventions in conjunction with joint mobilization/manipulation because most of the studies were designed to determine whether adding mobilization/manipulation to other interventions enhances outcomes. The question more relevant to this issue would be whether adding other interventions to joint mobilization/manipulation enhances outcomes compared with mobilization/manipulation alone.

MOBILIZATION/MANIPULATION MUSINGS

What Causes Joints to Crack?

Manipulation procedures applied to joint structures sometimes are accompanied by a cracking noise, or *cavitation*. The best evidence suggests that this noise occurs as the volume of the intra-articular space increases, and synovial fluid changes from a liquid to a gaseous state, or from the snapping of ligaments as the joint capsule changes shape. This increase in intra-articular space might explain the temporary increase in range of motion that occurs after manipulation techniques. Since the gas takes time to reabsorb, joints are not likely to crack again immediately after having been cracked.[39]

Some clinicians believe that producing an audible crack during a manipulation procedure maximizes the therapeutic effect of the intervention. The available research to date has not shown this to be the case. In one study, 71 subjects with nonradicular low back pain were treated with a grade V spinal manipulation technique. Investigators noted which of these subjects experienced an audible crack during this intervention. Subjects were followed for improvements in range of motion, pain, and disability. There was no difference in any of these outcomes based on whether an audible crack occurred with the manipulation procedure.[40]

Common folklore suggests that habitual self-cracking might result in osteoarthritic changes. In two separate studies in which investigators compared the prevalence of osteoarthritis among subjects with a history of habitual joint cracking, no such relationship was found.[41,42] In one of these studies, however, habitual knuckle cracking was associated with hand swelling and a decrease in hand strength.[42]

Should Children Be Treated with Joint Mobilization/Manipulation Techniques?

Children are less likely to have injuries resulting in joint stiffness than adults, in part because of the increased mobility of their joints, and because children are often naturally more mobile. Nevertheless, situations arise in which joint stiffness results from a musculoskeletal injury in childhood. Furthermore, in children with neuromuscular conditions, such as cerebral palsy, muscle shortening or weakness often causes capsular restrictions. In these situations, the clinician must make a determination as to whether intervention with joint mobilization/manipulation techniques is appropriate. Although no research has been performed showing that joint mobilization/manipulation is harmful to children, the clinician might want to consider the relative risks and benefits of this intervention in the presence of immature growth plates.

CONCLUSION

Harris[43] listed six criteria for evaluating the scientific merit of an intervention, as follows:
1. The theories underlying the treatment approach are supported by valid anatomical and physiological evidence.
2. The treatment approach is designed for a specific type of patient population.
3. Potential side effects of the treatment are presented.
4. Studies from peer-reviewed journals are provided that support the treatment's efficacy.
5. Peer-reviewed studies include well-designed, randomized controlled clinical trials or well-designed single-subject experimental studies.
6. The proponents of the treatment approach are open and willing to discuss its limitations.

These criteria can be analyzed in relation to joint mobilization/manipulation evaluation and intervention. Although the theoretical basis on which mobilization/manipulation is based is incomplete, studies have provided support for the premise that this intervention increases range of motion, decreases pain, and improves muscle performance. The type of patient who is most likely to benefit from joint mobilization/manipulation techniques has been identified, and information regarding potential side effects has been disseminated in the clinical literature. Numerous efficacy studies have been published, although they do not cover the wide range of issues involving joint mobilization/manipulation evaluation and intervention, and many of the studies that do exist have methodological flaws. Finally, many of the clinicians who advocate the use of joint mobilization/manipulation are willing to acknowledge the potential and actual limitations of this technique.

Harris's[43] criteria do not address several concerns that have relevance to determining the scientific merit of joint mobilization/manipulation. One of these concerns involves issues related to the reliability of joint mobilization/manipulation evaluation procedures. In regard to individual examination techniques involving joint position or motion, reliability is fair to poor. There is some evidence, however, that the reliability of various measures of spinal joint impairments improves to acceptable levels when a patient shows more than one indication of that spinal joint impairment (see Chapter 14).

Another concern involves the validity of techniques to determine the appropriate direction of force for glide mobilizations/manipulations. This is especially relevant when addressing decreases in passive range of motion. The two generally accepted methods to determine the optimal direction of glide mobilization/manipulations are the use of convex-concave rules and a comparison of the excursion in affected joints with that in unaffected joints. Neither of these techniques has been shown to be valid, although based on the premise that the reliability of determining hypomobility can improve with training, the better method most likely entails a comparison with unaffected joints. Nevertheless, this issue of determining the optimal glide technique for a specific range of motion impairment has not yet been resolved.

Although mobilization/manipulation examination, evaluation, and intervention have scientific merit, additional investigation of this technique is warranted. This is also the case with numerous other medical interventions that are commonly used to treat musculoskeletal pain and functional limitations. In the case of joint mobilization/manipulation, the best evidence suggests that it is an effective intervention for joint and periarticular impairments. Additional studies are warranted to refine our understanding of this discipline and increase the efficacy of treatment.

REFERENCES

1. Kaltenborn FM: Manual Mobilization of the Joints: The Kaltenborn Method of Joint Examination and Treatment, Vol I: The Extremities, 6th ed. Oslo, Norway, Norli, 2002.
2. Arvidsson I: The hip joint: forces needed for distraction and appearance of the vacuum phenomenon. Scand J Rehab Med 1990;22:157-162.
3. Kavanagh J: Is there a positional fault at the inferior tibiofibular joint in patients with acute or chronic ankle sprains compared to normals? Manual Ther 1999;4:19-24.
4. Roubal PJ, Dobritt D, Placzek JD: Glenohumeral gliding manipulation following interscalene brachial plexus block in patients with adhesive capsulitis. J Orthop Sports Phys Ther 1996;24:66-77.
5. Hsu A-T, Ho L, Ho S, et al: Immediate response of glenohumeral abduction range of motion to a caudally directed translational mobilization: a fresh cadaver simulation. Arch Phys Med Rehab 2000;81:1511-1516.
6. Hsu A-T, Headman T, Chang JH, et al: Changes in abduction and rotation range of motion in response to simulated dorsal and anterior translational mobilization of the glenohumeral joint. Phys Ther 2002;82:544-556.
7. Hjelm R, Draper C, Spencer S: Anterior-inferior capsular length insufficiency in the painful shoulder. J Orthop Sports Phys Ther 1996;23:216-222.
8. Hsu A-T, Ho L, Ho S, et al: Joint position during anterior-posterior glide mobilization: its effect on glenohumeral abduction range of motion. Arch Phys Med Rehab 2000;81:210-214.
9. Baeyens J-P, Van Roy P, Clarys JP: Intra-articular kinematics of the normal glenohumeral joint in the late preparatory phase of throwing: Kaltenborn's rule revisited. Ergonomics 2000;43:1726-1737.
10. Cyriax J: Textbook of Orthopaedic Medicine, Vol 1: Diagnosis of Soft Tissue Lesions, 8th ed. London, Bailliere Tindall, 1982.
11. Hayes KW, Petersen C, Falconer J: An examination of Cyriax's passive motion tests with patients having osteoarthritis of the knee. Phys Ther 1994;74:697-709.
12. Fritz JM, Delitto A, Erhard RE, et al: An examination of the selective tissue tension scheme, with evidence for the concept of a capsular pattern of the knee. Phys Ther 1998;78:1046-1061.
13. Klassbo M, Harms-Ringdahl K: Examination of passive ROM and capsular patterns in the hip. Physiother Res Int 2003;8:1-12.
14. Maitland GD: Vertebral Manipulation, 5th ed. London, Butterworth, 1986.
15. Matyas TA, Bach TM: The reliability of selected techniques in clinical arthrometrics. Aust J Physiother 1985;31:175-199.
16. Mootz RD, et al: Intra- and interobserver reliability of passive motion palpation of the lumbar spine. J Manip Physiol Therap 1989;12:440-445.
17. Binkley J, Stratford PW, Gill C: Interrater reliability of lumbar accessory motion mobility testing. Phys Ther 1995;75:786-795.
18. Keating J, et al: The effect of training on physical therapists' ability to apply specified forces of palpation. Phys Ther 1993;73:38-46.

19. Lee M, Moseley A, Refshauge K: Effect of feedback on learning a vertebral joint mobilization skill. Phys Ther 1990;70:97-104.

20. Gonnella C, Paris SV, Kutner M: Reliability in evaluating passive intervertebral motion. Phys Ther 1982;62:436-444.

21. Jull G, Bogduk N, Marsland A: The accuracy of manual diagnosis for cervical zygapophysial joint pain syndromes. Med J Aust 1988;148;233-236.

22. McQuade KJ, Shelley I, Cvitkovic J: Patterns of stiffness during clinical examination of the glenohumeral joint. Clin Biomech 1999;14:620-627.

23. Maitland GD: Peripheral Manipulation, 3rd ed. London, Butterworth-Heinemann, 1991.

24. Hsu A-T, Ho L, Chang J-H, et al: Characterization of tissue resistance during a dorsally directed translational mobilization of the glenohumeral joint. Arch Phys Med Rehab 2002;83:360-366.

25. Nwuga VCB: Relative therapeutic efficacy of vertebral manipulation and conventional treatment in back pain management. Am J Phys Med 1982;61:273-278.

26. Nicholson GG: The effects of passive joint mobilization on pain and hypomobility associated with adhesive capsulitis of the shoulder. J Orthop Sports Phys Ther 1985;6:238-246.

27. Wilson F: Manual therapy versus traditional exercises in mobilization of the ankle post-ankle fracture: a pilot study. N Z J Physiother 1991;19:11-16.

28. Randall T, Portney L, Harris BA: Effects of joint mobilization on joint stiffness and active motion of the metacarpophalangeal joint. J Orthop Sports Phys Ther 1992;16:30-36.

29. Gross AR, Aker PD, Goldsmith CH, Peloso P: Conservative management of mechanical neck disorders: a systematic overview and meta-analysis. Online Journal of Current Clinical Trials 1994;3.

30. Gross AR, Aker PD, Quartly C: Manual therapy in the treatment of neck pain. Musculoskel Med 1996;22:579-598.

31. Hurwitz EL, Aker PD, Adams AH, et al: Manipulation and mobilization of the cervical spine: a systematic review of the literature. Spine 1996;21:1746-1760.

32. Drechsler WI, Knarr JF, Snyder-Mackler L: A comparison of two treatment regimens for lateral epicondylitis: a randomized trial of clinical interventions. J Sport Rehab 1997;6:226-234.

33. Conroy DE, Hayes KW: The effect of joint mobilization as a component of comprehensive treatment for primary shoulder impingement syndrome. J Orthop Sports Phys Ther 1998;28:3-14.

34. Bang MD, Deyle GD: Comparison of supervised exercise with and without manual physical therapy for patients with shoulder impingement syndrome. J Orthop Sports Phys Ther 2000;30:126-137.

35. Deyle GD, Henderson NE, Matekel RL, et al: Effectiveness of manual physical therapy and exercise in osteoarthritis of the knee. Ann Intern Med 2000;132:173-181.

36. Crossley K, Bennell K, Green S, et al: Physical therapy for patellofemoral pain: a randomized, double-blinded, placebo-controlled trial. Am J Sports Med 2002;30:857-865.

37. Cleland JA, Whitman JM, Fritz JM: Effectiveness of manual physical therapy to the cervical spine in the management of lateral epicondylalgia: a retrospective analysis. J Orthop Sports Phys Ther 2004;34:713-721.

38. UK BEAM Team Trial: UK Back Pain Exercise and Manipulation (BEAM) randomized trial: effectiveness of physical treatments for back pain in primary care. BMJ 2004;329:1377-1380.

39. Brodeur R: The audible release associated with joint manipulation. J Manip Physiol Therap 1995;18:155-164.

40. Flynn TW, Fritz JM, Wainner RS, et al: The audible pop is not necessary for successful spinal high-velocity thrust manipulation in individuals with low back pain. Arch Phys Med Rehab 2003;84:1057-1060.

41. Swezey RL, Swezey SE: The consequences of habitual knuckle cracking. West J Med 1975;122:377-379.

42. Castellanos J, Axelrod D: Effect of habitual knuckle cracking on hand function. Ann Rheum Dis 1990;49:308-309.

43. Harris S: How should treatments be critiqued for scientific merit? Phys Ther 1996;76:175-181.

Section II

The Appendicular Skeletal System

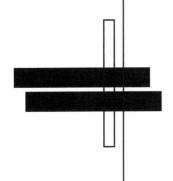

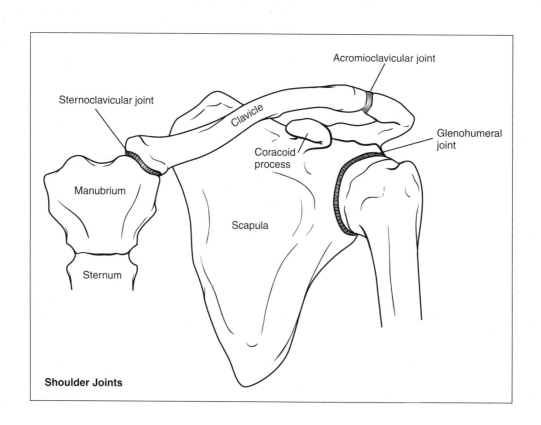

Sternoclavicular joint

Acromioclavicular joint

Clavicle

Coracoid process

Glenohumeral joint

Manubrium

Scapula

Sternum

Shoulder Joints

CHAPTER 3

The Shoulder

BASICS

The shoulder complex comprises four joints, all of which contribute to attaining full range of motion at the shoulder: the glenohumeral joint, scapulothoracic joint, sternoclavicular joint, and acromioclavicular joint. Approximately 120 degrees of motion into flexion and abduction must occur at the shoulder complex for most functional activities to occur.

Glenohumeral Joint

The glenohumeral articulation is the most mobile joint in the human body. This mobility is achieved in part because the humeral head is much larger than its articulating counterpart, the glenoid cavity. The sole attachment of the shoulder complex to the axial skeletal system at the sternoclavicular joint also contributes to its mobility. Many conditions affecting the shoulder can be attributable to its large arc of motion.

The inferior folds of the glenohumeral joint capsule, present when the shoulder is in the anatomical position, unfold as shoulder elevation occurs. When the shoulder is immobilized in adduction, these folds often adhere to one another.

Scapulothoracic Joint

Scapulothoracic lateral rotation and elevation are components of shoulder abduction, whereas scapulothoracic lateral rotation and protraction accompany shoulder flexion. With activities involving shoulder abduction, there is variability as to the amount of glenohumeral versus scapulothoracic motion. During the first 30 degrees of motion, the scapula attempts to stabilize itself against the thorax. In this phase, a greater proportion of the motion occurs at the glenohumeral joint. After this phase, several patterns of scapulohumeral rhythm have been reported; however, in most individuals, scapular motion predominates in the middle ranges of abduction, and glenohumeral motion predominates at the end ranges.

Sternoclavicular and Acromioclavicular Joints

Movement at the sternoclavicular and acromioclavicular joints accompanies shoulder elevation. As the scapula elevates and laterally rotates, the clavicle rotates on its longitudinal axis, contributing to full shoulder elevation range of motion.

SPECIFIC PATHOLOGY AND SHOULDER JOINT MOBILIZATION/ MANIPULATION

Musculoskeletal shoulder conditions are often multifaceted. For example, while the etiology of adhesive capsulitis is unknown, it has been attributed to such diverse causes as self-imposed immobilization after a minor shoulder injury, psychosocial profiles, joint hypomobility, periarticular muscle imbalances, and impaired posture. Patients with the same shoulder condition often present with diverse physical findings. In the absence of information obtained from radiography or surgical arthroscopy, there is no single consistent or commonly used criterion for diagnosing shoulder conditions. Nevertheless, in some of the research involving mobilization/manipulation interventions for shoulder joint impairments, an attempt was made to distinguish between different pathologies. The uncertainty of the diagnostic criteria could have easily influenced study conclusions regarding the efficacy of joint mobilization/manipulation.

Adhesive Capsulitis

Evidence suggests that mobilization/manipulation of the glenohumeral joint, combined with other interventions commonly used to treat patients with musculoskeletal conditions, is effective in increasing range of motion when the follow-up period is short term. In one of these studies, subjects were randomly assigned to receive mobilization and exercise or exercise alone. There was an increase in range of motion in the mobilization group, but no significant differences in pain between the two groups.[1] Another study showed a significant increase in range of motion with physical therapy and a steroid injection compared with physical therapy alone and a steroid injection alone. Physical therapy consisted of joint mobilization and range of motion exercises.[2] Several other studies have shown greater short-term benefits, however, from steroid injections compared with either mobilization or manipulation.[3-5] In studies that followed subjects for longer periods (6-12 months), differences in outcomes attributable to any intervention were not apparent.[2,3,6]

Impingement Syndrome

Two randomized trials specifically addressed the effectiveness of joint mobilization in the treatment of impingement syndrome. One study of 14 subjects compared intervention consisting of moist heat, range of motion, stretching, strengthening, soft tissue mobilization, and patient education with the same intervention with the addition of joint mobilization.[7] The other study, which consisted of 54 subjects, compared a stretching and strengthening program with the same intervention with the addition of joint mobilization.[8] In both studies, subjects receiving joint mobilization had greater improvements than the group that did not receive joint mobilization. Outcome measures included decreased pain,[7,8] improvement in function,[8] and increased strength.[8]

Nonspecific Shoulder Pain

One study of the effects of joint mobilization consisted of 66 subjects with painful stiff shoulders. The subjects were randomly assigned to receive a corticosteroid injection, physical therapy that included joint mobilization, or both. Improvements were identical in all three groups. The investigators also concluded that the steroid injections were more cost-effective than physical therapy.[9]

Decreased Glenohumeral Joint Range of Motion

Numerous studies, performed on cadavers and on live subjects, support the use of joint mobilization/manipulation for increasing glenohumeral joint range of motion. Various glide techniques performed with sufficient force to take the joint through tissue resistance increased motion in shoulder flexion, abduction, and rotation.[10-14] These studies are described in greater detail in Chapter 2.

GLENOHUMERAL JOINT

Osteokinematic motions:
  Flexion/extension
  Abduction/adduction
  Medial/lateral rotation
  Horizontal abduction/adduction
Ligaments:
  Superior glenohumeral ligament
  Middle glenohumeral ligament
  Inferior glenohumeral ligament
  Coracohumeral ligament
  Coracoacromial ligament
Joint orientation:
  Glenoid: lateral, anterior, inferior
  Humerus: medial, posterior, superior
Concave joint surface:
  Glenoid

Type of joint:
   Synovial
Resting position:
   55 degrees of abduction and 30 degrees of horizontal adduction (55 degrees of scaption), slight lateral rotation[15]
   30 to 40 degrees of abduction, no flexion, neutral rotation[16]
Close-packed position:
   Full elevation[15]
Capsular pattern of restriction:
   Lateral rotation more limited than abduction, which is more limited than medial rotation[17]

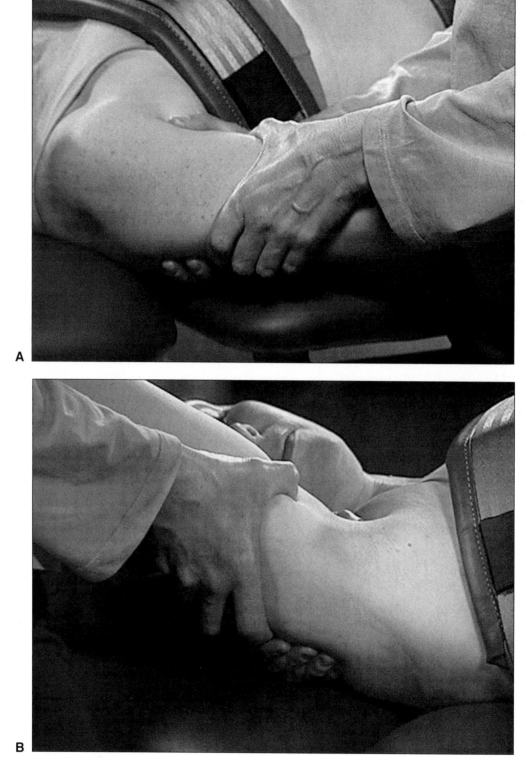

FIG. 3-1. Distraction. **A,** Distraction performed in the resting position. **B,** Distraction performed approximating the restricted range of motion into flexion.

DISTRACTION (Fig. 3-1)

Purpose

- To examine for glenohumeral joint impairment
- To increase accessory motion into glenohumeral joint distraction
- To increase range of motion at the glenohumeral joint
- To decrease pain
- To improve periarticular muscle performance

Positioning

1. The patient is supine.
2. The glenohumeral joint is placed in the resting position if conservative techniques are indicated or approximating restricted range of motion if more aggressive techniques are indicated.
3. The clinician can use a belt to hold the patient's scapula against the trunk, especially in the presence of scapulothoracic hypermobility or an increase in movement at the scapulothoracic joint with shoulder elevation.
4. The clinician is at the patient's side facing the glenohumeral joint.
5. The clinician can support the patient's forearm and hand by positioning them between the clinician's upper arm and trunk.
6. Both hands grip the proximal humerus as close to the axilla as possible from the medial and lateral side.

Procedure

1. Both hands move the humeral head lateral, anterior, and inferior, perpendicular to the glenoid joint surface (see Fig. 3-1).

Particulars

1. When the glenohumeral joint is positioned such that the long axis of the humerus is perpendicular to the flattened-out concave surface of the glenoid, this technique can be performed by pulling on the upper arm.

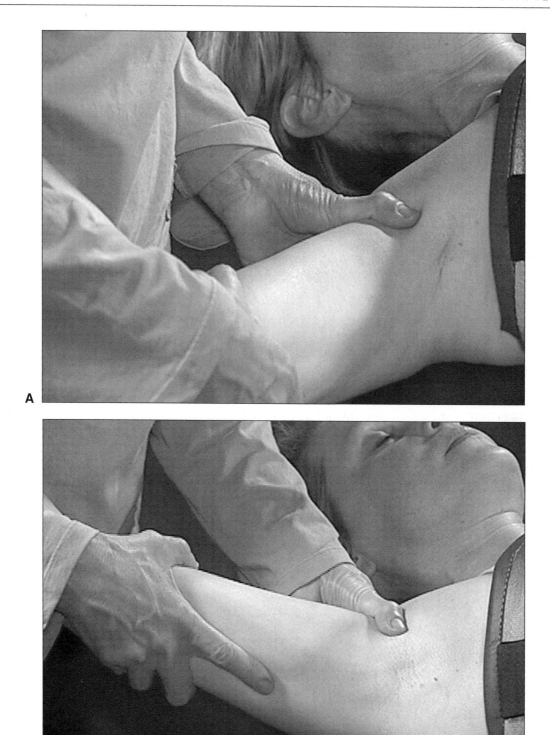

FIG. 3-2. Inferior glide. **A,** Inferior glide performed in the resting position. **B,** Inferior glide performed approximating the restricted range of motion into abduction.

INFERIOR GLIDE (Fig. 3-2)

Purpose
- To examine for glenohumeral joint impairment
- To increase accessory motion into glenohumeral joint inferior glide
- To increase range of motion at the glenohumeral joint
- To decrease pain
- To improve periarticular muscle performance

Positioning
1. The patient is supine.
2. The glenohumeral joint is placed in the resting position if conservative techniques are indicated or approximating restricted range of motion if more aggressive techniques are indicated.
3. The clinician can use a belt to hold the patient's scapula against the trunk.
4. The clinician is at the patient's head facing the glenohumeral joint.
5. The clinician can support the patient's forearm and hand by positioning them between the clinician's upper arm and trunk.
6. The mobilizing/manipulating hand is positioned with the web space over the superior surface of the proximal humerus.
7. The guiding hand supports the upper limb from the medial side of the distal humerus.

Procedure
1. The clinician applies a grade I traction to the joint.
2. The mobilizing/manipulating hand glides the humerus in an inferior direction.
3. The guiding hand controls the position of the humerus (see Fig. 3-2).

Particulars
1. This technique might be especially effective for increasing range of motion into glenohumeral joint abduction.

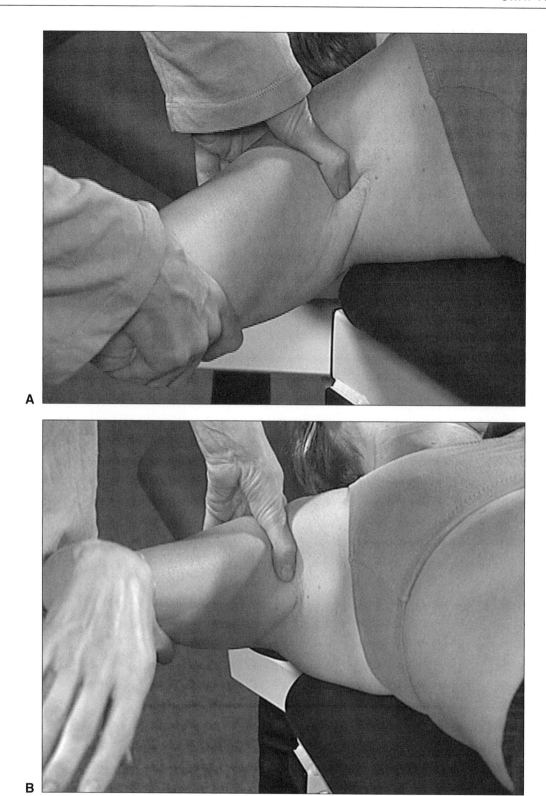

FIG. 3-3. Posterior glide. **A,** Posterior glide performed in the resting position. **B,** Posterior glide performed approximating the restricted range of motion into medial rotation.

POSTERIOR GLIDE (Fig. 3-3)

Purpose

- To examine for glenohumeral joint impairment
- To increase accessory motion into glenohumeral joint posterior glide
- To increase range of motion at the glenohumeral joint
- To decrease pain
- To improve periarticular muscle performance

Positioning

1. The patient is supine with the humerus positioned off the edge of the treatment table.
2. The glenohumeral joint is placed in the resting position if conservative techniques are indicated or approximating restricted range of motion if more aggressive techniques are indicated.
3. The clinician is at the patient's side facing the patient.
4. The clinician can support the patient's forearm and hand by positioning them between the clinician's upper arm and trunk.
5. The mobilizing/manipulating hand is positioned over the anterior surface of the proximal humerus.
6. The guiding hand supports the upper limb from the posterior side of the distal humerus.

Procedure

1. The clinician applies a grade I traction to the joint.
2. The mobilizing/manipulating hand glides the humerus in a posterior direction.
3. The guiding hand controls the position of the humerus (see Fig. 3-3).
4. When approximating the restricted range of motion for horizontal adduction, if the shoulder joint can be positioned in at least 90 degrees of horizontal adduction, the posterior glide can be directed through the shaft of the humerus.

Particulars

1. This technique might be especially effective for increasing range of motion into glenohumeral joint medial rotation, flexion, and horizontal adduction.

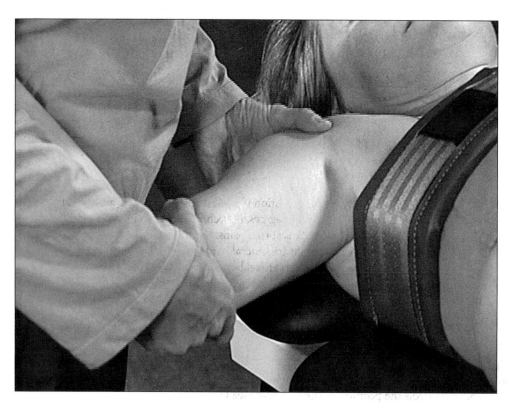

FIG. 3-4. Anterior glide: first technique.

ANTERIOR GLIDE: FIRST TECHNIQUE (Fig. 3-4)

Purpose
- To examine for glenohumeral joint impairment
- To increase accessory motion into glenohumeral joint anterior glide
- To increase range of motion at the glenohumeral joint
- To decrease pain
- To improve periarticular muscle performance

Positioning
1. The patient is supine.
2. The glenohumeral joint is placed in the resting position if conservative techniques are indicated or approximating restricted range of motion if more aggressive techniques are indicated.
3. The clinician can use a belt to hold the patient's scapula against the trunk.
4. The clinician is at the patient's side facing the glenohumeral joint.
5. The clinician can support the patient's forearm and hand by positioning them between the clinician's upper arm and trunk.
6. The mobilizing/manipulating hand is positioned over the posterior surface of the proximal humerus.
7. The guiding hand supports the upper limb from the anterior and posterior sides of the distal humerus.

Procedure
1. The clinician applies a grade I traction to the joint.
2. The mobilizing/manipulating hand glides the humerus in an anterior direction.
3. The guiding hand controls the position of the humerus (see Fig. 3-4).

Particulars
1. The clinician should use caution in performing this technique because this motion might be hypermobile. If it is, performing an anterior glide mobilization/manipulation technique might cause the humerus to dislocate.
2. This position requires that the clinician work against gravity and should be used only when the mobilization/manipulation technique is to be performed for a short amount of time.
3. This technique might be especially effective for increasing range of motion into glenohumeral joint lateral rotation, extension, and horizontal abduction.

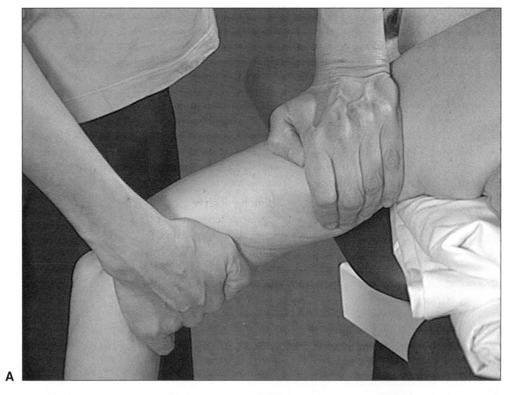

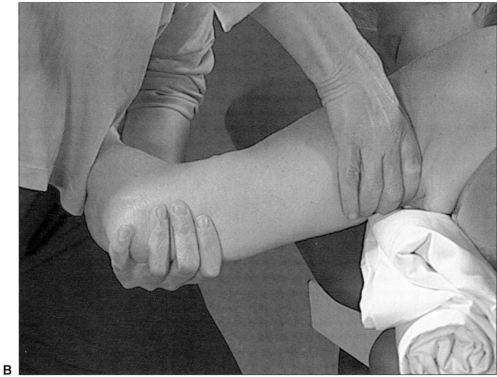

FIG. 3-5. Anterior glide: second technique. **A,** Anterior glide performed in the resting position. **B,** Anterior glide performed approximating the restricted range of motion into lateral rotation.

ANTERIOR GLIDE: SECOND TECHNIQUE (Fig. 3-5)

Purpose

- To examine for glenohumeral joint impairment
- To increase accessory motion into glenohumeral joint anterior glide
- To increase range of motion at the glenohumeral joint
- To decrease pain
- To improve periarticular muscle performance

Positioning

1. The patient is prone with the humerus positioned off the edge of the treatment table and a pillow supporting the coracoid process.
2. The glenohumeral joint is placed in the resting position if conservative techniques are indicated or approximating restricted range of motion if more aggressive techniques are indicated.
3. The clinician can use a belt to hold the patient's scapula against the trunk.
4. The clinician is at the patient's side facing the glenohumeral joint.
5. The mobilizing/manipulating hand is positioned over the posterior surface of the proximal humerus.
6. The guiding hand supports the upper limb from the anterior side of the distal humerus.

Procedure

1. The clinician applies a grade I traction to the joint.
2. The mobilizing/manipulating hand glides the humerus in an anterior direction.
3. The guiding hand controls the position of the humerus (see Fig. 3-5).

Particulars

1. The clinician should use caution in performing this technique because this motion might be hypermobile. If it is, performing an anterior glide mobilization/manipulation technique might cause the humerus to dislocate.
2. This technique might be especially effective for increasing range of motion into glenohumeral joint lateral rotation, extension, and horizontal abduction.

SCAPULOTHORACIC JOINT

Osteokinematic motions:
> Protraction/retraction
> Elevation/depression (these two motions are accompanied by upward and downward rotation)

Ligaments:
> None

Joint orientation:
> Thorax: posterior, lateral, superior
> Scapula: anterior, medial, inferior

Concave joint surface:
> Scapula

Type of joint:
> Functional articulation

Resting position:
> Not described by Kaltenborn

Close-packed position:
> None; not a synovial joint

Capsular pattern of restriction:
> None; not a synovial joint

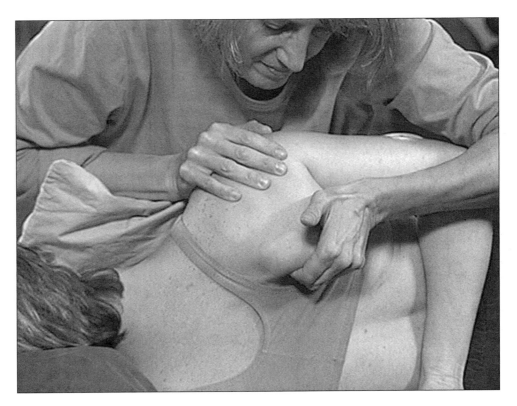

FIG. 3-6. Distraction.

DISTRACTION (Fig. 3-6)

Purpose

- To examine for scapulothoracic joint impairment
- To increase accessory motion into scapulothoracic joint distraction
- To increase range of motion at the shoulder complex
- To decrease pain
- To improve periarticular muscle performance

Positioning

1. The patient is lying on the side with the posterior surface of the hand positioned on the sacrum if shoulder range of motion allows.
2. The clinician is either in front or behind the patient facing the patient's shoulder.
3. If the clinician is positioned in front of the patient, a pillow should separate the patient's chest from the clinician.
4. The mobilizing hand is positioned over the acromion.
5. The guiding hand is positioned adjacent to the inferior angle of the scapula.

Procedure

1. The mobilizing hand moves the scapula medially and inferiorly over the guiding hand.
2. The guiding hand lifts the scapula away from the ribs (see Fig. 3-6).

Particulars

1. This joint can be difficult to mobilize, as it might take a great deal of effort on the part of the clinician to maneuver the hand between the scapula and thorax.
2. This is not a grade V manipulation technique.

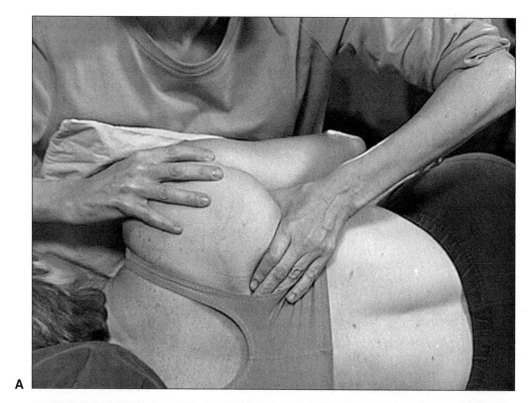

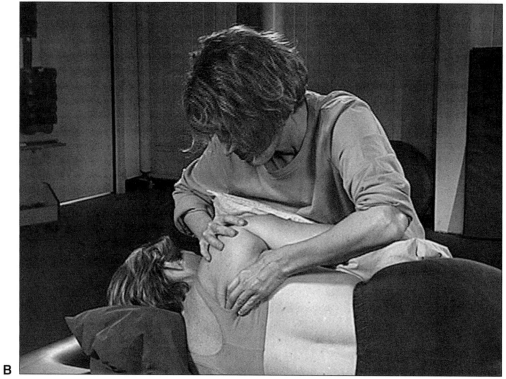

FIG. 3-7. Superior glide.

SUPERIOR GLIDE (Fig. 3-7)

Purpose

- To examine for scapulothoracic joint impairment
- To increase accessory motion into scapulothoracic superior glide
- To increase range of motion at the shoulder complex
- To decrease pain
- To improve periarticular muscle performance

Positioning

1. The patient is lying on the side with the arm in a neutral position.
2. The clinician is in front of the patient facing the patient's shoulder.
3. A pillow should separate the patient's chest from the clinician.
4. The mobilizing hand is positioned adjacent to the inferior angle of the scapula.
5. The guiding hand is positioned over the acromion.

Procedure

1. The clinician applies a grade I traction to the joint.
2. The mobilizing hand glides the scapula in a superior direction.
3. The guiding hand controls the position of the scapula (see Fig. 3-7).

Particulars

1. This is not a grade V manipulation technique.
2. This technique might be especially effective for increasing range of motion into scapulothoracic joint elevation and lateral rotation.

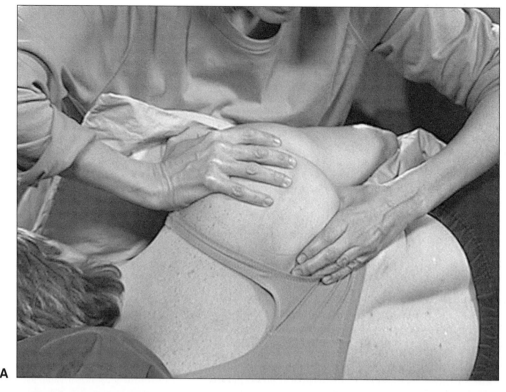

A

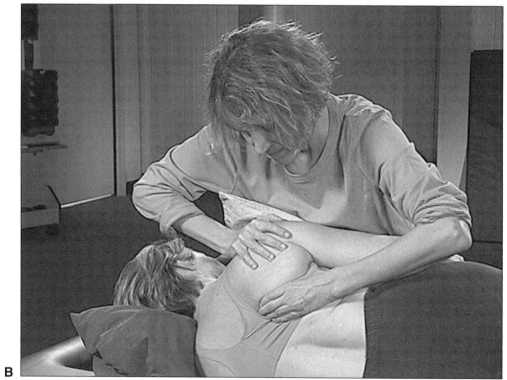

B

FIG. 3-8. Inferior glide.

INFERIOR GLIDE (Fig. 3-8)

Purpose

- To examine for scapulothoracic joint impairment
- To increase accessory motion into scapulothoracic inferior glide
- To increase range of motion at the shoulder complex
- To decrease pain
- To improve periarticular muscle performance

Positioning

1. The patient is lying on the side with the arm in a neutral position.
2. The clinician is in front of the patient facing the patient's shoulder.
3. A pillow should separate the patient's chest from the clinician.
4. The mobilizing hand is positioned over the acromion.
5. The guiding hand is positioned over the inferior angle of the scapula.

Procedure

1. The clinician applies a grade I traction to the joint.
2. The mobilizing hand glides the acromion in an inferior direction.
3. The guiding hand controls the position of the scapula (see Fig. 3-8).

Particulars

1. This is not a grade V manipulation technique.
2. This technique might be especially effective for increasing range of motion into scapulothoracic joint depression and medial rotation.

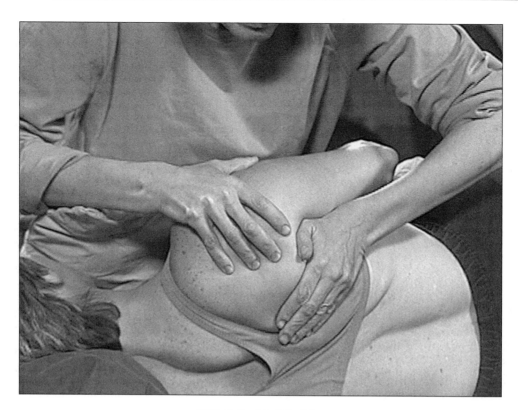

FIG. 3-9. Medial glide.

MEDIAL GLIDE (Fig. 3-9)

Purpose

- To examine for scapulothoracic joint impairment
- To increase accessory motion into scapulothoracic medial glide
- To increase range of motion at the shoulder complex
- To decrease pain
- To improve periarticular muscle performance

Positioning

1. The patient is lying on the side with the arm in a neutral position.
2. The clinician is in front of the patient facing the patient's shoulder.
3. A pillow should separate the patient's chest from the clinician.
4. Both hands are positioned over the lateral surface of the scapula, one hand over the axillary border and the other hand over the acromion.

Procedure

1. Both hands glide the scapula in a medial direction (see Fig. 3-9).

Particulars

1. This is not a grade V manipulation technique.
2. This technique might be especially effective for increasing range of motion into scapulothoracic joint retraction, depression, and medial rotation.

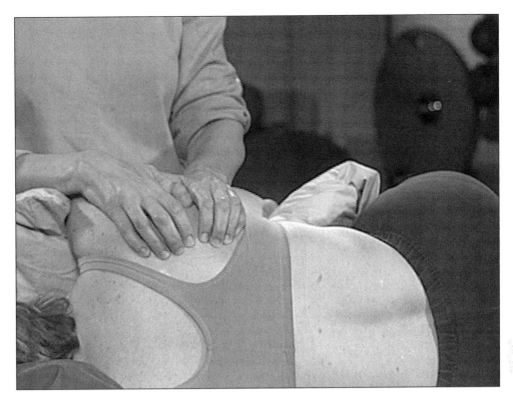

FIG. 3-10. Lateral glide.

LATERAL GLIDE (Fig. 3-10)

Purpose
- To examine for scapulothoracic joint impairment
- To increase accessory motion into scapulothoracic lateral glide
- To increase range of motion at the shoulder complex
- To decrease pain
- To improve periarticular muscle performance

Positioning
1. The patient is lying on the side with the arm in a neutral position.
2. The clinician is in front of the patient facing the patient's shoulder.
3. A pillow should separate the patient's chest from the clinician.
4. Both hands are positioned with the fingertips over the vertebral border of the scapula.

Procedure
1. Both hands glide the scapula in a lateral direction (see Fig. 3-10).

Particulars
1. This is not a grade V manipulation technique.
2. The clinician should use caution in performing this technique because this motion might be hypermobile, especially among patients with posture impairments involving the shoulder.
3. This technique might be especially effective for increasing range of motion into scapulothoracic joint protraction, elevation, and lateral rotation.

STERNOCLAVICULAR JOINT

Osteokinematic motions:
   Elevation/depression
   Protraction/retraction
Ligaments:
   Costoclavicular ligament
   Interclavicular ligament
   Posterior sternoclavicular ligament
   Anterior sternoclavicular ligament
Joint orientation:
   Manubrium: lateral, superior
   Clavicle: medial, inferior
Concave joint surface:
   Sternum concave superior to inferior
   Clavicle concave anterior to posterior
Type of joint:
   Synovial
Resting position:
   Not described by Kaltenborn
Close-packed position:
   Arm fully elevated[15]
Capsular pattern of restriction:
   Pain at the end of range of shoulder motion[17]

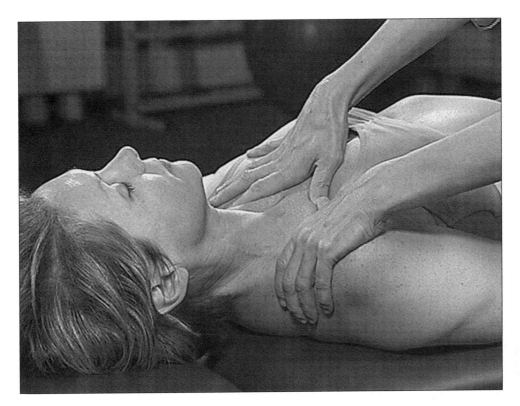

FIG. 3-11. Superior glide.

SUPERIOR GLIDE (Fig. 3-11)

Purpose
- To examine for sternoclavicular joint impairment
- To increase accessory motion into sternoclavicular superior glide
- To increase range of motion at the shoulder complex
- To decrease pain
- To improve periarticular muscle performance

Positioning
1. The patient is supine with the arm resting at the side.
2. The clinician is at the patient's side facing the sternoclavicular joint.
3. The mobilizing/manipulating hand is positioned with the thumb over the thumb of the guiding hand.
4. The guiding hand is positioned with the thumb over the inferior surface of the clavicle about 3 cm lateral to the most medial surface.

Procedure
1. The mobilizing/manipulating hand glides the clavicle in a superior direction.
2. The guiding hand controls the position of the mobilizing/manipulating hand (see Fig. 3-11).

Particulars
1. The clinician should use caution in performing this technique because this motion might be hypermobile.

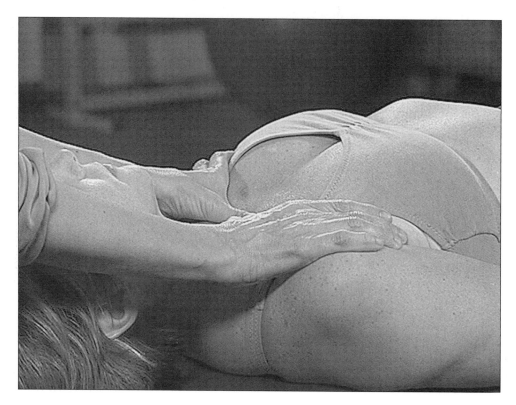

FIG. 3-12. Inferior glide.

INFERIOR GLIDE (Fig. 3-12)

Purpose

- To examine for sternoclavicular joint impairment
- To increase accessory motion into sternoclavicular inferior glide
- To increase range of motion at the shoulder complex
- To decrease pain
- To improve periarticular muscle performance

Positioning

1. The patient is supine with the arm resting at the side.
2. The clinician is at the patient's head facing the sternoclavicular joint.
3. The mobilizing/manipulating hand is positioned with the thumb over the thumb of the guiding hand.
4. The guiding hand is positioned with the thumb over the superior surface of the clavicle about 3 cm lateral to the most medial surface.

Procedure

1. The mobilizing/manipulating hand glides the clavicle in an inferior direction.
2. The guiding hand controls the position of the mobilizing/manipulating hand (see Fig. 3-12).

Particulars

1. The clinician should use caution in performing this technique because this motion might be hypermobile.

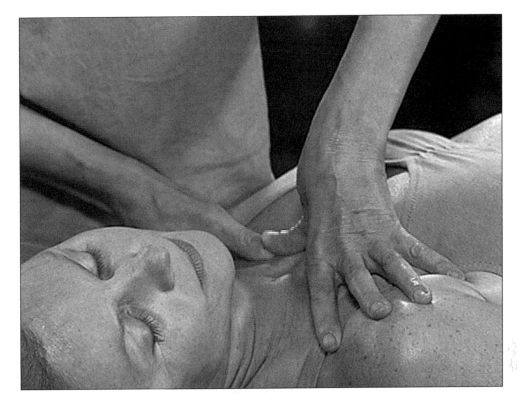

FIG. 3-13. Posterior glide.

POSTERIOR GLIDE (Fig. 3-13)

Purpose

- To examine for sternoclavicular joint impairment
- To increase accessory motion into sternoclavicular posterior glide
- To increase range of motion at the shoulder complex
- To decrease pain
- To improve periarticular muscle performance

Positioning

1. The patient is supine with the arm resting at the side.
2. The clinician is at the patient's head facing the sternoclavicular joint.
3. The mobilizing/manipulating hand is positioned with the thumb over the thumb of the guiding hand.
4. The guiding hand is positioned with the thumb over the anterior surface of the clavicle about 3 cm lateral to the most medial surface.

Procedure

1. The mobilizing/manipulating hand glides the clavicle in a posterior direction.
2. The guiding hand controls the position of the mobilizing/manipulating hand (see Fig. 3-13).

Particulars

1. The clinician should use caution in performing this technique because this motion might be hypermobile.

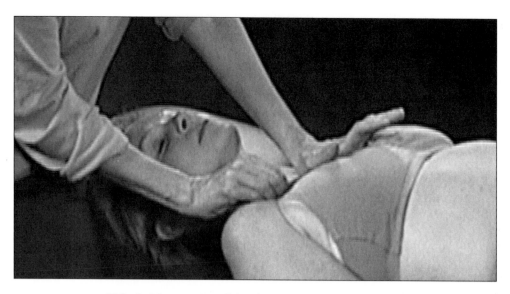

FIG. 3-14. Anterior glide of the clavicle on the sternum.

ANTERIOR GLIDE OF THE CLAVICLE ON THE STERNUM (Fig. 3-14)

Purpose

- To examine for sternoclavicular joint impairment
- To increase accessory motion into sternoclavicular anterior glide
- To increase range of motion at the shoulder complex
- To decrease pain
- To improve periarticular muscle performance

Positioning

1. The patient is supine with the arm resting at the side.
2. The clinician is at the patient's head facing the sternoclavicular joint.
3. The stabilizing hand grips around the clavicle superiorly and inferiorly as close to the posterior surface as possible with the fingers.
4. The mobilizing/manipulating hand is positioned over the patient's sternum.

Procedure

1. The stabilizing hand holds the clavicle in position.
2. The mobilizing/manipulating hand glides the sternum in a posterior direction, imparting an anterior force to the clavicle on the sternum (see Fig. 3-14).

Particulars

1. The clinician should use caution in performing this technique because this motion might be hypermobile.
2. The clinician should be aware that the grip on the clavicle might be uncomfortable for the patient.

ACROMIOCLAVICULAR JOINT

Osteokinematic motions:
   Elevation/depression
   Protraction/retraction
Ligaments:
   Superior acromioclavicular ligament
   Inferior acromioclavicular ligament
   Coracoclavicular ligaments (conoid and trapezoid)
Joint orientation:
   Acromion: superior, medial, anterior
   Clavicle: inferior, lateral, posterior
Concave joint surface:
   Acromion
Type of joint:
   Synovial
Resting position:
   Not described by Kaltenborn
Close-packed position:
   90 degrees of abduction[15]
Capsular pattern of restriction:
   Pain at the end of range of shoulder motion[17]

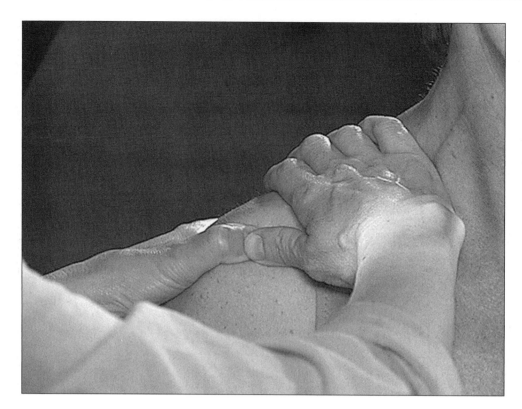

FIG. 3-15. Posterior glide.

POSTERIOR GLIDE (Fig. 3-15)

Purpose
- To examine for acromioclavicular joint impairment
- To increase accessory motion into acromioclavicular posterior glide
- To increase range of motion at the shoulder complex
- To decrease pain
- To improve periarticular muscle performance

Positioning
1. The patient is sitting with the arm resting at the side.
2. The clinician is in front of the patient facing the anterior surface of the acromioclavicular joint.
3. The stabilizing hand is positioned over the posterior surface of the scapula.
4. The mobilizing/manipulating hand is positioned with the thumb over the thumb of the guiding hand.
5. The guiding hand, which is the same hand as the stabilizing hand, is positioned with the thumb over the anterolateral surface of the clavicle.

Procedure
1. The stabilizing hand holds the scapula in position.
2. The mobilizing/manipulating hand glides the clavicle in a posterior direction.
3. The guiding hand controls the position of the mobilizing/manipulating hand (see Fig. 3-15).

Particulars
1. The clinician should use caution in performing this technique because this motion might be hypermobile.

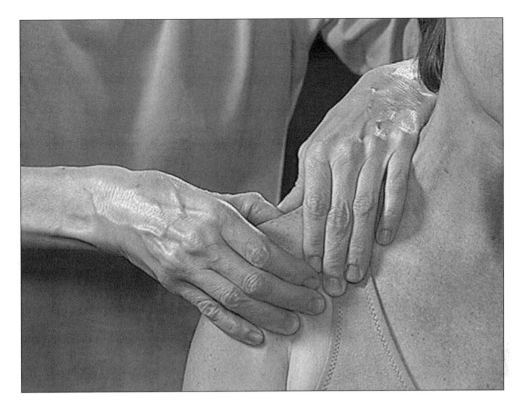

FIG. 3-16. Anterior glide.

ANTERIOR GLIDE (Fig. 3-16)

Purpose

- To examine for acromioclavicular joint impairment
- To increase accessory motion into acromioclavicular anterior glide
- To increase range of motion at the shoulder complex
- To decrease pain
- To improve periarticular muscle performance

Positioning

1. The patient is sitting with the arm resting at the side.
2. The clinician is behind the patient facing the posterior surface of the acromioclavicular joint.
3. The stabilizing hand is positioned over the anterior acromion and over the anterior surface of the proximal humerus.
4. The mobilizing/manipulating hand is positioned with the thumb over the thumb of the guiding hand.
5. The guiding hand, which is the same hand as the stabilizing hand, is positioned with the thumb over the posterolateral surface of the clavicle.

Procedure

1. The stabilizing hand holds the acromion in position.
2. The mobilizing/manipulating hand glides the clavicle in an anterior direction.
3. The guiding hand controls the position of the mobilizing/manipulating hand (see Fig. 3-16).

Particulars

1. The clinician should use caution in performing this technique because this motion might be hypermobile.

SUPERIOR GLIDE OF THE ACROMION ON THE CLAVICLE/MANIPULATION
(Fig. 3-17)

Purpose

- To increase accessory motion at the acromioclavicular joint
- To increase range of motion at the shoulder complex
- To decrease pain
- To improve periarticular muscle performance

Positioning

1. The patient is sitting with the upper arm at the side and the elbow bent.
2. The clinician is behind the patient with the arm of the manipulating hand reaching across the patient's trunk toward the elbow.
3. The manipulating hand is positioned over the guiding hand.
4. The guiding hand is positioned over the patient's elbow.

Procedure

1. The manipulating hand moves the humerus in a superior direction toward the shelf of the acromion, indirectly gliding the acromion superiorly on the clavicle.
2. The guiding hand controls the position of the humerus (see Fig. 3-17).

Particulars

1. It is important to screen for glenohumeral joint impairments before performing this technique.
2. The clinician should use caution in performing this technique because this motion might be hypermobile.
3. This technique should be performed using grade V manipulations.
4. This technique is helpful for treating acromioclavicular impairments when the acromioclavicular joint is tender to palpation.

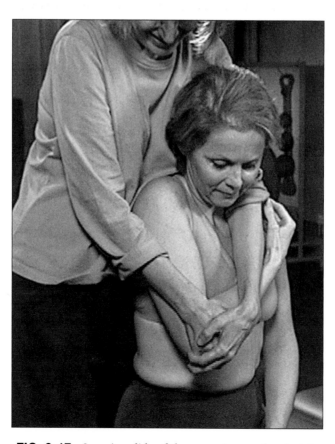

FIG. 3-17. Superior glide of the acromion on the clavicle.

REFERENCES

1. Nicholson GG: The effects of passive joint mobilization on pain and hypomobility associated with adhesive capsulitis of the shoulder. J Orthop Sports Phys Ther 1985;6:238-246.
2. Carette S, Moffet H, Tardif J, et al: Intraarticular corticosteroids, supervised physiotherapy, or a combination of the two in the treatment of adhesive capsulitis of the shoulder. Arthritis Rheum 2003;48:829-838.
3. Bulgin DY, Binder AI, Hazleman BL, et al: Frozen shoulder: prospective clinical study with an evaluation of three treatment regimens. Ann Rheum Dis 1984;43:353-360.
4. Winters JC, Sobel JS, Groenier KH, et al: Comparison of physiotherapy, manipulation, and corticosteroid injection for treating shoulder complaints in general practice: randomized, single blind study. BMJ 1997;314:1320-1325.
5. Van der Windt DAWM, Koes BW, Deville W, et al: Effectiveness of corticosteroid injections versus physiotherapy for treatment of painful stiff shoulder in primary care: randomized trial. BMJ 1998;317:1292-1296.
6. Binder AI, Bulgin DY, Hazleman BL, et al: Frozen shoulder: a long-term prospective study. Ann Rheum Dis 1984;43:361-364.
7. Conroy DE, Hayes KW: The effect of joint mobilization as a component of comprehensive treatment for primary shoulder impingement syndrome. J Orthop Sports Phys Ther 1998;28:3-14.
8. Bang MD, Deyle GD: Comparison of supervised exercise with and without manual physical therapy for patients with shoulder impingement syndrome. J Orthop Sports Phys Ther 2000;30:126-137.
9. Dacre JE, Beeney N, Scott DL: Injections and physiotherapy for the painful stiff shoulder. Ann Rheum Dis 1989;48:322-325.
10. Hjelm R, Draper C, Spencer S: Anterior-inferior capsular length insufficiency in the painful shoulder. J Orthop Sports Phys Ther 1996;23:216-222.
11. Roubal PJ, Dobritt D, Placzek JD: Glenohumeral gliding manipulation following interscalene brachial plexus block in patients with adhesive capsulitis. J Orthop Sports Phys Ther 1996;24:66-77.
12. Hsu A-T, Ho L, Ho S, et al: Immediate response of glenohumeral abduction range of motion to a caudally directed translational mobilization: a fresh cadaver simulation. Arch Phys Med Rehabil 2000;81:1511-1516.
13. Hsu A-T, Ho L, Ho S, et al: Joint position during anterior-posterior glide mobilization: its effect on glenohumeral abduction range of motion. Arch Phys Med Rehabil 2000;81:210-214.
14. Hsu A-T, Headman T, Chang JH, et al: Changes in abduction and rotation range of motion in response to simulated dorsal and anterior translational mobilization of the glenohumeral joint. Phys Ther 2002;82:544-556.
15. Kaltenborn FM: Manual Mobilization of the Joints: The Kaltenborn Method of Joint Examination and Treatment, Vol I: The Extremities, 6th ed. OPTP, Oslo, Norway, Norli, 2002.
16. Lind T, Blyme PJH, Strange-Vognsen HH, et al: Pressure-position relations in the glenohumeral joint. Acta Orthop Belg 1992;58:81-83.
17. Cyriax J: Textbook of Orthopaedic Medicine, Vol 1: Diagnosis of Soft Tissue Lesions, 8th ed. London, Bailliere Tindall, 1982.

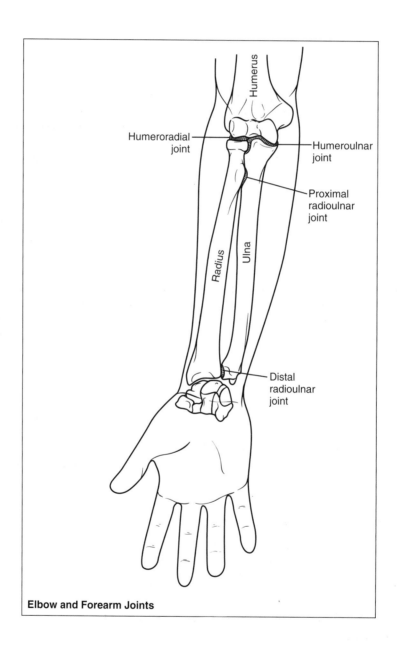

Elbow and Forearm Joints

CHAPTER 4

The Elbow and Forearm

BASICS

The elbow complex comprises three distinct articulations: the humeroulnar and humeroradial joints and the proximal radioulnar joint. Flexion and extension occur at the humeroulnar and humeroradial joints. Pronation and supination are considered motions of the forearm and occur at the humeroradial joint, the proximal and distal radioulnar joints, and the ulnomeniscotriquetral joint of the wrist. Most functional activities occur between 30 and 130 degrees of elbow flexion and between 50 degrees of pronation and 50 degrees of supination.

Humeroulnar Joint

The humeroulnar joint is classified as a hinge joint. The ulnar concave articular surface has a larger curvature than most joint surfaces. Posterior and anterior glides might be ineffective at this joint because the two joint surfaces are likely to jam together when these glide techniques are attempted. Assuming this is the case, humeroulnar joint techniques are limited to distraction and medial and lateral gliding and gapping.

   Distraction techniques for all joints are performed such that the bone being mobilized/manipulated is moved in a direction perpendicular to the treatment plane. Since the proximal ulna is angulated 45 degrees anterior to the shaft of the ulna, the shaft of the ulna is not perpendicular to the treatment plane, and humeroulnar distraction mobilization/manipulation occurs at an angle that is 45 degrees less flexion than the position of the shaft of the ulna (see Fig. 2-3).

Humeroradial Joint

Positional faults are believed to be a fairly common occurrence at the humeroradial joint. Compression positional faults can be caused by a fall on an outstretched arm, causing the humerus to move closer to the radius, whereas distraction positional faults can occur when the arm is pulled, which causes the opposite alignment impairment to occur. Distraction positional faults are especially common in young children. This condition is called a *pulled elbow*.

Proximal and Distal Radioulnar Joints

Motion into pronation and supination occurs simultaneously at the proximal and distal radioulnar joints. When the ulna is stationary, the radius rotates anteriorly and medially with pronation and posteriorly and laterally with supination. The radius also spins on the humerus during these two motions.

SPECIFIC PATHOLOGY AND ELBOW AND FOREARM JOINT MOBILIZATION/MANIPULATION

Lateral Epicondylalgia

Several studies have addressed the efficacy of elbow mobilization/manipulation in the treatment of lateral epicondylalgia. In one randomized study of 18 subjects with lateral epicondylalgia, joint mobilization to the radial head combined with neuromobilization to the radial nerve was compared with a program consisting of ultrasound, friction massage, and strengthening and stretching exercises. At 3-month follow-up, only the group receiving joint and neuromobilization interventions had improved.[1]

In another study, the effects of a Mulligan mobilization with movement technique were assessed on a sample of 24 subjects with chronic lateral epicondylalgia. These subjects were assigned to receive mobilization with movement to the elbow, a placebo treatment, or no treatment in random order. The treatment involved a lateral glide of the ulna on the humerus, painlessly applied and sustained for approximately 6 seconds while the subject performed a pain-free gripping action. The gliding pressure was maintained until the subject completely released the grip. Outcome measures included pain-free grip force and pressure pain threshold, measured in affected and unaffected arms. Results showed an increase in pain-free grip force and pressure pain threshold in the affected arm after mobilization compared with the other two conditions. There were no significant changes in the unaffected arm.[2]

The same mobilization intervention was investigated in a follow-up study of 24 subjects, also with chronic lateral epicondylalgia. The design of this study was similar to that of the first study except that outcomes were measured only on the affected limb, and thermal pain threshold and several measures of sympathetic nervous system activity were assessed. Results showed an increase in pain-free grip force, pressure pain threshold, and several measures of sympathetic nervous system activity, but no change in thermal pain threshold in the mobilization condition compared with the other two conditions.[3]

Several articles addressing elbow joint pathology have advocated using a Mills manipulation to treat lateral epicondylalgia. This technique entails first positioning the patient with the elbow slightly flexed, forearm pronated, and wrist flexed. The clinician applies a grade V anterior manipulation to the distal humerus, while extending the elbow and flexing the wrist.[4] The efficacy of this technique has not been researched.

Myositis Ossificans

One concern with performing mobilization/manipulation techniques, particularly on the elbow joint, is the development of myositis ossificans. Myositis ossificans is a condition characterized by heterotopic cartilage and bone formation in the soft tissues around the joint and in the area of damaged muscle.[5] This condition has been shown to produce periarticular pain and a decrease in joint range of motion in affected joints. Some clinicians believe that myositis ossificans is caused by passive stretching, including joint mobilization/manipulation techniques, especially if bony damage has occurred.[6] One study reported an onset of myositis ossificans in rabbits after experimentally induced muscle necrosis by repeated forced passive exercise.[5] These study results suggest that aggressive stretching techniques, including joint mobilization/manipulation, might trigger the onset of myositis ossificans. Conversely, in a case series report of subjects with head trauma and myositis ossificans who were treated with manipulation under anesthesia, manipulation did not seem to cause the ossification process to progress. Instead, it helped maintain joint motion and prevent bony ankylosis.[7] It is unclear from the results of these two studies what effect joint mobilization/manipulation techniques have on the onset and development of myositis ossificans.

HUMEROULNAR JOINT

Osteokinematic motion:
  Flexion/extension
Ligaments:
  Ulnar collateral ligament
Joint orientation:
  Humerus: inferior, posterior
  Ulna: superior, anterior
  Note: The flattened-out concave joint surface (the treatment plane) of the ulna forms a 45-degree angle with the
    shaft of the ulna
Concave joint surface:
  Ulna
Type of joint:
  Synovial
Resting position:
  70 degrees flexion, 10 degrees supination[8]
Close-packed position:
  Full extension and supination[8]
Capsular pattern of restriction:
  Flexion is more limited than extension[9]

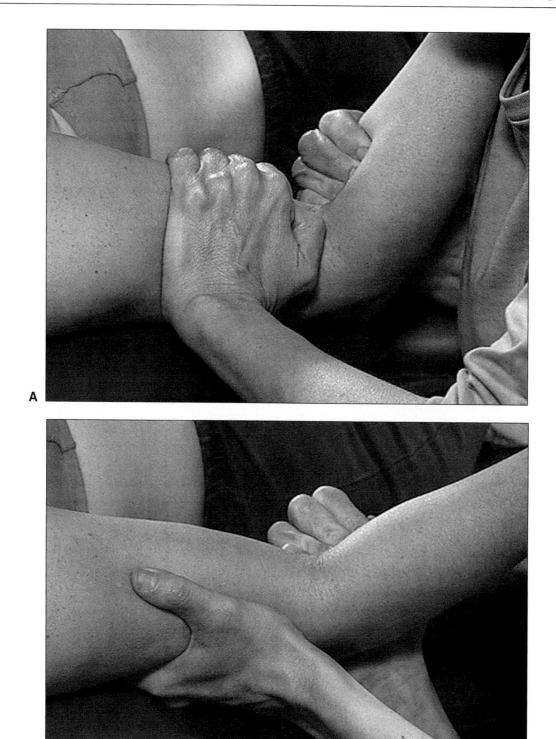

FIG. 4-1. Distraction. **A,** Distraction performed in the resting position. **B,** Distraction performed approximating the restricted range of motion into extension.

DISTRACTION (Fig. 4-1)

Purpose

- To examine for humeroulnar joint impairment
- To increase accessory motion into humeroulnar joint distraction
- To increase range of motion at the elbow joint
- To decrease pain
- To improve periarticular muscle performance

Positioning

1. The patient is supine.
2. The humeroulnar joint is placed in the resting position if conservative techniques are indicated or approximating restricted range of motion if more aggressive techniques are indicated.
3. The clinician is at the patient's hip facing the humeroulnar joint, with the patient's upper arm resting on the treatment table, the elbow joint positioned off the edge of the table, and the distal forearm resting on the clinician's shoulder.
4. The stabilizing hand grips the distal humerus from the anterior side.
5. Instead of or in addition to the stabilizing hand, the clinician can use a belt to hold the patient's humerus to the treatment table.
6. The mobilizing/manipulating hand grips the proximal ulna from the anterior side, avoiding contact with the radius.

Procedure

1. The stabilizing hand holds the distal humerus against the treatment table.
2. The mobilizing/manipulating hand moves the proximal ulna in a direction perpendicular to the ulnar joint surface, which is at an angle that is in 45 degrees less flexion than the position of the ulnar shaft (see Fig. 2-3 and Fig. 4-1).

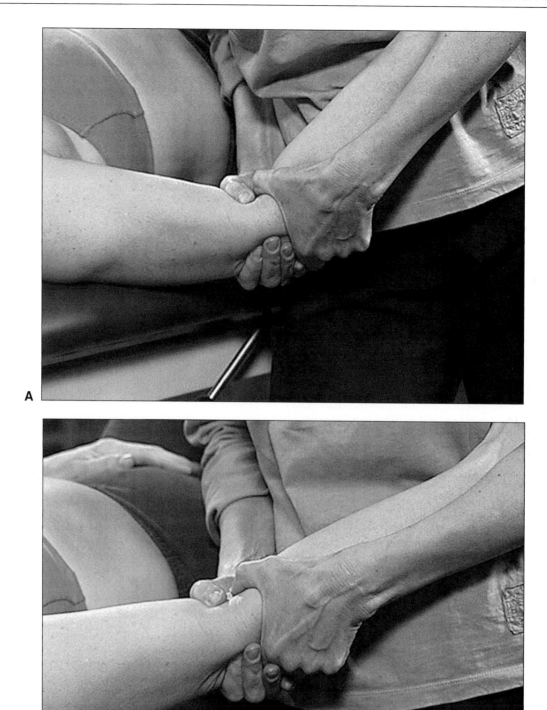

FIG. 4-2. Medial glide. **A,** Medial glide performed in the resting position. **B,** Medial glide performed approximating the restricted range of motion into extension.

MEDIAL GLIDE (Fig. 4-2)

Purpose

- To examine for humeroulnar joint impairment
- To increase accessory motion into humeroulnar medial glide
- To increase range of motion at the elbow joint
- To decrease pain
- To improve periarticular muscle performance

Positioning

1. The patient is supine.
2. The humeroulnar joint is placed in the resting position if conservative techniques are indicated or approximating restricted range of motion if more aggressive techniques are indicated.
3. The clinician is facing the patient between the patient's arm and trunk with the patient's forearm between the clinician's upper arm and trunk.
4. The stabilizing hand grips the distal humerus from the medial side.
5. The mobilizing/manipulating hand grips the proximal radius from the lateral side.

Procedure

1. The clinician applies a grade I traction to the joint.
2. The stabilizing hand holds the humerus in position.
3. The mobilizing/manipulating hand glides the proximal ulna in a medial direction indirectly through the radius while the clinician's trunk guides the motion (see Fig. 4-2).

Particulars

1. This technique is commonly performed with the elbow in slight flexion using a grade V manipulation and when performed in this manner is considered to be effective in treating medial epicondylalgia.

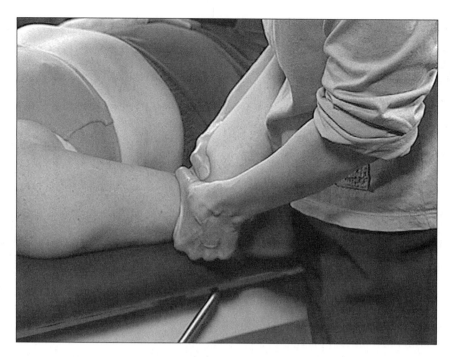

FIG. 4-3. Lateral glide.

LATERAL GLIDE (Fig. 4-3)

Purpose

- To examine for humeroulnar joint impairment
- To increase accessory motion into humeroulnar lateral glide
- To increase range of motion at the elbow joint
- To decrease pain
- To improve periarticular muscle performance

Positioning

1. The patient is supine.
2. The humeroulnar joint is placed in the resting position if conservative techniques are indicated or approximating restricted range of motion if more aggressive techniques are indicated.
3. The clinician is at the patient's side facing the humeroulnar joint with the patient's forearm between the clinician's upper arm and trunk.
4. The stabilizing hand grips the distal humerus from the lateral side.
5. The mobilizing/manipulating hand grips the proximal ulna from the medial side.

Procedure

1. The clinician applies a grade I traction to the joint.
2. The stabilizing hand holds the humerus in position.
3. The mobilizing/manipulating hand glides the proximal ulna in a lateral direction while the clinician's trunk guides the motion (see Fig. 4-3).

Particulars

1. A variation of this technique, using mobilization with movement, has been shown to be effective in treating lateral epicondylalgia. In the study, a lateral glide, painlessly applied and sustained for approximately 6 seconds while the subject performed a pain-free gripping action, and maintained until the subject completely released the grip, was performed.[2,3]
2. This technique is commonly performed with the elbow in slight flexion using a grade V manipulation and when performed in this manner is considered to be effective in treating lateral epicondylalgia.

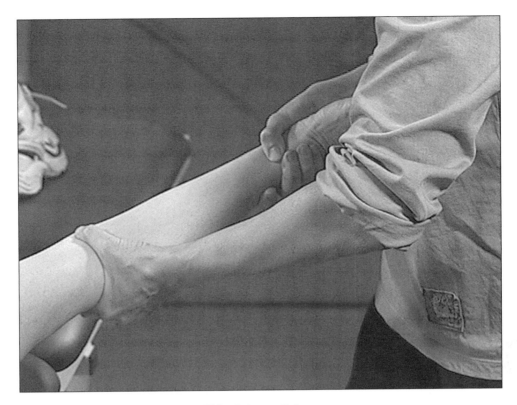

FIG. 4-4. Medial gap.

MEDIAL GAP (Fig. 4-4)

Purpose

- To examine for humeroulnar joint impairment
- To increase accessory motion into humeroulnar medial gap
- To increase range of motion at the elbow joint
- To decrease pain
- To improve periarticular muscle performance

Positioning

1. The patient is supine.
2. The humeroulnar joint is positioned in slight flexion.
3. The clinician is at the patient's side facing the humeroulnar joint with the patient's forearm between the clinician's upper arm and trunk.
4. The stabilizing hand supports the forearm from the medial (ulnar) side and holds it against the clinician's trunk.
5. The mobilizing/manipulating hand grips the lateral side of the elbow at the joint line.

Procedure

1. The stabilizing hand holds the forearm in position.
2. The mobilizing/manipulating hand moves the elbow at the lateral joint line in a medial direction, creating a gapping at the medial joint line (see Fig. 4-4).

Particulars

1. The clinician should use caution in performing this technique because this motion might be hypermobile, especially if the patient sprained the medial collateral ligament of the elbow.
2. This technique is commonly performed using a grade V manipulation and is considered to be effective in treating medial epicondylalgia.

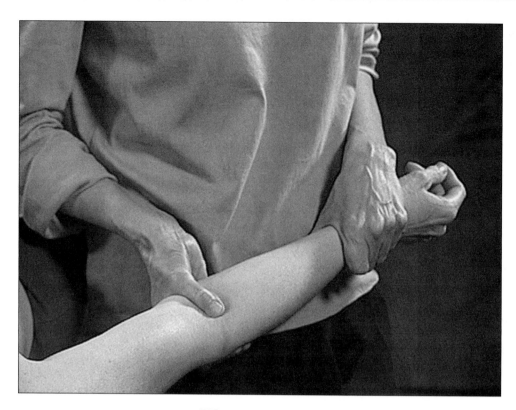

FIG. 4-5. Lateral gap.

LATERAL GAP (Fig. 4-5)

Purpose

- To examine for humeroulnar joint impairment
- To increase accessory motion into humeroulnar lateral gap
- To increase range of motion at the elbow joint
- To decrease pain
- To improve periarticular muscle performance

Positioning

1. The patient is supine.
2. The humeroulnar joint is positioned in slight flexion.
3. The clinician is facing the patient between the patient's arm and trunk with the patient's forearm between the clinician's upper arm and trunk.
4. The stabilizing hand supports the forearm from the lateral (radial) side and holds it against the clinician's trunk.
5. The mobilizing/manipulating hand grips the medial side of the elbow at the joint line.

Procedure

1. The stabilizing hand holds the forearm in position.
2. The mobilizing/manipulating hand moves the elbow at the medial joint line in a lateral direction, creating a gapping at the lateral joint line (see Fig. 4-5).

Particulars

1. The clinician should use caution in performing this technique because this motion might be hypermobile, especially if the patient sprained the lateral collateral ligament of the elbow.
2. This technique is commonly performed using a grade V manipulation and is considered to be effective in treating lateral epicondylalgia.

HUMERORADIAL JOINT

Osteokinematic motions:
   Flexion/extension
   Pronation/supination
Ligaments:
   Radial collateral ligament
Type of joint:
   Synovial
Joint orientation:
   Humerus: inferior
   Radius: superior
Concave joint surface:
   Radius
Resting position:
   Full extension and supination[8]
Close-packed position:
   90 degrees flexion, 5 degrees supination[8]
Capsular pattern of restriction:
   Flexion is more limited than extension[9]

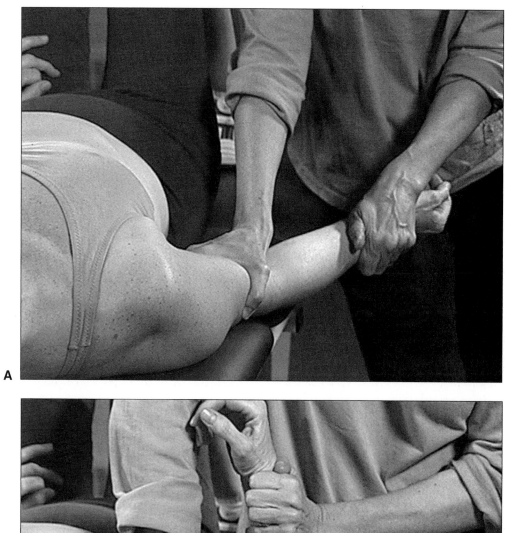

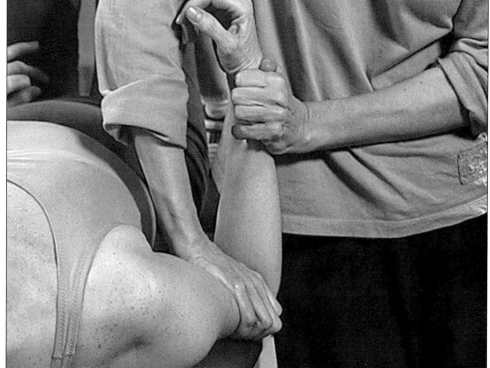

FIG. 4-6. Distraction. **A,** Distraction performed in the resting position. **B,** Distraction performed approximating the restricted range of motion into flexion.

DISTRACTION (Fig. 4-6)

Purpose

- To examine for humeroradial joint impairment
- To increase accessory motion into humeroradial joint distraction
- To increase range of motion at the elbow joint
- To decrease pain
- To improve periarticular muscle performance

Positioning

1. The patient is supine.
2. The humeroradial joint is placed in the resting position if conservative techniques are indicated, or approximating restricted range of motion if more aggressive techniques are indicated.
3. The clinician is at the patient's side facing the humeroradial joint.
4. The stabilizing hand grips the distal humerus from the anterior side.
5. The mobilizing/manipulating hand grips the distal radius, avoiding contact with the ulna.

Procedure

1. The stabilizing hand holds the humerus in position.
2. The mobilizing/manipulating hand moves the radial head distally perpendicular to the radial joint surface (see Fig. 4-6).

Particulars

1. This technique might be effective in correcting a humeroradial joint compression positional fault.

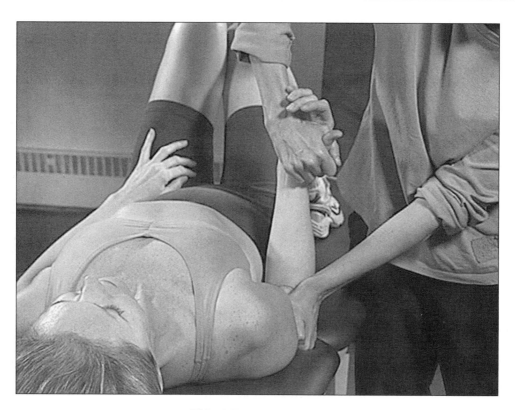

FIG. 4-7. Compression.

COMPRESSION (Fig. 4-7)

Purpose

- To correct a humeroradial joint distraction positional fault

Positioning

1. The patient is supine.
2. The elbow joint is positioned in 90 degrees of flexion with the forearm in full supination.
3. The clinician is at the patient's side facing the humeroradial joint.
4. The stabilizing hand supports the distal humerus.
5. The mobilizing/manipulating hand grips the patient's hand.

Procedure

1. The stabilizing hand holds the humerus in position.
2. The mobilizing/manipulating hand moves the shaft of the radius downward toward the humerus indirectly through the wrist (see Fig. 4-7).

Particulars

1. It is important to screen for wrist joint impairments before performing this technique.

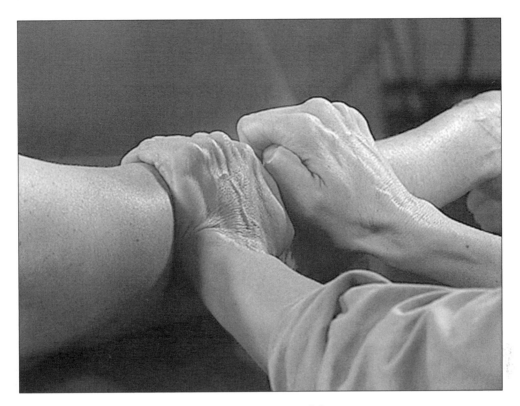

FIG. 4-8. Posterior glide.

POSTERIOR GLIDE (Fig. 4-8)

Purpose

- To examine for humeroradial joint impairment
- To increase accessory motion into humeroradial posterior glide
- To increase range of motion at the elbow joint
- To decrease pain
- To improve periarticular muscle performance

Positioning

1. The patient is supine with the shoulder medially rotated.
2. The humeroradial joint is placed in the resting position if conservative techniques are indicated or approximating restricted range of motion if more aggressive techniques are indicated.
3. The clinician is at the patient's side facing the humeroradial joint.
4. The stabilizing hand grips the distal humerus from the posterior side.
5. The mobilizing/manipulating hand grips the proximal radius from the anterior side.

Procedure

1. The clinician applies a grade I traction to the joint.
2. The stabilizing hand holds the humerus in position.
3. The mobilizing/manipulating hand glides the proximal radius in a posterior direction (see Fig. 4-8).

Particulars

1. The clinician should use caution in performing this technique because this motion might be hypermobile.
2. This technique might be especially effective for increasing range of motion into elbow joint extension.

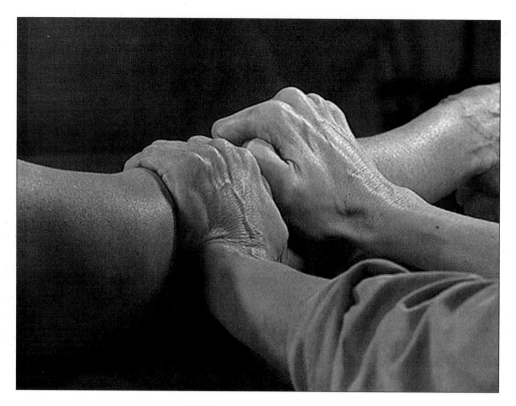

FIG. 4-9. Anterior glide.

ANTERIOR GLIDE (Fig. 4-9)

Purpose

- To examine for humeroradial joint impairment
- To increase accessory motion into humeroradial anterior glide
- To increase range of motion at the elbow joint
- To decrease pain
- To improve periarticular muscle performance

Positioning

1. The patient is supine with the shoulder medially rotated.
2. The humeroradial joint is placed in the resting position if conservative techniques are indicated or approximating restricted range of motion if more aggressive techniques are indicated.
3. The clinician is at the patient's side facing the humeroradial joint.
4. The stabilizing hand grips the distal humerus from the anterior side.
5. The mobilizing/manipulating hand grips the proximal radius from the posterior side.

Procedure

1. The clinician applies a grade I traction to the joint.
2. The stabilizing hand holds the humerus in position.
3. The mobilizing/manipulating hand glides the proximal radius in an anterior direction (see Fig. 4-9).

Particulars

1. The clinician should use caution in performing this technique because this motion might be hypermobile.
2. This technique might be especially effective for increasing range of motion into elbow joint flexion.

PROXIMAL RADIOULNAR JOINT

Osteokinematic motion:
  Pronation/supination
Ligaments:
  Annular ligament
  Quadrate ligament
  Interosseous membrane
Joint orientation:
  Ulna: lateral, anterior
  Radius: medial, posterior
Concave joint surface:
  Ulna
Type of joint:
  Synovial
Resting position:
  35 degrees of flexion, 70 degrees of supination[8]
Close-packed position:
  Full supination or full pronation[8]
Capsular pattern of restriction:
  Pain at the end of the range of motion for pronation or supination or both[9]

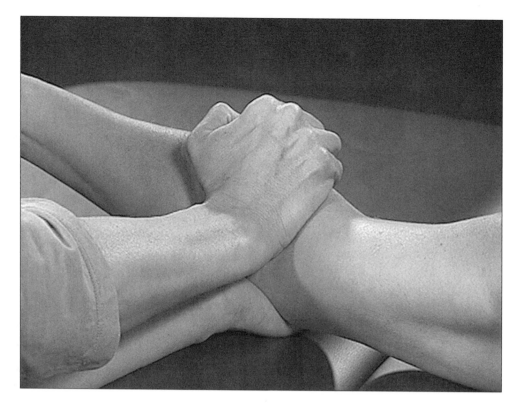

FIG. 4-10. Posterior glide of the radial head.

POSTERIOR GLIDE OF THE PROXIMAL RADIUS (Fig. 4-10)

Purpose

- To examine for proximal radioulnar joint impairment
- To increase accessory motion into proximal radioulnar posterior glide
- To increase range of motion at the forearm
- To decrease pain
- To improve periarticular muscle performance

Positioning

1. The patient is sitting with the forearm resting on the treatment table.
2. The proximal radioulnar joint is placed in the resting position if conservative techniques are indicated or approximating restricted range of motion if more aggressive techniques are indicated.
3. The clinician is at the patient's side facing the proximal radioulnar joint.
4. The stabilizing hand grips the proximal ulna from the posterior surface.
5. The mobilizing/manipulating hand grips the radial head anteriorly.

Procedure

1. The stabilizing hand holds the ulna in position.
2. The mobilizing/manipulating hand glides the radial head in a posterior direction (see Fig. 4-10).

Particulars

1. This technique might be especially effective for increasing range of motion into forearm pronation.

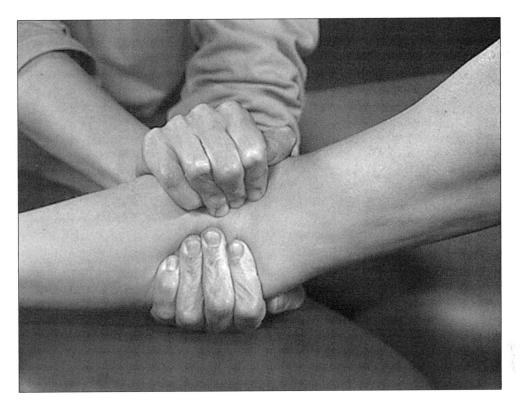

FIG. 4-11. Anterior glide of the radial head.

ANTERIOR GLIDE OF THE PROXIMAL RADIUS (Fig. 4-11)

Purpose
- To examine for proximal radioulnar joint impairment
- To increase accessory motion into proximal radioulnar anterior glide
- To increase range of motion at the forearm
- To decrease pain
- To improve periarticular muscle performance

Positioning
1. The patient is sitting with the forearm resting on the treatment table.
2. The proximal radioulnar joint is placed in the resting position if conservative techniques are indicated or approximating restricted range of motion if more aggressive techniques are indicated.
3. The clinician is at the patient's side facing the proximal radioulnar joint.
4. The stabilizing hand grips the proximal ulna from the anterior surface.
5. The mobilizing/manipulating hand grips the radial head posteriorly.

Procedure
1. The stabilizing hand holds the ulna in position.
2. The mobilizing/manipulating hand glides the radial head in an anterior direction (see Fig. 4-11).

Particulars
1. This technique might be especially effective for increasing range of motion into forearm supination.

DISTAL RADIOULNAR JOINT

Osteokinematic motion:
Pronation/supination
Ligaments:
Anterior radioulnar ligament
Posterior radioulnar ligament
Interosseous membrane
Joint orientation:
Ulna: lateral
Radius: medial
Concave joint surface:
Radius
Type of joint:
Synovial
Resting position:
10 degrees supination[8]
Close-packed position:
Full supination or full pronation[8]
Capsular pattern of restriction:
Pain at the end of the range of motion for pronation or supination or both[9]

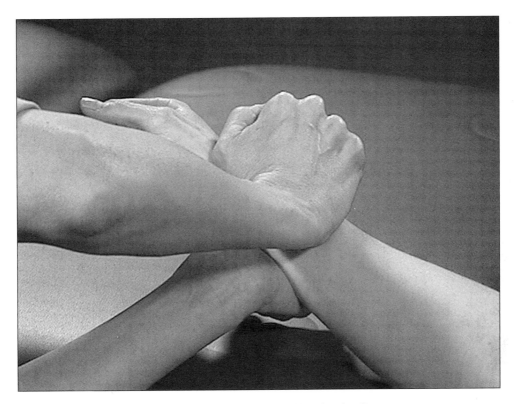

FIG. 4-12. Posterior glide of the distal radius.

POSTERIOR GLIDE OF THE DISTAL RADIUS (Fig. 4-12)

Purpose
- To examine for distal radioulnar joint impairment
- To increase accessory motion into distal radioulnar posterior glide
- To increase range of motion at the forearm
- To decrease pain
- To improve periarticular muscle performance

Positioning
1. The patient is sitting with the forearm resting on the treatment table.
2. The distal radioulnar joint is placed in the resting position if conservative techniques are indicated or approximating restricted range of motion if more aggressive techniques are indicated.
3. The clinician is at the patient's side facing the distal radioulnar joint.
4. The stabilizing hand grips the distal ulna from the posterior surface.
5. The mobilizing/manipulating hand grips the distal radius anteriorly.

Procedure
1. The stabilizing hand holds the ulna in position.
2. The mobilizing/manipulating hand glides the distal radius in a posterior direction (see Fig. 4-12).

Particulars
1. This technique might be especially effective for increasing range of motion into forearm supination.

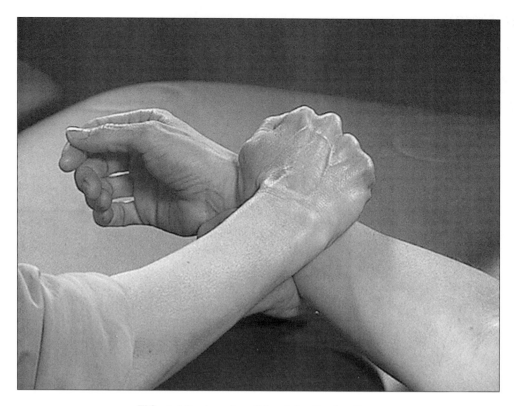

FIG. 4-13. Anterior glide of the distal radius.

ANTERIOR GLIDE OF THE DISTAL RADIUS (Fig. 4-13)

Purpose
- To examine for distal radioulnar joint impairment
- To increase accessory motion into distal radioulnar anterior glide
- To increase range of motion at the forearm
- To decrease pain
- To improve periarticular muscle performance

Positioning
1. The patient is sitting with the forearm resting on the treatment table.
2. The distal radioulnar joint is placed in the resting position if conservative techniques are indicated or approximating restricted range of motion if more aggressive techniques are indicated.
3. The clinician is at the patient's side facing the distal radioulnar joint.
4. The stabilizing hand grips the distal ulna from the anterior surface.
5. The mobilizing/manipulating hand grips the distal radius posteriorly.

Procedure
1. The stabilizing hand holds the ulna in position.
2. The mobilizing/manipulating hand glides the distal radius in an anterior direction (see Fig. 4-13).

Particulars
1. This technique might be especially effective for increasing range of motion into forearm pronation.

REFERENCES

1. Drechsler WI, Knarr JF, Snyder-Mackler L: A comparison of two treatment regimens for lateral epicondylitis: a randomized trial of clinical interventions. J Sport Rehabil 1997;6:226-234.
2. Vicenzino B, Paungmali A, Buratowski S, et al: Specific manipulative therapy treatment for chronic lateral epicondylalgia produces uniquely characteristic hypoalgesia. Manual Ther 2001;6:205-212.
3. Paungmali A, O'Leary S, Souvlis T, et al: Hypoalgesic and sympathoexcitatory effects of mobilization with movement for lateral epicondylalgia. Phys Ther 2003;83:374-383.
4. Kaufman RL: Conservative chiropractic care of lateral epicondylitis. J Manip Physiol Therap 2000;23:619-622.
5. Michelsson JE, Rauschning W: Pathogenesis of experimental heterotopic bone formation following temporary forcible exercising of immobilized joints. Clin Orthop 1983;176:265-272.
6. Stoddard A: Manipulation of the elbow. Physiotherapy 1971;57:259-260.
7. Garland DE, Razza BE, Waters RL: Forceful joint manipulation in head-injured adults with heterotopic ossification. Clin Orthop 1982;169:133-138.
8. Kaltenborn FM: Manual Mobilization of the Joints: The Kaltenborn Method of Joint Examination and Treatment, Vol I: The Extremities, 6th ed. Oslo, Norway, Norli, 2002.
9. Cyriax J: Textbook of Orthopaedic Medicine, Vol 1: Diagnosis of Soft Tissue Lesions, 8th ed. London, Bailliere Tindall, 1982.

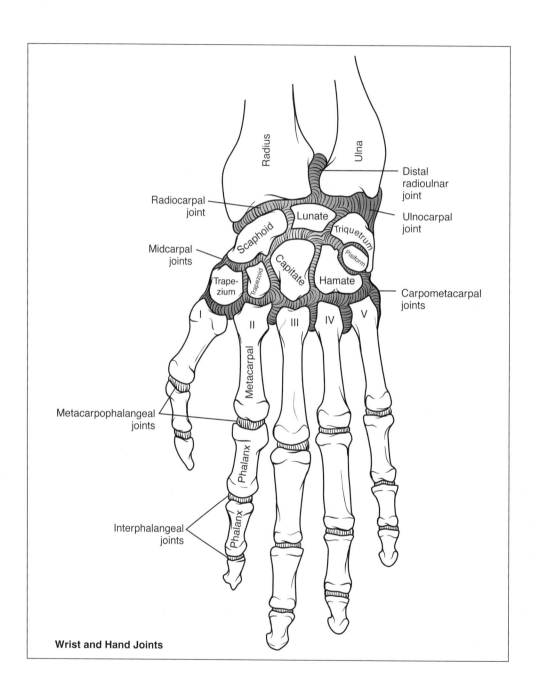

Wrist and Hand Joints

The Wrist and Hand

BASICS

The wrist and hand comprise numerous small joints that are located in close proximity to one another. This proximity allows the individual to perform a wide variety of skilled activities.

Wrist Joint

The wrist comprises the radiocarpal and ulnocarpal joints, the triquetrum-pisiform articulation, and the midcarpal joints. Wrist range of motion is considered functional if 10 degrees of flexion and 35 degrees of extension are present because this amount of motion allows the wrist to position the hand for skilled activities.

Intermetacarpal Joints

The metacarpals are capable of gliding on one another, causing the arch of the hand to increase and decrease. The axis for this motion is the third metacarpal.

Thumb and Finger Joints

There is a relatively large amount of motion at the thumb and finger joints, allowing for a wide variety of functional hand movements. The amount of range of motion considered functional depends on the specific task being performed.

Of all the joints in the human body, the trapeziometacarpal joint is considered the most important because it allows an individual to grasp objects. The trapezium is flexed, abducted, and medially rotated in relation to the other carpal bones; therefore it does not lie in the same plane as the joints of the fingers. Flexion and extension occur in a plane parallel to the plane of the palm of the hand, and abduction and adduction occur in a plane perpendicular to this plane. Opposition occurs at the trapeziometacarpal and metacarpophalangeal articulations, although most of this motion occurs at the trapeziometacarpal joint. Movement into opposition, a prerequisite for grasping motion, combines trapeziometacarpal flexion, abduction, and rotation. A fair amount of ligamentous laxity at the trapeziometacarpal joint must be present for functional opposition to occur.

SPECIFIC PATHOLOGY AND WRIST AND HAND JOINT MOBILIZATION/ MANIPULATION

Carpal Tunnel Syndrome

One study addressed the efficacy of carpal joint mobilization as an intervention for carpal tunnel syndrome. In this study, 21 subjects were randomly assigned to receive carpal joint mobilization, neural mobilization, or no intervention. Outcomes included active range of motion, pain, function, and whether the subject eventually required surgery. Subjects receiving joint mobilization and neural mobilization demonstrated better outcomes than subjects who received no treatment; however the small sample size precluded drawing conclusions regarding the relative efficacy of joint vs. neural mobilization.[1]

Lateral Epicondylalgia

In a small clinical trial, 31 subjects with lateral epicondylalgia were randomly assigned to receive wrist manipulation or combined therapy consisting of ultrasound, friction massage, progressive muscle strengthening and stretching exercises, and a home exercise program. The manipulation technique consisted of an anteriorly directed grade V manipulation of the scaphoid while performing either passive or resistive wrist extension. Outcomes were measured at 3 and 6 weeks after the intervention and consisted of a subjective rating of overall improvement, pain and inconvenience, wrist range of motion, grip force, and pain pressure threshold. The subjective rating of overall improvement was significantly increased at 3-week follow-up, and pain was significantly decreased at 6-week follow-up in the group receiving manipulation.[2]

Decreased Metacarpophalangeal Joint Range of Motion

In two different studies, there was a significant increase in range of motion in the metacarpophalangeal joints after joint mobilization/manipulation. In one study, subjects who had sustained a metacarpophalangeal fracture received either a home exercise program or a home exercise program with the addition of joint mobilization intervention. The mobilization and exercise group experienced a significant increase in range of motion compared with the exercise-alone group.[3] In the other study, the relative effect of joint mobilization was compared with that of grade V manipulation in a sample of normal subjects. The group receiving manipulation experienced a significant increase in range of motion compared with the mobilization group.[4] These studies are described in greater detail in Chapter 1.

RADIOCARPAL AND ULNOCARPAL JOINTS

Osteokinematic motions:
   Flexion/extension
   Radial/ulnar deviation
   Pronation/supination
Ligaments:
   Ulnar collateral ligament
   Radial collateral ligament
   Transverse carpal ligament
   Palmar radiocarpal ligaments
   Dorsal radiocarpal ligaments
   Intercarpal ligaments
Joint orientation:
   Radius and ulna: inferior, anterior, medial (in an ulnar direction)
   Carpals: superior, posterior, lateral (in a radial direction)
Concave joint surface:
   Radius and ulna
Type of joint:
   Synovial
Resting position:
   Slight flexion and ulnar deviation[5]
Close-packed position:
   Full extension[5]
Capsular pattern of restriction:
   Flexion and extension equally limited[6]

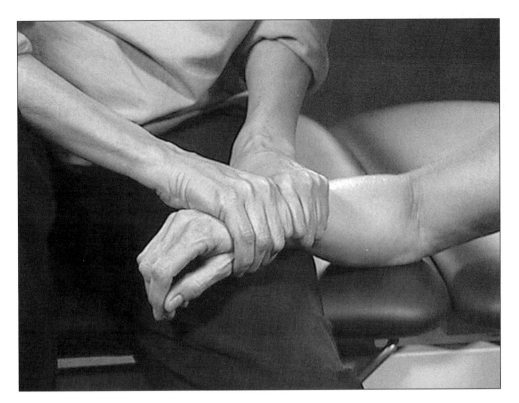

FIG. 5-1. Distraction.

DISTRACTION (Fig. 5-1)

Purpose

- To examine for radiocarpal and ulnocarpal joint impairment
- To increase accessory motion into radiocarpal and ulnocarpal joint distraction
- To increase range of motion at the wrist joint
- To decrease pain
- To improve periarticular muscle performance

Positioning

1. The patient is sitting with the anterior surface of the forearm on the treatment table and the hand off the table.
2. The radiocarpal and ulnocarpal joints are placed in the resting position if conservative techniques are indicated or approximating restricted range of motion if more aggressive techniques are indicated.
3. The clinician is facing the radiocarpal and ulnocarpal joints.
4. The stabilizing hand grips the distal radius and ulna from the posterior side.
5. The mobilizing/manipulating hand grips the proximal row of carpals from the posterior side.

Procedure

1. The stabilizing hand holds the radius and ulna to the treatment table.
2. The mobilizing/manipulating hand moves the proximal row of carpals distally perpendicular to the radioulnar joint surface (see Fig. 5-1).

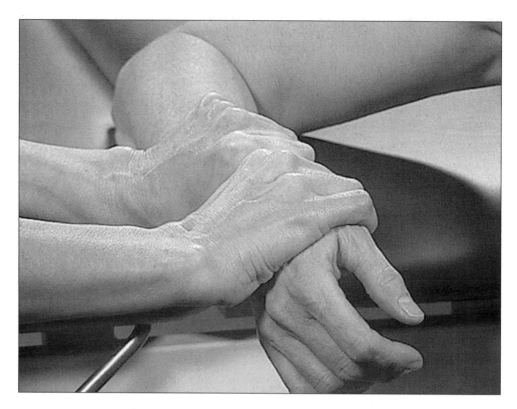

FIG. 5-2. Posterior glide.

POSTERIOR GLIDE (Fig. 5-2)

Purpose

- To examine for radiocarpal and ulnocarpal joint impairment
- To increase accessory motion into radiocarpal and ulnocarpal joint posterior glide
- To increase range of motion at the wrist joint
- To decrease pain
- To improve periarticular muscle performance

Positioning

1. The patient is sitting with the medial (ulnar) surface of the forearm on the treatment table and the hand off the table.
2. The radiocarpal and ulnocarpal joints are placed in the resting position if conservative techniques are indicated or approximating restricted range of motion if more aggressive techniques are indicated.
3. The clinician is facing the radiocarpal and ulnocarpal joints.
4. The stabilizing hand grips the distal radius and ulna from the posterior side.
5. The mobilizing/manipulating hand grips the proximal row of carpals from the posterior side.

Procedure

1. The clinician applies a grade I traction to the joint.
2. The stabilizing hand holds the radius and ulna to the treatment table.
3. The mobilizing/manipulating hand glides the proximal row of carpals in a posterior direction (see Fig. 5-2).

Particulars

1. This technique might be especially effective for increasing range of motion into wrist joint flexion.

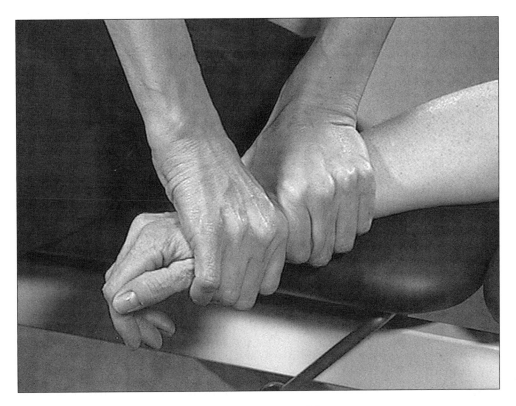

FIG. 5-3. Anterior glide.

ANTERIOR GLIDE (Fig. 5-3)

Purpose
- To examine for radiocarpal and ulnocarpal joint impairment
- To increase accessory motion into radiocarpal and ulnocarpal joint anterior glide
- To increase range of motion at the wrist joint
- To decrease pain
- To improve periarticular muscle performance

Positioning
1. The patient is sitting with the anterior surface of the forearm on the treatment table and the hand off the table.
2. The radiocarpal and ulnocarpal joints are placed in the resting position if conservative techniques are indicated or approximating restricted range of motion if more aggressive techniques are indicated.
3. The clinician is facing the radiocarpal and ulnocarpal joints.
4. The stabilizing hand grips the distal radius and ulna from the posterior side.
5. The mobilizing/manipulating hand grips the proximal row of carpals from the posterior side.

Procedure
1. The clinician applies a grade I traction to the joint.
2. The stabilizing hand holds the radius and ulna to the treatment table.
3. The mobilizing/manipulating hand glides the proximal row of carpals in an anterior direction (see Fig. 5-3).

Particulars
1. This technique might be especially effective for increasing range of motion into wrist joint extension.

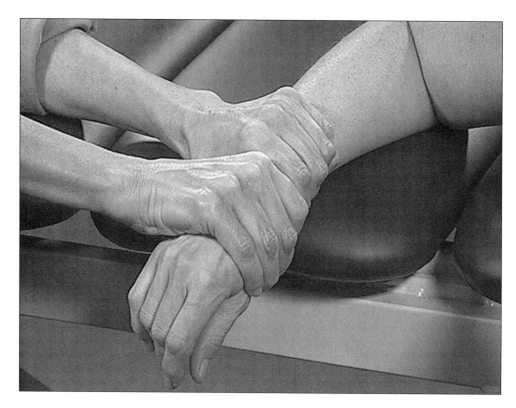

FIG. 5-4. Lateral (radial) glide.

LATERAL (RADIAL) GLIDE (Fig. 5-4)

Purpose

- To examine for radiocarpal and ulnocarpal joint impairment
- To increase accessory motion into radiocarpal and ulnocarpal joint lateral (radial) glide
- To increase range of motion at the wrist joint
- To decrease pain
- To improve periarticular muscle performance

Positioning

1. The patient is sitting with the anterior surface of the forearm on the treatment table and the hand off the table.
2. The radiocarpal and ulnocarpal joints are placed in the resting position if conservative techniques are indicated or approximating restricted range of motion if more aggressive techniques are indicated.
3. The clinician is facing the radiocarpal and ulnocarpal joints.
4. The stabilizing hand grips the distal radius and ulna from the posterior side.
5. The mobilizing/manipulating hand grips the proximal row of carpals from the medial (ulnar) side.

Procedure

1. The clinician applies a grade I traction to the joint.
2. The stabilizing hand holds the radius and ulna to the treatment table.
3. The mobilizing/manipulating hand glides the proximal row of carpals in a lateral (radial) direction (see Fig. 5-4).

Particulars

1. This technique might be especially effective for increasing range of motion into wrist joint ulnar deviation.

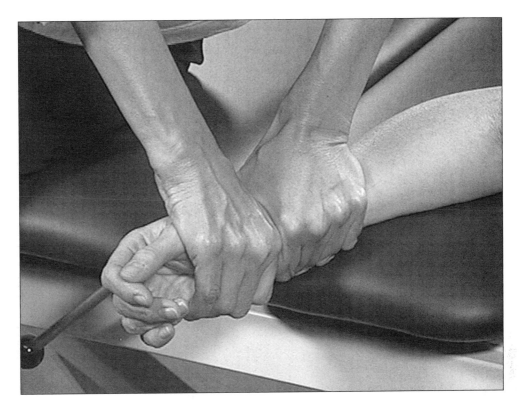

FIG. 5-5. Medial (ulnar) glide.

MEDIAL (ULNAR) GLIDE (Fig. 5-5)

Purpose

- To examine for radiocarpal and ulnocarpal joint impairment
- To increase accessory motion into radiocarpal and ulnocarpal joint medial (ulnar) glide
- To increase range of motion at the wrist joint
- To decrease pain
- To improve periarticular muscle performance

Positioning

1. The patient is sitting with the medial (ulnar) surface of the forearm on the treatment table and the hand off the table.
2. The radiocarpal and ulnocarpal joints are placed in the resting position if conservative techniques are indicated or approximating restricted range of motion if more aggressive techniques are indicated.
3. The clinician is facing the radiocarpal and ulnocarpal joints.
4. The stabilizing hand grips the distal radius and ulna from the anterior side.
5. The mobilizing/manipulating hand grips the proximal row of carpals from the lateral (radial) side.

Procedure

1. The clinician applies a grade I traction to the joint.
2. The stabilizing hand holds the radius and ulna to the treatment table.
3. The mobilizing/manipulating hand glides the proximal row of carpals in a medial (ulnar) direction (see Fig. 5-5).

Particulars

1. This technique might be especially effective for increasing range of motion into wrist joint radial deviation.

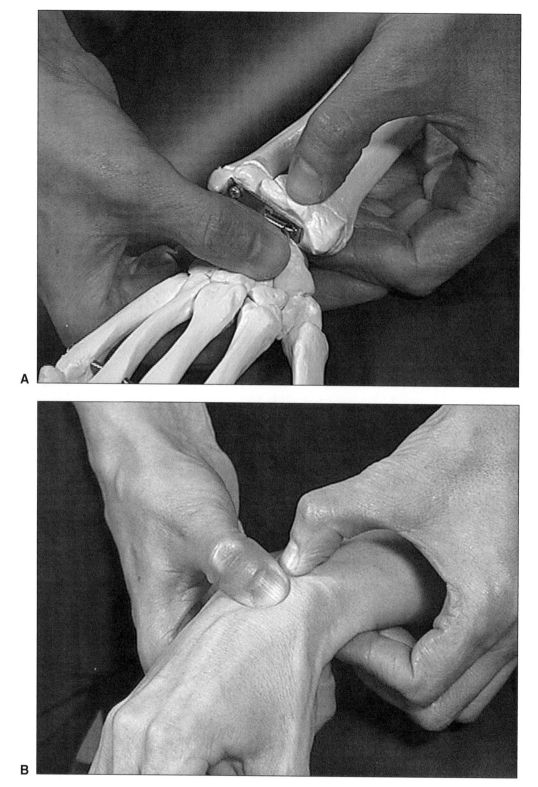

FIG. 5-6. Specific radiocarpal and ulnocarpal joint posterior glide mobilizations/manipulations.

SPECIFIC RADIOCARPAL AND ULNOCARPAL JOINT POSTERIOR GLIDE MOBILIZATIONS/MANIPULATIONS (Fig. 5-6)

Purpose

- To examine for radiocarpal and ulnocarpal joint impairment
- To increase accessory motion into radiocarpal and ulnocarpal joint posterior glide
- To increase range of motion at the wrist joint
- To decrease pain
- To improve periarticular muscle performance

Positioning

1. The patient is sitting with the anterior surface of the forearm on the treatment table and the hand off the table.
2. The radiocarpal and ulnocarpal joints are placed in the resting position if conservative techniques are indicated or approximating restricted range of motion if more aggressive techniques are indicated.
3. The clinician is facing the radiocarpal and ulnocarpal joints.
4. The stabilizing hand grips the distal radius or ulna with the thumb on the posterior surface and the index finger on the anterior surface.
5. The mobilizing/manipulating hand grips the proximal row carpal bone with the thumb on the posterior surface and the index finger on the anterior surface.

Procedure

1. The stabilizing hand holds the radius or ulna in position.
2. The mobilizing/manipulating hand glides the scaphoid in a posterior direction on the radius, the lunate in a posterior direction on the radius, and the triquetrum in a posterior direction on the ulna (see Fig. 5-6).

Particulars

1. The clinician should use caution in performing these techniques because some of these motions might be hypermobile.
2. These techniques might be especially effective for increasing range of motion into wrist joint flexion.

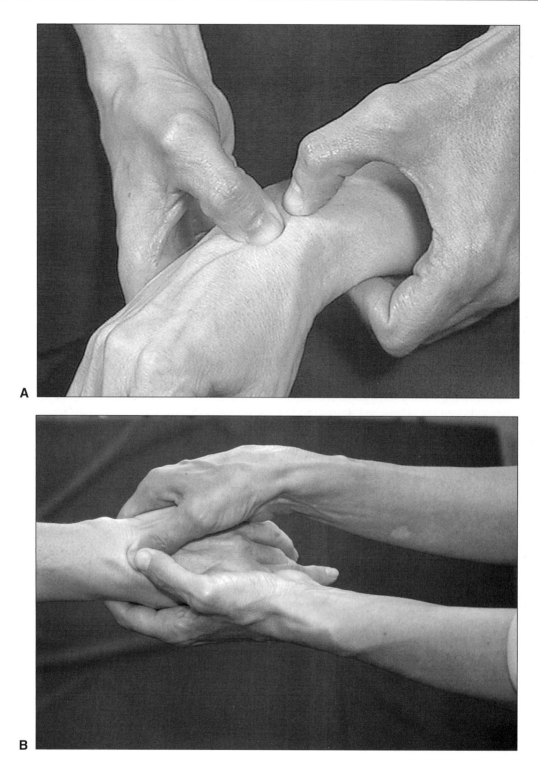

FIG. 5-7. Specific radiocarpal and ulnocarpal joint anterior glide mobilizations/manipulations.

SPECIFIC RADIOCARPAL AND ULNOCARPAL JOINT ANTERIOR GLIDE MOBILIZATIONS/MANIPULATIONS (Fig. 5-7)

Purpose

- To examine for radiocarpal and ulnocarpal joint impairment
- To increase accessory motion into radiocarpal and ulnocarpal joint anterior glide
- To increase range of motion at the wrist joint
- To decrease pain
- To improve periarticular muscle performance

Positioning

1. The patient is sitting with the anterior surface of the forearm on the treatment table and the hand off the table.
2. The radiocarpal and ulnocarpal joints are placed in the resting position if conservative techniques are indicated or approximating the restricted range of motion if more aggressive techniques are indicated.
3. The clinician is facing the radiocarpal and ulnocarpal joints.
4. The stabilizing hand grips the distal radius or ulna with the thumb on the posterior surface and the index finger on the anterior surface.
5. The mobilizing/manipulating hand grips the proximal row carpal bone with the thumb on the posterior surface and the index finger on the anterior surface.

Procedure

1. The stabilizing hand holds the radius or ulna in position.
2. The mobilizing/manipulating hand glides the scaphoid in an anterior direction on the radius, the lunate in an anterior direction on the radius, and the triquetrum in an anterior direction on the ulna (see Fig. 5-7A).

Particulars

1. The clinician should use caution in performing these techniques because some of these motions might be hypermobile.
2. A variation of this technique, using mobilization with movement (in this case "manipulation" with movement), has been shown to be effective in treating lateral epicondylalgia. In the study, an anterior glide grade V manipulation was performed on the scaphoid, while performing either passive or resistive wrist extension exercises.[2]
3. Gliding the lunate on the radius commonly is performed using a grade V manipulation and can be performed with both of the clinician's thumbs on the lunate (see Fig. 5-7B).
4. The radiolunate technique might be effective in correcting a radiolunate joint positional fault.
5. These techniques might be especially effective for increasing range of motion into wrist joint extension.

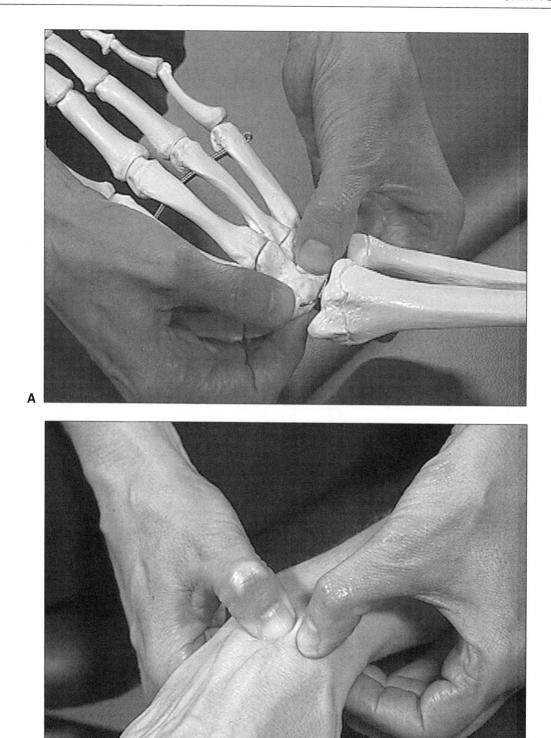

FIG. 5-8. Specific proximal row carpal joint posterior glide mobilizations/manipulations.

SPECIFIC PROXIMAL ROW CARPAL JOINT POSTERIOR GLIDE MOBILIZATIONS/MANIPULATIONS (Fig. 5-8)

Purpose

- To examine for proximal row carpal joint impairment
- To increase accessory motion into proximal row carpal joint posterior glide
- To increase range of motion at the wrist joint
- To decrease pain
- To improve periarticular muscle performance

Positioning

1. The patient is sitting with the anterior surface of the forearm on the treatment table and the hand off the table.
2. The radiocarpal, ulnocarpal, and midcarpal joints are placed in the resting position if conservative techniques are indicated or approximating restricted range of motion if more aggressive techniques are indicated.
3. The clinician is facing the proximal row of carpal joints.
4. The stabilizing hand grips the one carpal bone with the thumb on the posterior surface and the index finger on the anterior surface.
5. The mobilizing/manipulating hand grips the other carpal bone with the thumb on the posterior surface and the index finger on the anterior surface.

Procedure

1. The stabilizing hand holds the one carpal bone in position.
2. The mobilizing/manipulating hand glides the scaphoid in a posterior direction on the lunate and the triquetrum in a posterior direction on the lunate (see Fig. 5-8).

Particulars

1. The clinician should use caution in performing these techniques because some of these motions might be hypermobile.

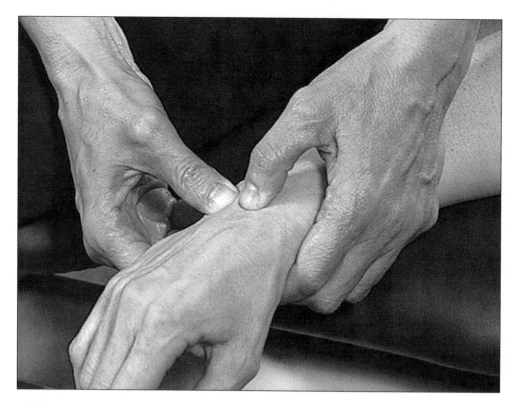

FIG. 5-9. Specific proximal row carpal joint anterior glide mobilizations/manipulations.

SPECIFIC PROXIMAL ROW CARPAL JOINT ANTERIOR GLIDE MOBILIZATIONS/MANIPULATIONS (Fig. 5-9)

Purpose

- To examine for proximal row carpal joint impairment
- To increase accessory motion into proximal row carpal joint anterior glide
- To increase range of motion at the wrist joint
- To decrease pain
- To improve periarticular muscle performance

Positioning

1. The patient is sitting with the anterior surface of the forearm on the treatment table and the hand off the table.
2. The radiocarpal, ulnocarpal, and midcarpal joints are placed in the resting position if conservative techniques are indicated or approximating restricted range of motion if more aggressive techniques are indicated.
3. The clinician is facing the proximal row of carpal joints.
4. The stabilizing hand grips the one carpal bone with the thumb on the posterior surface and the index finger on the anterior surface.
5. The mobilizing/manipulating hand grips the other carpal bone with the thumb on the posterior surface and the index finger on the anterior surface.

Procedure

1. The stabilizing hand holds the one carpal bone in position.
2. The mobilizing/manipulating hand glides the scaphoid in an anterior direction on the lunate and the triquetrum in an anterior direction on the lunate (see Fig. 5-9).

Particulars

1. The clinician should use caution in performing these techniques because some of these motions might be hypermobile.

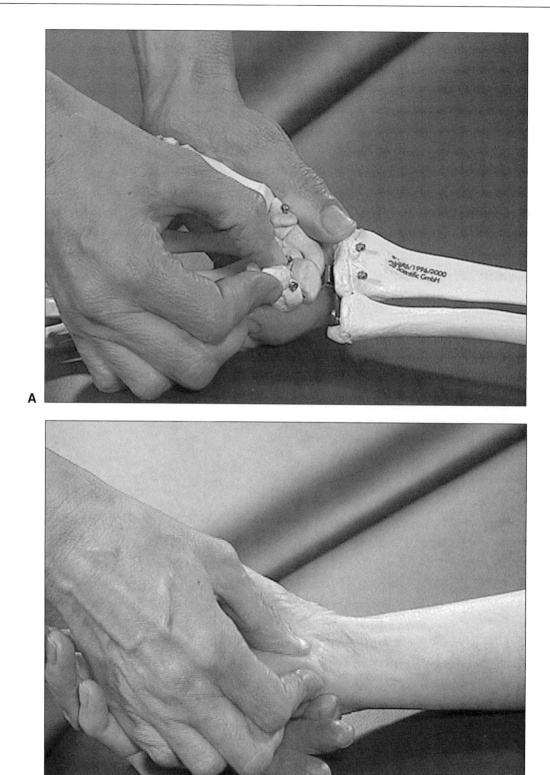

FIG. 5-10. Specific triquetrum-pisiform joint lateral (radial) and medial (ulnar) glide mobilizations/manipulations.

SPECIFIC TRIQUETRUM-PISIFORM JOINT LATERAL (RADIAL) AND MEDIAL (ULNAR) GLIDE MOBILIZATIONS/MANIPULATIONS (Fig. 5-10)

Purpose
- To examine for triquetrum-pisiform joint impairment
- To increase accessory motion into triquetrum-pisiform lateral (radial) and medial (ulnar) glide
- To decrease pain
- To improve periarticular muscle performance

Positioning
1. The patient is sitting with the posterior surface of the forearm, wrist, and hand on the treatment table.
2. The radiocarpal, ulnocarpal, and midcarpal joints are placed in the resting position if conservative techniques are indicated or approximating restricted range of motion if more aggressive techniques are indicated.
3. The clinician is facing the pisiform.
4. The stabilizing hand grips the lateral (radial) and medial (ulnar) surfaces of the wrist with the thumb and index finger.
5. The mobilizing/manipulating hand grips the lateral (radial) and medial (ulnar) surfaces of the pisiform with the thumb and index finger.

Procedure
1. The stabilizing hand holds the scaphoid, lunate, and triquetrum in position.
2. The mobilizing/manipulating hand glides the pisiform in a lateral (radial) direction on the triquetrum and the pisiform in a medial (ulnar) direction on the triquetrum (see Fig. 5-10).

Particulars
1. The clinician should use caution in performing this technique because this motion might be hypermobile (especially if the patient is a therapist who frequently performs spinal mobilization/manipulation techniques with the pisiform).

MIDCARPAL JOINTS

Osteokinematic motions:
    Flexion/extension
    Radial/ulnar deviation
Ligaments:
    Radial collateral ligament
    Dorsal radiocarpal ligament
    Volar radiocarpal ligament
    Intercarpal ligament
Joint orientation:
    Proximal row: inferior
    Distal row: superior
Concave joint surface:
    Varies, depending on the specific joint
Type of joint:
    Synovial
Resting position:
    Slight flexion and ulnar deviation[5]
Close-packed position:
    Full extension[5]
Capsular pattern of restriction:
    Flexion and extension are equally limited[6]

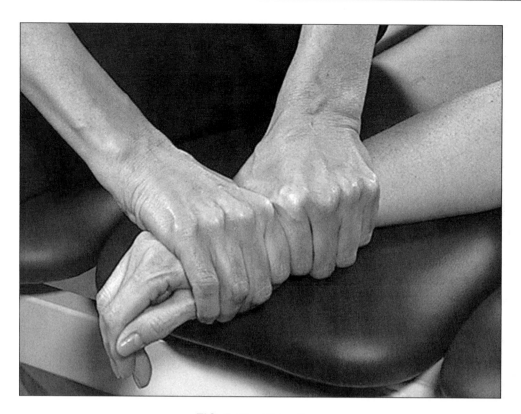

FIG. 5-11. Distraction.

DISTRACTION (Fig. 5-11)

Purpose

- To examine for midcarpal joint impairment
- To increase accessory motion into midcarpal joint distraction
- To increase range of motion at the wrist joint
- To decrease pain
- To improve periarticular muscle performance

Positioning

1. The patient is sitting with the anterior surface of the forearm on the treatment table and the hand off the table.
2. The midcarpal joints are placed in the resting position if conservative techniques are indicated or approximating restricted range of motion if more aggressive techniques are indicated.
3. The clinician is facing the midcarpal joints.
4. The stabilizing hand grips the proximal row of carpals from the posterior side.
5. The mobilizing/manipulating hand grips the distal row of carpals from the posterior side.

Procedure

1. The stabilizing hand holds the proximal row of carpals to the treatment table.
2. The mobilizing/manipulating hand moves the distal row of carpals distally perpendicular to the proximal carpal row joint surface (see Fig. 5-11).

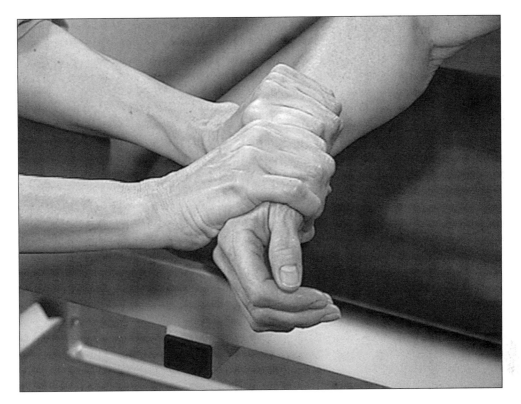

FIG. 5-12. Posterior glide.

POSTERIOR GLIDE (Fig. 5-12)

Purpose
- To examine for midcarpal joint impairment
- To increase accessory motion into midcarpal joint posterior glide
- To increase range of motion at the wrist joint
- To decrease pain
- To improve periarticular muscle performance

Positioning
1. The patient is sitting with the medial (ulnar) surface of the forearm on the treatment table and the hand off the table.
2. The midcarpal joints are placed in the resting position if conservative techniques are indicated or approximating the restricted range of motion if more aggressive techniques are indicated.
3. The clinician is facing the midcarpal joints.
4. The stabilizing hand grips the proximal row of carpals from the posterior side.
5. The mobilizing/manipulating hand grips the distal row of carpals from the posterior side.

Procedure
1. The clinician applies a grade I traction to the joint.
2. The stabilizing hand holds the proximal row of carpals to the treatment table.
3. The mobilizing/manipulating hand glides the distal row of carpals in a posterior direction (see Fig. 5-12).

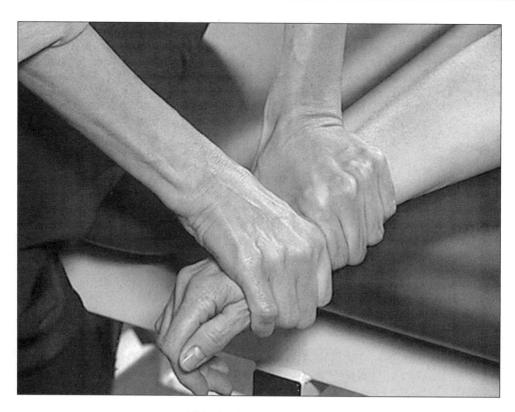

FIG. 5-13. Anterior glide.

ANTERIOR GLIDE (Fig. 5-13)

Purpose
- To examine for midcarpal joint impairment
- To increase accessory motion into midcarpal joint anterior glide
- To increase range of motion at the wrist joint
- To decrease pain
- To improve periarticular muscle performance

Positioning
1. The patient is sitting with the anterior surface of the forearm on the treatment table and the hand off the table.
2. The midcarpal joints are placed in the resting position if conservative techniques are indicated or approximating restricted range of motion if more aggressive techniques are indicated.
3. The clinician is facing the midcarpal joints.
4. The stabilizing hand grips the proximal row of carpals from the posterior side.
5. The mobilizing/manipulating hand grips the distal row of carpals from the posterior side.

Procedure
1. The clinician applies a grade I traction to the joint.
2. The stabilizing hand holds the proximal row of carpals to the treatment table.
3. The mobilizing/manipulating hand glides the distal row of carpals in an anterior direction (see Fig. 5-13).

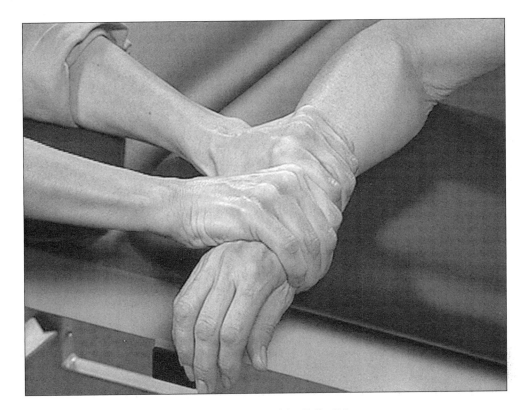

FIG. 5-14. Lateral (radial) glide.

LATERAL (RADIAL) GLIDE (Fig. 5-14)

Purpose
- To examine for midcarpal joint impairment
- To increase accessory motion into midcarpal joint lateral (radial) glide
- To increase range of motion at the wrist joint
- To decrease pain
- To improve periarticular muscle performance

Positioning
1. The patient is sitting with the anterior surface of the forearm on the treatment table and the hand off the table.
2. The midcarpal joints are placed in the resting position if conservative techniques are indicated or approximating restricted range of motion if more aggressive techniques are indicated.
3. The clinician is facing the midcarpal joints.
4. The stabilizing hand grips the proximal row of carpals from the posterior side.
5. The mobilizing/manipulating hand grips the distal row of carpals from the medial (ulnar) side.

Procedure
1. The clinician applies a grade I traction to the joint.
2. The stabilizing hand holds the proximal row of carpals to the treatment table.
3. The mobilizing/manipulating hand glides the distal row of carpals in a lateral (radial) direction (see Fig. 5-14).

Particulars
1. This technique might be especially effective for increasing range of motion into wrist joint ulnar deviation.

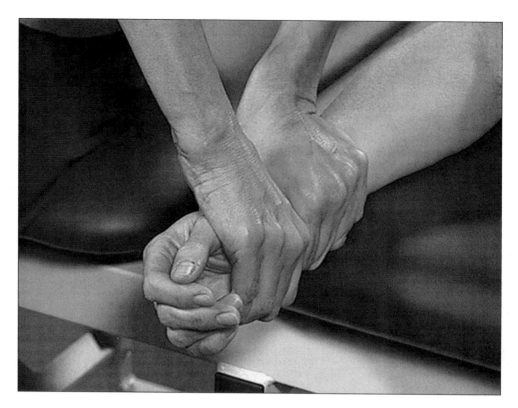

FIG. 5-15. Medial (ulnar) glide.

MEDIAL (ULNAR) GLIDE (Fig. 5-15)

Purpose

- To examine for midcarpal joint impairment
- To increase accessory motion into midcarpal joint medial (ulnar) glide
- To increase range of motion at the wrist joint
- To decrease pain
- To improve periarticular muscle performance

Positioning

1. The patient is sitting with the medial (ulnar) surface of the forearm on the treatment table and the hand off the table.
2. The midcarpal joints are placed in the resting position if conservative techniques are indicated or approximating restricted range of motion if more aggressive techniques are indicated.
3. The clinician is facing the midcarpal joints.
4. The stabilizing hand grips the proximal row of carpals from the anterior side.
5. The mobilizing/manipulating hand grips the distal row of carpals from the lateral (radial) side.

Procedure

1. The clinician applies a grade I traction to the joint.
2. The stabilizing hand holds the proximal row of carpals to the treatment table.
3. The mobilizing/manipulating hand glides the distal row of carpals in a medial (ulnar) direction (see Fig. 5-15).

Particulars

1. This technique might be especially effective for increasing range of motion into wrist joint radial deviation.

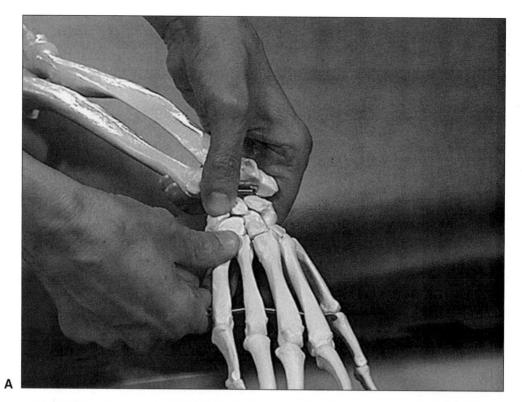

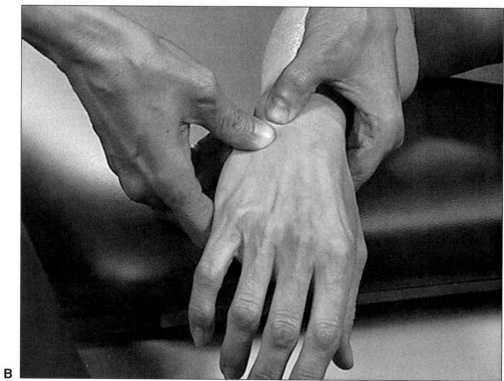

FIG. 5-16. Specific midcarpal joint posterior glide mobilizations/manipulations.

SPECIFIC MIDCARPAL JOINT POSTERIOR GLIDE MOBILIZATIONS/ MANIPULATIONS (Fig. 5-16)

Purpose

- To examine for midcarpal joint impairment
- To increase accessory motion into midcarpal joint posterior glide
- To increase range of motion at the wrist joint
- To decrease pain
- To improve periarticular muscle performance

Positioning

1. The patient is sitting with the anterior surface of the forearm on the treatment table and the hand off the table.
2. The midcarpal joints are placed in the resting position if conservative techniques are indicated or approximating restricted range of motion if more aggressive techniques are indicated.
3. The clinician is facing the midcarpal joints.
4. The stabilizing hand grips the proximal row carpal bone with the thumb on the posterior surface and the index finger on the anterior surface.
5. The mobilizing/manipulating hand grips the distal row carpal bone with the thumb on the posterior surface and the index finger on the anterior surface.

Procedure

1. The stabilizing hand holds the proximal row carpal bone in position.
2. The mobilizing/manipulating hand glides the trapezium and trapezoid in a posterior direction on the scaphoid, the capitate in a posterior direction on the lunate, and the hamate in a posterior direction on the triquetrum (see Fig. 5-16).

Particulars

1. The clinician should use caution in performing these techniques because these motions might be hypermobile.

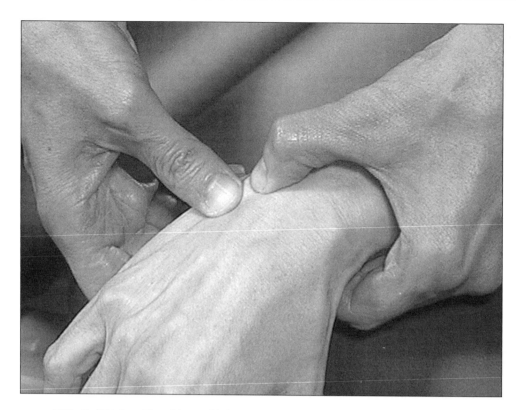

FIG. 5-17. Specific midcarpal joint anterior glide mobilizations/manipulations.

SPECIFIC MIDCARPAL JOINT ANTERIOR GLIDE MOBILIZATIONS/ MANIPULATIONS (Fig. 5-17)

Purpose

- To examine for midcarpal joint impairment
- To increase accessory motion into midcarpal joint anterior glide
- To increase range of motion at the wrist joint
- To decrease pain
- To improve periarticular muscle performance

Positioning

1. The patient is sitting with the anterior surface of the forearm on the treatment table and the hand off the table.
2. The midcarpal joints are placed in the resting position if conservative techniques are indicated or approximating restricted range of motion if more aggressive techniques are indicated.
3. The clinician is facing the midcarpal joints.
4. The stabilizing hand grips the proximal row carpal bone with the thumb on the posterior surface and the index finger on the anterior surface.
5. The mobilizing/manipulating hand grips the distal row carpal bone with the thumb on the posterior surface and the index finger on the anterior surface.

Procedure

1. The stabilizing hand holds the proximal row carpal bone in position.
2. The mobilizing/manipulating hand glides the trapezium and trapezoid in an anterior direction on the scaphoid, the capitate in an anterior direction on the lunate, and the hamate in an anterior direction on the triquetrum (see Fig. 5-17).

Particulars

1. The clinician should use caution in performing these techniques because these motions might be hypermobile.
2. Gliding the capitate on the lunate commonly is performed using a grade V manipulation.
3. The lunate-capitate technique might be effective in correcting a lunate-capitate joint positional fault.

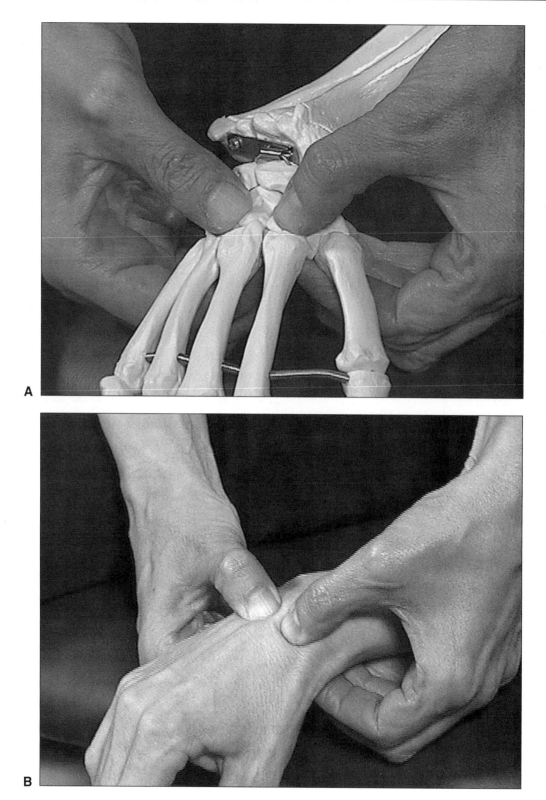

FIG. 5-18. Specific distal row carpal joint posterior glide mobilizations/manipulations.

SPECIFIC DISTAL ROW CARPAL JOINT POSTERIOR GLIDE MOBILIZATIONS/ MANIPULATIONS (Fig. 5-18)

Purpose

- To examine for distal row carpal joint impairment
- To increase accessory motion into distal row carpal joint posterior glide
- To increase range of motion at the wrist joint
- To decrease pain
- To improve periarticular muscle performance

Positioning

1. The patient is sitting with the anterior surface of the forearm on the treatment table and the hand off the table.
2. The midcarpal joints are placed in the resting position if conservative techniques are indicated or approximating restricted range of motion if more aggressive techniques are indicated.
3. The clinician is facing the distal row of carpal joints.
4. The stabilizing hand grips the one carpal bone with the thumb on the posterior surface and the index finger on the anterior surface.
5. The mobilizing/manipulating hand grips the other carpal bone with the thumb on the posterior surface and the index finger on the anterior surface.

Procedure

1. The stabilizing hand holds the one carpal bone in position.
2. The mobilizing/manipulating hand glides the trapezoid in a posterior direction on the capitate and the hamate in a posterior direction on the capitate (see Fig. 5-18).

Particulars

1. The clinician should use caution in performing these techniques because these motions might be hypermobile.

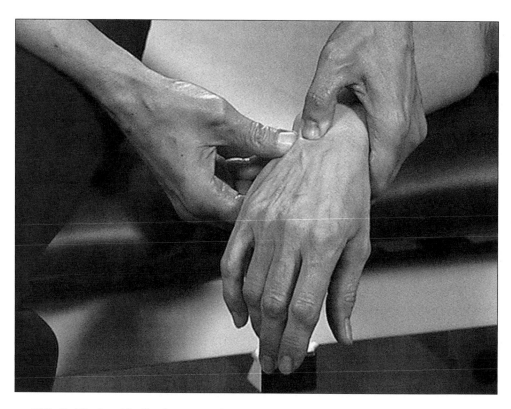

FIG. 5-19. Specific distal row carpal joint anterior glide mobilizations/manipulations.

SPECIFIC DISTAL ROW CARPAL JOINT ANTERIOR GLIDE MOBILIZATIONS/ MANIPULATIONS (Fig. 5-19)

Purpose
- To examine for distal row carpal joint impairment
- To increase accessory motion into distal row carpal joint anterior glide
- To increase range of motion at the wrist joint
- To decrease pain
- To improve periarticular muscle performance

Positioning
1. The patient is sitting with the anterior surface of the forearm on the treatment table and the hand off the table.
2. The midcarpal joints are placed in the resting position if conservative techniques are indicated or approximating restricted range of motion if more aggressive techniques are indicated.
3. The clinician is facing the distal row of carpal joints.
4. The stabilizing hand grips the one carpal bone with the thumb on the posterior surface and the index finger on the anterior surface.
5. The mobilizing/manipulating hand grips the other carpal bone with the thumb on the posterior surface and the index finger on the anterior surface.

Procedure
1. The stabilizing hand holds the one carpal bone in position.
2. The mobilizing/manipulating hand glides the trapezoid in an anterior direction on the capitate and the hamate in an anterior direction on the capitate (see Fig. 5-19).

Particulars
1. The clinician should use caution in performing these techniques because these motions might be hypermobile.

TRAPEZIOMETACARPAL JOINT

Osteokinematic motions:
  Flexion/extension
  Abduction/adduction
  Medial/lateral rotation
Ligament:
  Capsular ligament
Joint orientation:
  Trapezium: inferior, anterior, lateral
  Metacarpal: superior, posterior, medial
    *Note that the trapezium and first metacarpal are rotated approximately 90 degrees in relation to the palm of
      the hand.
Concave joint surface:
  Trapezium concave posterior to anterior
  First metacarpal concave lateral (radial) to medial (ulnar)
Type of joint:
  Synovial
Resting position:
  Midway between flexion and extension and abduction and adduction[5]
Close-packed position:
  Full opposition[5]
Capsular pattern of restriction:
  Limitation in abduction and extension and no limitation in flexion[6]

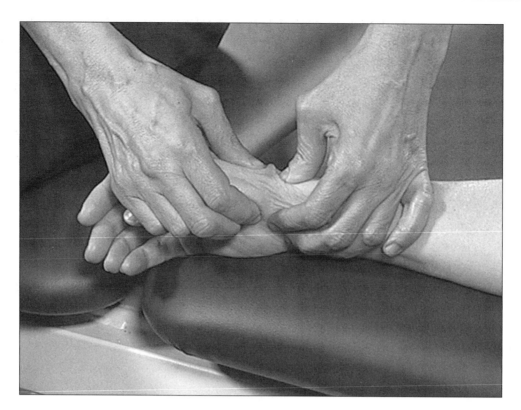

FIG. 5-20. Distraction.

DISTRACTION (Fig. 5-20)

Purpose

- To examine for trapeziometacarpal joint impairment
- To increase accessory motion into trapeziometacarpal joint distraction
- To increase range of motion at the trapeziometacarpal joint
- To decrease pain
- To improve periarticular muscle performance

Positioning

1. The patient is sitting with the medial (ulnar) surface of the forearm on the treatment table.
2. The trapeziometacarpal joint is placed in the resting position if conservative techniques are indicated or approximating restricted range of motion if more aggressive techniques are indicated.
3. The clinician is facing the trapeziometacarpal joint.
4. The stabilizing hand grips the trapezium with the thumb on the lateral (radial) surface and the index finger on the medial (ulnar) surface.
5. The mobilizing/manipulating hand grips the proximal metacarpal with the thumb on lateral (radial) surface (the back of the thumb) and the index finger on the medial (ulnar) surface (the front of the thumb).

Procedure

1. The stabilizing hand holds the trapezium in position.
2. The mobilizing/manipulating hand moves the metacarpal distally perpendicular to the trapezium and metacarpal joint surfaces (see Fig. 5-20).

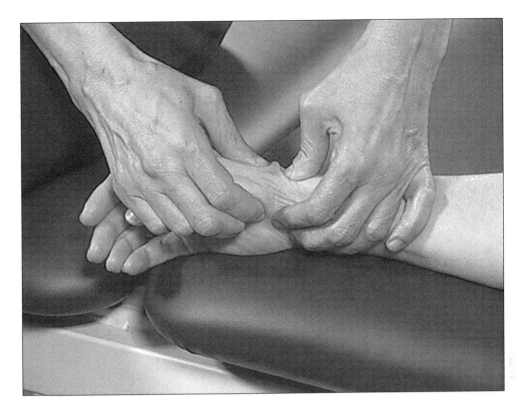

FIG. 5-21. Posterior glide.

POSTERIOR GLIDE (Fig. 5-21)

Purpose
- To examine for trapeziometacarpal joint impairment
- To increase accessory motion into trapeziometacarpal joint posterior glide
- To increase range of motion at the trapeziometacarpal joint
- To decrease pain
- To improve periarticular muscle performance

Positioning
1. The patient is sitting with the medial (ulnar) surface of the forearm on the treatment table.
2. The trapeziometacarpal joint is placed in the resting position if conservative techniques are indicated or approximating restricted range of motion if more aggressive techniques are indicated.
3. The clinician is facing the trapeziometacarpal joint.
4. The stabilizing hand grips the trapezium with the thumb as close to the posterior surface (the back of the hand) and index finger as close to the anterior surface (the palm of the hand) as possible.
5. The mobilizing/manipulating hand grips the proximal metacarpal with the thumb and index fingers on the posterior and anterior surfaces (sides) of the metacarpal.

Procedure
1. The clinician applies a grade I traction to the joint.
2. The stabilizing hand holds the trapezium in position.
3. The mobilizing/manipulating hand glides the metacarpal in a posterior direction (toward the back of the hand).

Particulars
1. This technique might be especially effective for increasing range of motion into trapeziometacarpal joint abduction.

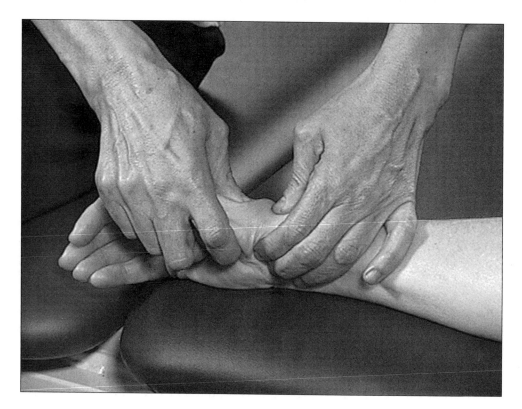

FIG. 5-22. Anterior glide.

ANTERIOR GLIDE (Fig. 5-22)

Purpose

- To examine for trapeziometacarpal joint impairment
- To increase accessory motion into trapeziometacarpal joint anterior glide
- To increase range of motion at the trapeziometacarpal joint
- To decrease pain
- To improve periarticular muscle performance

Positioning

1. The patient is sitting with the medial (ulnar) surface of the forearm on the treatment table.
2. The trapeziometacarpal joint is placed in the resting position if conservative techniques are indicated or approximating restricted range of motion if more aggressive techniques are indicated.
3. The clinician is facing the trapeziometacarpal joint.
4. The stabilizing hand grips the trapezium with the thumb as close to the posterior surface (the back of the hand) and the index finger as close to the anterior surface (the palm of the hand) as possible.
5. The mobilizing/manipulating hand grips the proximal metacarpal with the thumb and index fingers on the posterior and anterior surfaces (sides) of the metacarpal.

Procedure

1. The clinician applies a grade I traction to the joint.
2. The stabilizing hand holds the trapezium in position.
3. The mobilizing/manipulating hand glides the metacarpal in an anterior direction (toward the palm of the hand).

Particulars

1. This technique might be especially effective for increasing range of motion into trapeziometacarpal joint adduction.

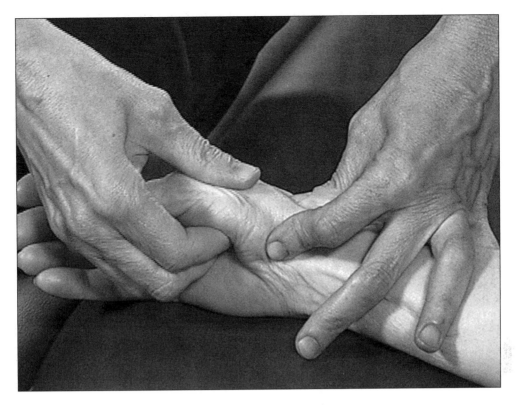

FIG. 5-23. Lateral (radial) glide.

LATERAL (RADIAL) GLIDE (Fig. 5-23)

Purpose

- To examine for trapeziometacarpal joint impairment
- To increase accessory motion into trapeziometacarpal joint lateral (radial) glide
- To increase range of motion at the trapeziometacarpal joint
- To decrease pain
- To improve periarticular muscle performance

Positioning

1. The patient is sitting with the medial (ulnar) surface of the forearm on the treatment table.
2. The trapeziometacarpal joint is placed in the resting position if conservative techniques are indicated or approximating restricted range of motion if more aggressive techniques are indicated.
3. The clinician is facing the trapeziometacarpal joint.
4. The stabilizing hand grips the trapezium with the thumb on the lateral (radial) and the index finger on the medial (ulnar) surface.
5. The mobilizing/manipulating hand grips the proximal metacarpal with the thumb on the lateral (radial) surface (the back of the thumb) and the index finger on the medial (ulnar) surface (the front of the thumb).

Procedure

1. The clinician applies a grade I traction to the joint.
2. The stabilizing hand holds the trapezium in position.
3. The mobilizing/manipulating hand glides the metacarpal in a lateral (radial) direction (toward the back of the metacarpal).

Particulars

1. This technique might be especially effective for increasing range of motion into trapeziometacarpal joint extension.

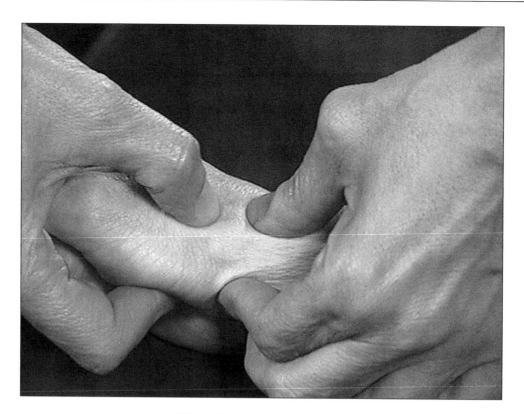

FIG. 5-24. Medial (ulnar) glide.

MEDIAL (ULNAR) GLIDE (Fig. 5-24)

Purpose

- To examine for trapeziometacarpal joint impairment
- To increase accessory motion into trapeziometacarpal joint medial (ulnar) glide
- To increase range of motion at the trapeziometacarpal joint
- To decrease pain
- To improve periarticular muscle performance

Positioning

1. The patient is sitting with the medial (ulnar) surface of the forearm on the treatment table.
2. The trapeziometacarpal joint is placed in the resting position if conservative techniques are indicated or approximating restricted range of motion if more aggressive techniques are indicated.
3. The clinician is facing the trapeziometacarpal joint.
4. The stabilizing hand grips the trapezium with the thumb on the lateral (radial) surface and the index finger on the medial (ulnar) surface.
5. The mobilizing/manipulating hand grips the proximal metacarpal with the thumb on the lateral (radial) surface (the back of the thumb) and the index finger on the medial (ulnar) surface (the front of the thumb).

Procedure

1. The clinician applies a grade I traction to the joint.
2. The stabilizing hand holds the trapezium in position.
3. The mobilizing/manipulating hand glides the metacarpal in a medial (ulnar) direction (toward the front of the metacarpal).

Particulars

1. This technique might be especially effective for increasing range of motion into trapeziometacarpal joint flexion.

INTERMETACARPAL JOINTS TWO THROUGH FIVE

Osteokinematic motion:
    Increasing/decreasing the arch of the hand
Ligaments:
    Palmar interosseous ligament
    Dorsal interosseous ligament
Joint orientation:
    Medial metacarpal: lateral
    Lateral metacarpal: medial
Concave joint surface:
    None; these are plane joints
Type of joint:
    Synarthrosis
Resting position:
    Unknown[5]
Close-packed position:
    Unknown[5]
Capsular pattern of restriction:
    None, not a synovial joint

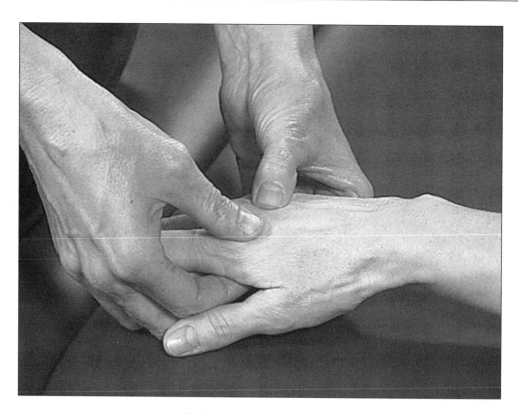

FIG. 5-25. Posterior glide.

POSTERIOR GLIDE (Fig. 5-25)

Purpose

- To examine for intermetacarpal joint impairment
- To increase accessory motion into intermetacarpal posterior glide, using the third metacarpal as a reference point
- To increase range of motion at the palm of the hand
- To decrease pain
- To improve periarticular muscle performance

Positioning

1. The patient is sitting with the palm down.
2. The hand is in a relaxed position.
3. The clinician is facing the intermetacarpal joints.
4. The stabilizing hand grips the midshaft of one metacarpal with the thumb on the posterior surface and the index finger on the anterior surface.
5. The mobilizing/manipulating hand grips the midshaft of the other metacarpal with the thumb on the posterior surface and the index finger on the anterior surface.

Procedure

1. The clinician applies a grade I traction to the joint.
2. The stabilizing hand holds one metacarpal in position.
3. The mobilizing/manipulating hand glides the second metacarpal in a posterior direction on the third metacarpal, the fourth metacarpal in a posterior direction on the third metacarpal, and the fifth metacarpal in a posterior direction on the fourth metacarpal (see Fig. 5-25).

Particulars

1. This technique might be especially effective for increasing range of motion into decreasing the arch of the hand.

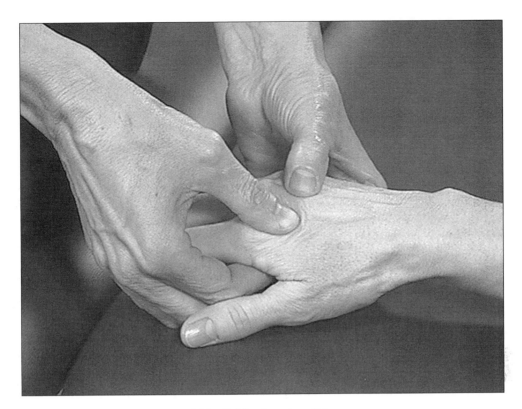

FIG. 5-26. Anterior glide.

ANTERIOR GLIDE (Fig. 5-26)

Purpose
- To examine for intermetacarpal joint impairment
- To increase accessory motion into intermetacarpal anterior glide, using the third metacarpal as a reference point
- To increase range of motion at the palm of the hand
- To decrease pain
- To improve periarticular muscle performance

Positioning
1. The patient is sitting with the palm down.
2. The hand is in a relaxed position.
3. The clinician is facing the intermetacarpal joints.
4. The stabilizing hand grips the midshaft of the one metacarpal with the thumb on the posterior surface and the index finger on the anterior surface.
5. The mobilizing/manipulating hand grips the midshaft of the other metacarpal with the thumb on the posterior surface and the index finger on the anterior surface.

Procedure
1. The clinician applies a grade I traction to the joint.
2. The stabilizing hand holds one metacarpal in position.
3. The mobilizing/manipulating hand glides the second metacarpal in an anterior direction on the third metacarpal, the fourth metacarpal in an anterior direction on the third metacarpal, and the fifth metacarpal in an anterior direction on the fourth metacarpal (see Fig. 5-26).

Particulars
1. This technique might be especially effective for increasing range of motion into increasing the arch of the hand.

FIRST METACARPOPHALANGEAL JOINT

Osteokinematic motion:
   Flexion/extension
Ligaments:
   Collateral ligament
   Palmar ligament
   Deep transverse ligament
Joint orientation:
   Metacarpals: inferior, anterior, lateral
   Phalanges: superior, posterior, medial
Concave joint surface:
   Phalanx
Type of joint:
   Synovial
Resting position:
   Slight flexion[5]
Close-packed position:
   Full extension[5]
Capsular pattern of restriction:
   Flexion is more limited than extension[6]

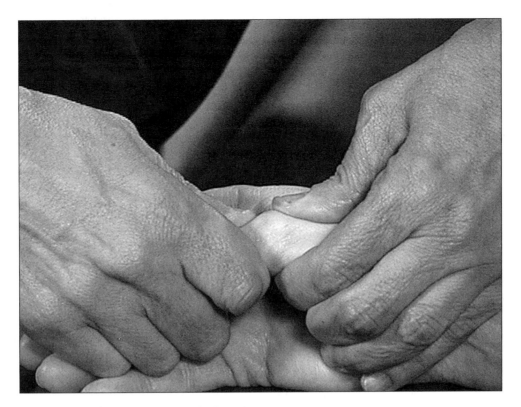

FIG. 5-27. Distraction.

DISTRACTION (Fig. 5-27)

Purpose
- To examine for thumb metacarpophalangeal joint impairment
- To increase accessory motion into thumb metacarpophalangeal joint distraction
- To increase range of motion at the metacarpophalangeal joint of the thumb
- To decrease pain
- To improve periarticular muscle performance

Positioning
1. The patient is sitting with the medial (ulnar) surface of the forearm on the treatment table.
2. The metacarpophalangeal joint of the thumb is placed in the resting position if conservative techniques are indicated or approximating restricted range of motion if more aggressive techniques are indicated.
3. The clinician is facing the metacarpophalangeal joint of the thumb.
4. The stabilizing hand grips the head of the first metacarpal with the thumb on the lateral (radial) surface and the index finger on the medial (ulnar) surface.
5. The mobilizing/manipulating hand grips the proximal end of the first proximal phalanx with the thumb on the lateral (radial) surface and the index finger on the medial (ulnar) surface.

Procedure
1. The stabilizing hand holds the metacarpal in position.
2. The mobilizing/manipulating hand moves the proximal phalanx distally perpendicular to the proximal phalanx joint surface (see Fig. 5-27).

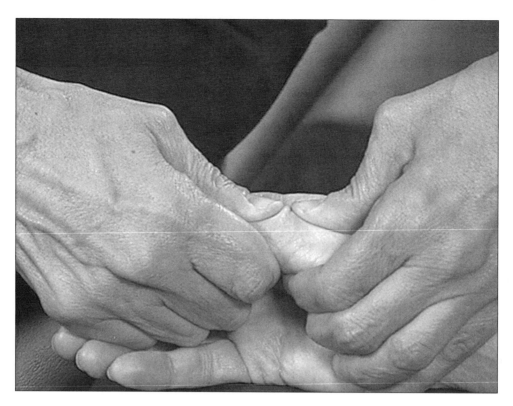

FIG. 5-28. Lateral (radial) glide.

LATERAL (RADIAL) GLIDE (Fig. 5-28)

Purpose

- To examine for thumb metacarpophalangeal joint impairment
- To increase accessory motion into thumb metacarpophalangeal joint lateral (radial) glide
- To increase range of motion at the metacarpophalangeal joint of the thumb
- To decrease pain
- To improve periarticular muscle performance

Positioning

1. The patient is sitting with the medial (ulnar) surface of the forearm on the treatment table.
2. The metacarpophalangeal joint of the thumb is placed in the resting position if conservative techniques are indicated or approximating restricted range of motion if more aggressive techniques are indicated.
3. The clinician is facing the metacarpophalangeal joint of the thumb.
4. The stabilizing hand grips the head of the first metacarpal with the thumb on the lateral (radial) surface and the index finger on the medial (ulnar) surface.
5. The mobilizing/manipulating hand grips the proximal end of the first proximal phalanx with the thumb on the lateral (radial) surface and the index finger on the medial (ulnar) surface.

Procedure

1. The clinician applies a grade I traction to the joint.
2. The stabilizing hand holds the metacarpal in position.
3. The mobilizing/manipulating hand glides the proximal phalanx in a lateral (radial) direction (see Fig. 5-28).

Particulars

1. This technique might be especially effective for increasing range of motion into first metacarpophalangeal joint extension.

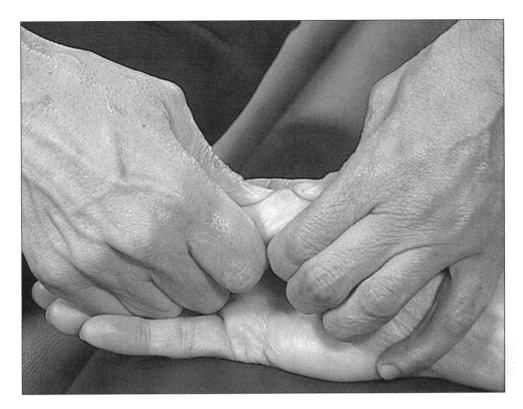

FIG. 5-29. Medial (ulnar) glide.

MEDIAL (ULNAR) GLIDE (Fig. 5-29)

Purpose
- To examine for thumb metacarpophalangeal joint impairment
- To increase accessory motion into thumb metacarpophalangeal joint medial (ulnar) glide
- To increase range of motion at the metacarpophalangeal joint of the thumb
- To decrease pain
- To improve periarticular muscle performance

Positioning
1. The patient is sitting with the medial (ulnar) surface of the forearm on the treatment table.
2. The metacarpophalangeal joint of the thumb is placed in the resting position if conservative techniques are indicated or approximating restricted range of motion if more aggressive techniques are indicated.
3. The clinician is facing the metacarpophalangeal joint of the thumb.
4. The stabilizing hand grips the head of the first metacarpal with the thumb on the lateral (radial) surface and the index finger on the medial (ulnar) surface.
5. The mobilizing/manipulating hand grips the proximal end of the first proximal phalanx with the thumb on the lateral (radial) surface and the index finger on the medial (ulnar) surface.

Procedure
1. The clinician applies a grade I traction to the joint.
2. The stabilizing hand holds the metacarpal in position.
3. The mobilizing/manipulating hand glides the proximal phalanx in a medial (ulnar) direction (see Fig. 5-29).

Particulars
1. This technique might be especially effective for increasing range of motion into first metacarpophalangeal joint flexion.

METACARPOPHALANGEAL JOINTS TWO THROUGH FIVE

Osteokinematic motions:
    Flexion/extension
    Radial/ulnar deviation
Ligaments:
    Collateral ligament
    Palmar ligament
    Deep transverse ligament
Joint orientation:
    Metacarpals: inferior
    Phalanges: superior
Concave joint surface:
    Phalanx
Type of joint:
    Synovial
Resting position:
    Slight flexion and slight ulnar deviation[5]
Close-packed position:
    Full flexion[5]
Capsular pattern of restriction:
    Flexion more limited than extension[6]

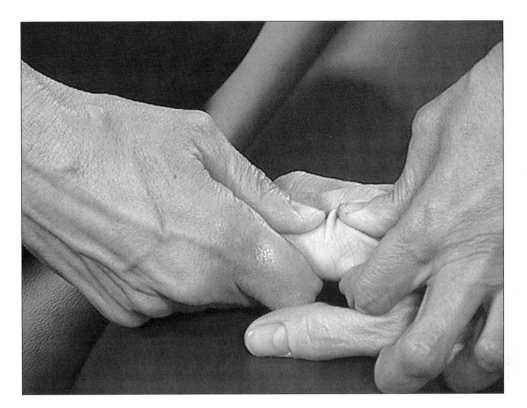

FIG. 5-30. Distraction.

DISTRACTION (Fig. 5-30)

Purpose

- To examine for digits two through five metacarpophalangeal joint impairment
- To increase accessory motion into metacarpophalangeal joint distraction of digits two through five
- To increase range of motion at the metacarpophalangeal joints of digits two through five
- To decrease pain
- To improve periarticular muscle performance

Positioning

1. The patient is sitting with the palm down.
2. The metacarpophalangeal joints of digits two through five are placed in the resting position if conservative techniques are indicated or approximating restricted range of motion if more aggressive techniques are indicated.
3. The clinician is facing the metacarpophalangeal joints of digits two through five.
4. The stabilizing hand grips the head of the metacarpal with the thumb on the posterior surface and the index finger on the anterior surface.
5. The mobilizing/manipulating hand grips the proximal end of the proximal phalanx with the thumb on the posterior surface and the index finger on the anterior surface.

Procedure

1. The stabilizing hand holds the metacarpal in position.
2. The mobilizing/manipulating hand moves the proximal phalanx distally perpendicular to the proximal phalanx joint surface (see Fig. 5-30).

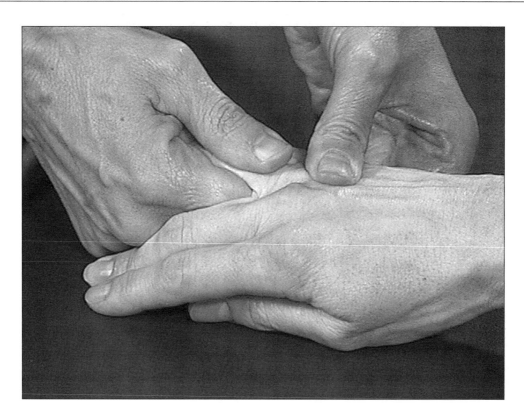

FIG. 5-31. Posterior glide.

POSTERIOR GLIDE (Fig. 5-31)

Purpose
- To examine for digits two through five metacarpophalangeal joint impairment
- To increase accessory motion into digits two through five metacarpophalangeal joint posterior glide
- To increase range of motion at the metacarpophalangeal joints of digits two through five
- To decrease pain
- To improve periarticular muscle performance

Positioning
1. The patient is sitting with the palm down.
2. The metacarpophalangeal joints of digits two through five are placed in the resting position if conservative techniques are indicated or approximating restricted range of motion if more aggressive techniques are indicated.
3. The clinician is facing the metacarpophalangeal joints of digits two through five.
4. The stabilizing hand grips the head of the metacarpal with the thumb on the posterior surface and the index finger on the anterior surface.
5. The mobilizing/manipulating hand grips the proximal end of the proximal phalanx with the thumb on the posterior surface and the index finger on the anterior surface.

Procedure
1. The clinician applies a grade I traction to the joint.
2. The stabilizing hand holds the metacarpal in position.
3. The mobilizing/manipulating hand glides the proximal phalanx in a posterior direction (see Fig. 5-31).

Particulars
1. This technique might be especially effective for increasing range of motion into digits two through five metacarpophalangeal joint extension.

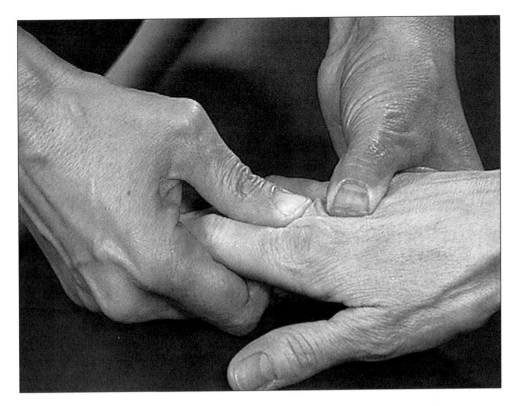

FIG. 5-32. Anterior glide.

ANTERIOR GLIDE (Fig. 5-32)

Purpose
- To examine for digits two through five metacarpophalangeal joint impairment
- To increase accessory motion into digits two through five metacarpophalangeal joint anterior glide
- To increase range of motion at the metacarpophalangeal joints of digits two through five
- To decrease pain
- To improve periarticular muscle performance

Positioning
1. The patient is sitting with the palm down.
2. The metacarpophalangeal joints of digits two through five are placed in the resting position if conservative techniques are indicated or approximating restricted range of motion if more aggressive techniques are indicated.
3. The clinician is facing the metacarpophalangeal joints of digits two through five.
4. The stabilizing hand grips the head of the metacarpal with the thumb on the posterior surface and the index finger on the anterior surface.
5. The mobilizing/manipulating hand grips the proximal end of the proximal phalanx with the thumb on the posterior surface and the index finger on the anterior surface.

Procedure
1. The clinician applies a grade I traction to the joint.
2. The stabilizing hand holds the metacarpal in position.
3. The mobilizing/manipulating hand glides the proximal phalanx in an anterior direction (see Fig. 5-32).

Particulars
1. This technique might be especially effective for increasing range of motion into digits two through five metacarpophalangeal joint flexion.

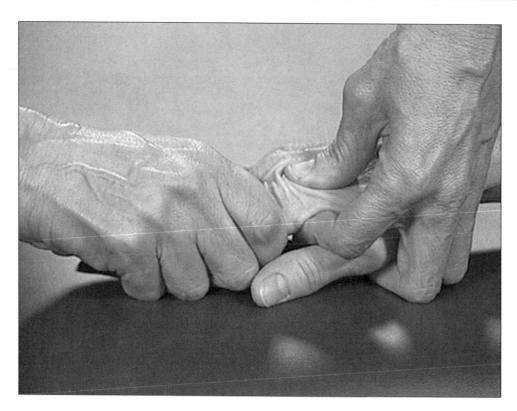

FIG. 5-33. Lateral (radial) glide.

LATERAL (RADIAL) GLIDE (Fig. 5-33)

Purpose

- To examine for digits two through five metacarpophalangeal joint impairment
- To increase accessory motion into digits two through five metacarpophalangeal joint lateral (radial) glide
- To increase range of motion at the metacarpophalangeal joints of digits two through five
- To decrease pain
- To improve periarticular muscle performance

Positioning

1. The patient is sitting with the palm down.
2. The metacarpophalangeal joints of digits two through five are placed in the resting position if conservative techniques are indicated or approximating restricted range of motion if more aggressive techniques are indicated.
3. The clinician is facing the metacarpophalangeal joints of digits two through five.
4. The stabilizing hand grips the head of the metacarpal with the thumb on the posterolateral surface and the index finger on the anterolateral surface.
5. The mobilizing/manipulating hand grips the proximal end of the proximal phalanx on the lateral (radial) and medial (ulnar) surfaces.

Procedure

1. The clinician applies a grade I traction to the joint.
2. The stabilizing hand holds the metacarpal in position.
3. The mobilizing/manipulating hand glides the proximal phalanx in a lateral (radial) direction (see Fig. 5-33).

Particulars

1. This technique might be especially effective for increasing range of motion into digits two through five metacarpophalangeal joint radial deviation.

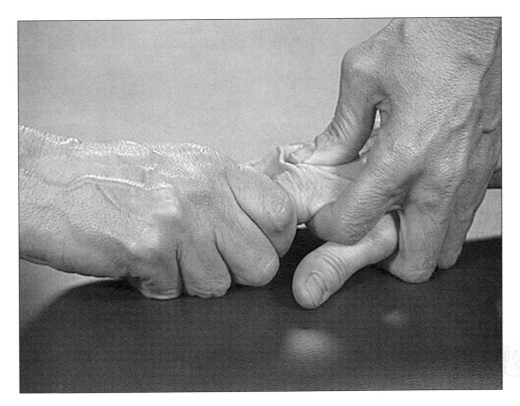

FIG. 5-34. Medial (ulnar) glide.

MEDIAL (ULNAR) GLIDE (Fig. 5-34)

Purpose

- To examine for digits two through five metacarpophalangeal joint impairment
- To increase accessory motion into digits two through five metacarpophalangeal joint medial (ulnar) glide
- To increase range of motion at the metacarpophalangeal joints of digits two through five
- To decrease pain
- To improve periarticular muscle performance

Positioning

1. The patient is sitting with the palm down.
2. The metacarpophalangeal joints of digits two through five are placed in the resting position if conservative techniques are indicated or approximating restricted range of motion if more aggressive techniques are indicated.
3. The clinician is facing the metacarpophalangeal joints of digits two through five.
4. The stabilizing hand grips the head of the metacarpal with the thumb on the posteromedial surface and the index finger on the anteromedial surface.
5. The mobilizing/manipulating hand grips the proximal end of the proximal phalanx on the lateral (radial) and medial (ulnar) surfaces.

Procedure

1. The clinician applies a grade I traction to the joint.
2. The stabilizing hand holds the metacarpal in position.
3. The mobilizing/manipulating hand glides the proximal phalanx in a medial (ulnar) direction (see Fig. 5-34).

Particulars

1. This technique might be especially effective for increasing range of motion into digits two through five metacarpophalangeal joint ulnar deviation.

INTERPHALANGEAL JOINTS OF FINGERS ONE THROUGH FIVE

Osteokinematic motion:
    Flexion/extension
Ligaments:
    Palmar ligament
    Medial collateral ligament
    Lateral collateral ligament
Joint orientation:
    Proximal phalanx: inferior
    Distal phalanx: superior
Concave joint surface:
    Distal phalanx
Type of joint:
    Synovial
Resting position:
    Slight flexion[5]
Close-packed position:
    Full extension[5]
Capsular pattern of restriction:
    Flexion is more limited than extension[6]

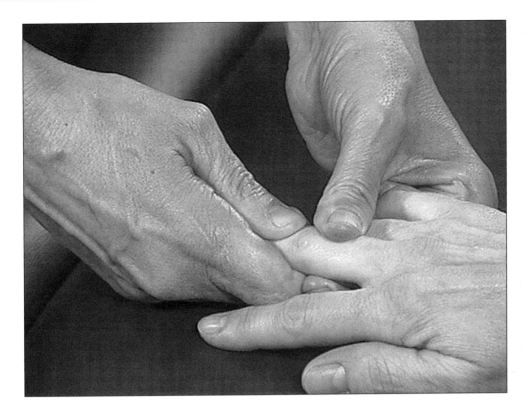

FIG. 5-35. Distraction.

DISTRACTION (Fig. 5-35)

Purpose

- To examine for finger interphalangeal joint impairment
- To increase accessory motion into finger interphalangeal joint distraction
- To increase range of motion at the interphalangeal joints of the fingers
- To decrease pain
- To improve periarticular muscle performance

Positioning

1. The patient is sitting with the palm down.
2. The interphalangeal joints are placed in the resting position if conservative techniques are indicated or approximating restricted range of motion if more aggressive techniques are indicated.
3. The clinician is facing the interphalangeal joints.
4. The stabilizing hand grips the distal end of the more proximal phalanx with the thumb on the posterior surface and the index finger on the anterior surface. If the thumb interphalangeal joint is being mobilized/manipulated, the clinician's thumb grips the lateral (radial) surface, and the index finger grips the medial (ulnar) surface.
5. The mobilizing/manipulating hand grips the proximal end of the more distal phalanx with the thumb on the posterior surface and the index finger on the anterior surface. If the thumb interphalangeal joint is being mobilized/manipulated, the clinician's thumb grips the lateral (radial) surface, and the index finger grips the medial (ulnar) surface.

Procedure

1. The stabilizing hand holds the proximal phalanx in position.
2. The mobilizing/manipulating hand moves the distal phalanx distally perpendicular to the distal phalanx joint surface (see Fig. 5-35).
3. The clinician could grip the patient's digit with a padded tongue depressor to assist in directing a more precise mobilization/manipulation.
4. The clinician could wear surgical gloves to reduce slippage against the patient's skin.

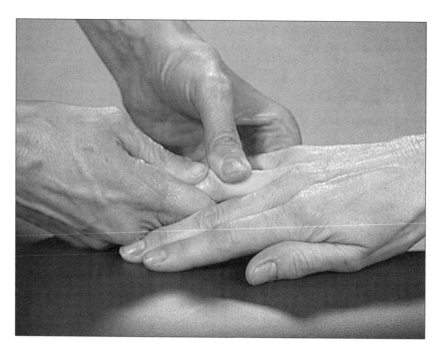

FIG. 5-36. Posterior glide.

POSTERIOR GLIDE (Fig. 5-36)

Purpose

- To examine for finger interphalangeal joint impairment
- To increase accessory motion into finger interphalangeal posterior glide
- To increase range of motion at the interphalangeal joints of the fingers
- To decrease pain
- To improve periarticular muscle performance

Positioning

1. The patient is sitting with the palm down.
2. The interphalangeal joints are placed in the resting position if conservative techniques are indicated or approximating restricted range of motion if more aggressive techniques are indicated.
3. The clinician is facing the interphalangeal joints.
4. The stabilizing hand grips the distal end of the more proximal phalanx with the thumb on the posterior surface and the index finger on the anterior surface. If the thumb interphalangeal joint is being mobilized/manipulated, the clinician's thumb grips the lateral (radial) surface, and the index finger grips the medial (ulnar) surface.
5. The mobilizing/manipulating hand grips the proximal end of the more distal phalanx with the thumb on the posterior surface and the index finger on the anterior surface. If the thumb interphalangeal joint is being mobilized/manipulated, the clinician's thumb grips the lateral (radial) surface, and the index finger grips the medial (ulnar) surface.

Procedure

1. The clinician applies a grade I traction to the joint.
2. The stabilizing hand holds the proximal phalanx in position.
3. The mobilizing/manipulating hand glides the distal phalanx in a posterior direction. If the thumb interphalangeal joint is being mobilized/manipulated, the distal phalanx is glided in a lateral (radial) direction (see Fig. 5-36).
4. The clinician could grip the patient's digit with a padded tongue depressor to assist in directing a more precise mobilization/manipulation.
5. The clinician could wear surgical gloves to reduce slippage against the patient's skin.

Particulars

1. This technique might be especially effective for increasing range of motion into interphalangeal joint extension.

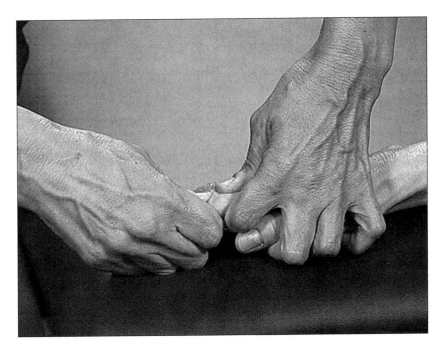

FIG. 5-37. Anterior glide.

ANTERIOR GLIDE (Fig. 5-37)

Purpose

- To examine for finger interphalangeal joint impairment
- To increase accessory motion into finger interphalangeal anterior glide
- To increase range of motion at the interphalangeal joints of the fingers
- To decrease pain
- To improve periarticular muscle performance

Positioning

1. The patient is sitting with the palm down.
2. The interphalangeal joints are placed in the resting position if conservative techniques are indicated or approximating restricted range of motion if more aggressive techniques are indicated.
3. The clinician is facing the interphalangeal joints.
4. The stabilizing hand grips the distal end of the more proximal phalanx with the thumb on the posterior surface and the index finger on the anterior surface. If the thumb interphalangeal joint is being mobilized/manipulated, the clinician's thumb grips the lateral (radial) surface, and the index finger grips the medial (ulnar) surface.
5. The mobilizing/manipulating hand grips the proximal end of the more distal phalanx with the thumb on the posterior surface and the index finger on the anterior surface. If the thumb interphalangeal joint is being mobilized/manipulated, the clinician's thumb grips the lateral (radial) surface, and the index finger grips the medial (ulnar) surface.

Procedure

1. The clinician applies a grade I traction to the joint.
2. The stabilizing hand holds the proximal phalanx in position.
3. The mobilizing/manipulating hand glides the distal phalanx in an anterior direction. If the thumb interphalangeal joint is being mobilized/manipulated, the distal phalanx is glided in a medial (ulnar) direction (see Fig. 5-37).
4. The clinician could grip the patient's digit with a padded tongue depressor to assist in directing a more precise mobilization/manipulation.
5. The clinician could wear surgical gloves to reduce slippage against the patient's skin.

Particulars

1. This technique might be especially effective for increasing range of motion into interphalangeal joint flexion.

REFERENCES

1. Tal-Akabi A, Rushton A: An investigation to compare the effectiveness of carpal bone mobilisation and neurodynamic mobilisation as methods of treatment for carpal tunnel syndrome. Manual Ther 2000;5:214-222.
2. Struijs PAA, Damen P-J, Bakker EWP, et al: Manipulation of the wrist for management of lateral epicondylitis: a randomized pilot study. Phys Ther 2003;83:608-616.
3. Randall T, Portney L, Harris BA: Effects of joint mobilization on joint stiffness and active motion of the metacarpophalangeal joint. J Orthop Sports Phys Ther 1992;16:30-36.
4. Mierau D, Cassidy JD, Bowen V, et al: Manipulation and mobilization of the third metacarpophalangeal joint: a quantitative radiographic and range of motion study. Manual Med 1988;3:135-140.
5. Kaltenborn FM: Manual Mobilization of the Joints: The Kaltenborn Method of Joint Examination and Treatment, Vol I: The Extremities, 6th ed. Oslo, Norway, Norli, 2002.
6. Cyriax J: Textbook of Orthopaedic Medicine, Vol 1: Diagnosis of Soft Tissue Lesions, 8th ed. London, Bailliere Tindall, 1982.

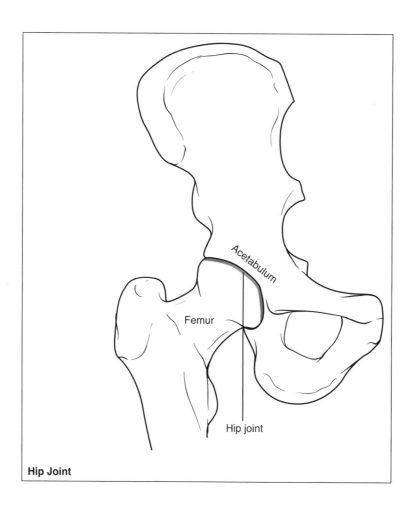

Hip Joint

CHAPTER 6

The Hip Joint

BASICS

Hip

The hip is a ball-and-socket joint with a compressed anterior to posterior diameter. Its construction is similar to that of the glenohumeral joint, but the hip is far more stable. This increased stability is due to negative intracapsular atmospheric pressure, a stronger joint capsule, a more spherical femoral head, and a deeper socket made even deeper by the labrum, which provides greater joint surface contact area than at the glenohumeral joint. Most functional activities occur between 0 and 120 degrees of hip flexion and between 0 and 20 degrees of lateral rotation and abduction.

SPECIFIC PATHOLOGY AND HIP JOINT MOBILIZATION/MANIPULATION

Hip Osteoarthritis

In a study investigating treatment for hip osteoarthritis, 109 subjects were randomly assigned to receive mobilization and manipulation to the hip joint or active exercises designed to improve strength and range of motion. Subjects were seen for nine visits over 5 weeks. At the end of the study, 81% of subjects receiving mobilization and manipulation reported improvement compared with 50% in the exercise group. The subjects receiving mobilization and manipulation also experienced a significant improvement in hip function and range of motion and a decrease in pain and stiffness compared with the exercise group. These improvements were present immediately after the treatment period and persisted at 29 weeks' follow-up.[1]

HIP JOINT

Osteokinematic motions:
    Flexion/extension
    Abduction/adduction
    Medial/lateral rotation
Ligaments:
    Iliofemoral (Y) ligament
    Ischiofemoral ligament
    Pubofemoral ligament
    Ligamentum teres
    Zona orbicularis
    Transverse ligament
Joint orientation:
    Acetabulum: inferior, lateral, anterior
    Femur: superior, medial, anterior
Concave joint surface:
    Acetabulum
Type of joint:
    Synovial

Resting position:
   30 degrees flexion, 30 degrees abduction, and slight lateral rotation[2]
Close-packed position:
   Full extension, abduction, and medial rotation[2]
Capsular pattern of restriction:
   Flexion, abduction, and medial rotation are grossly limited; extension is slightly limited[3]

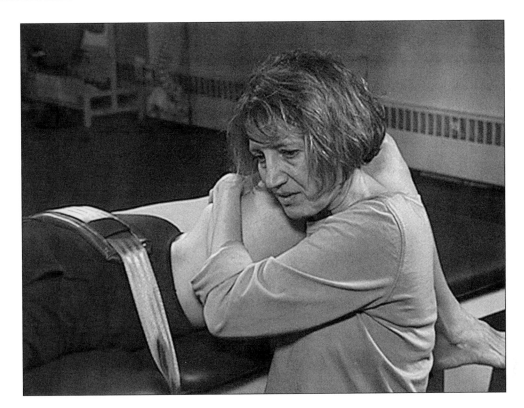

FIG. 6-1. Distraction.

DISTRACTION (Fig. 6-1)

Purpose
- To examine for hip joint impairment
- To increase accessory motion into hip joint distraction
- To increase range of motion at the hip joint
- To decrease pain
- To improve periarticular muscle performance

Positioning
1. The patient is supine with the leg positioned over the clinician's shoulder.
2. The clinician can wrap a belt around the patient's pelvis and the treatment table to help stabilize the pelvis.
3. The hip joint is placed as close to the resting position as possible if conservative techniques are indicated or approximating restricted range of motion if more aggressive techniques are indicated.
4. The clinician is at the patient's side facing the patient's hip.
5. Both hands are positioned on the medial surface of the proximal thigh.

Procedure
1. Both hands move the femoral head inferior, lateral, and anterior, while the clinician elevates the shoulder, moving the femur perpendicular to the joint surface of the acetabulum (see Fig. 6-1).

Particulars
1. This technique is commonly performed using a grade V manipulation.

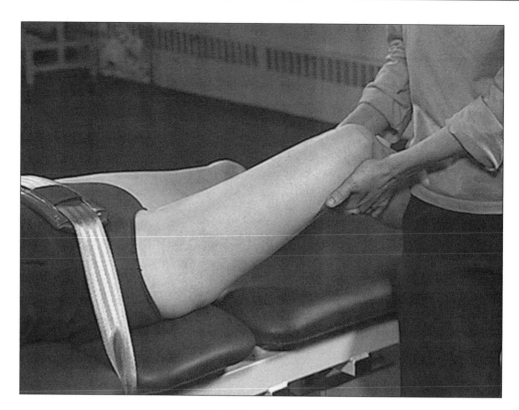

FIG. 6-2. Inferior glide.

INFERIOR GLIDE (Fig. 6-2)

Purpose

- To examine for hip joint impairment
- To increase accessory motion into hip joint inferior glide
- To increase range of motion at the hip joint
- To decrease pain
- To improve periarticular muscle performance

Positioning

1. The patient is supine.
2. The clinician can wrap a belt around the patient's pelvis and the treatment table to help stabilize the pelvis.
3. The hip joint is placed in the resting position if conservative techniques are indicated or approximating restricted range of motion if more aggressive techniques are indicated.
4. The clinician is at the patient's foot facing the patient's hip.
5. Both hands grip the distal thigh.

Procedure

1. The clinician applies a grade I traction to the joint.
2. Both hands glide the femoral head in an inferior direction as the clinician leans away from the joint (see Fig. 6-2).

Particulars

1. It is important to screen for sacroiliac joint impairments before performing this technique.
2. This technique is commonly performed using a grade V manipulation.
3. This technique is also called a *long axis distraction*.
4. This technique might be especially effective for increasing range of motion into hip joint abduction.

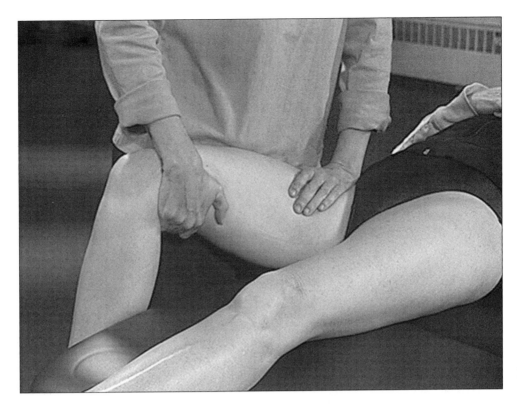

FIG. 6-3. Posterior glide.

POSTERIOR GLIDE (Fig. 6-3)

Purpose
- To examine for hip joint impairment
- To increase accessory motion into hip joint posterior glide
- To increase range of motion at the hip joint
- To decrease pain
- To improve periarticular muscle performance

Positioning
1. The patient is supine.
2. The hip joint is placed in the resting position if conservative techniques are indicated or approximating restricted range of motion if more aggressive techniques are indicated.
3. The clinician is at the patient's knee facing the patient's hip.
4. The mobilizing/manipulating hand is positioned on the anterior surface of the proximal thigh.
5. The guiding hand is positioned on the posterior surface of the distal thigh.

Procedure
1. The clinician applies a grade I traction to the joint.
2. The mobilizing/manipulating hand glides the femur in a posterior direction.
3. The guiding hand controls the position of the femur (see Fig. 6-3).

Particulars
1. It is important to screen for sacroiliac joint impairments before performing this technique.
2. This technique might be especially effective for increasing range of motion into hip joint flexion and medial rotation.

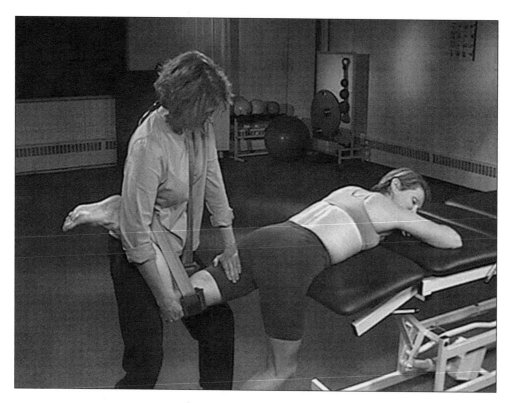

FIG. 6-4. Anterior glide: first technique.

ANTERIOR GLIDE: FIRST TECHNIQUE (Fig. 6-4)

Purpose

- To examine for hip joint impairment
- To increase accessory motion into hip joint anterior glide
- To increase range of motion at the hip joint
- To decrease pain
- To improve periarticular muscle performance

Positioning

1. The patient is prone with the pelvis on the treatment table and the legs off the end of the table.
2. The clinician can wrap a belt around the patient's thigh and the clinician's shoulder to help control the motion.
3. The hip joint is placed in the resting position if conservative techniques are indicated or approximating restricted range of motion if more aggressive techniques are indicated.
4. The clinician is at the foot of the treatment table facing the patient's hip.
5. The patient's leg is supported between the clinician's arm and trunk.
6. The mobilizing/manipulating hand is positioned on the posterior surface of the proximal thigh.
7. The guiding hand is positioned on the anterior surface of the distal thigh.

Procedure

1. The clinician applies a grade I traction to the joint.
2. The mobilizing/manipulating hand glides the femur in an anterior direction as the clinician leans on the patient's thigh.
3. The guiding hand controls the position of the thigh (see Fig. 6-4).

Particulars

1. It is important to screen for sacroiliac joint impairments before performing this technique.
2. This technique might be especially effective for increasing range of motion into hip joint extension and lateral rotation.

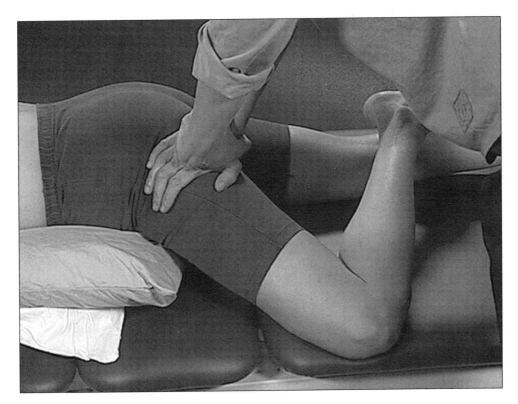

FIG. 6-5. Anterior glide: second technique.

ANTERIOR GLIDE: SECOND TECHNIQUE (Fig. 6-5)

Purpose

- To examine for hip joint impairment
- To increase accessory motion into hip joint anterior glide
- To increase range of motion at the hip joint
- To decrease pain
- To improve periarticular muscle performance

Positioning

1. The patient is prone with one or more pillows under the trunk and the hip positioned in abduction and lateral rotation.
2. The clinician is at the side of the treatment table facing the patient's hip.
3. The mobilizing/manipulating hand is positioned over the guiding hand.
4. The guiding hand is positioned on the posterolateral surface of the proximal thigh.

Procedure

1. The clinician applies a grade I traction to the joint.
2. The mobilizing/manipulating hand glides the femur in an anterior direction as the clinician leans on the patient's thigh.
3. The guiding hand controls the position of the mobilizing hand (see Fig. 6-5).

Particulars

1. This technique might be especially effective for increasing range of motion into hip joint extension and lateral rotation.

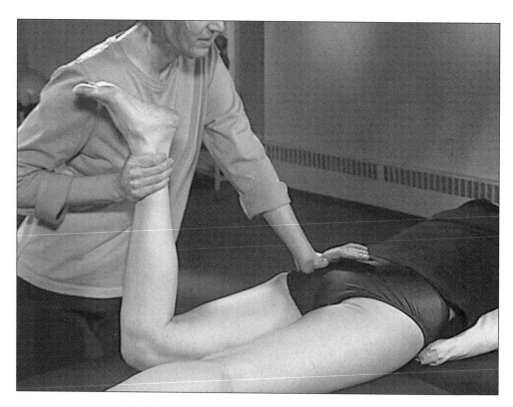

FIG. 6-6. Posterolateral glide of the femur on the pelvis.

POSTEROLATERAL GLIDE OF THE FEMUR ON THE PELVIS (Fig. 6-6)

Purpose

- To examine for hip joint impairment
- To increase accessory motion into hip joint posterolateral glide
- To increase range of motion at the hip joint
- To decrease pain
- To improve periarticular muscle performance

Positioning

1. The patient is prone with the knee on the side being treated flexed to 90 degrees.
2. The hip joint is placed in as close to resting position as possible if conservative techniques are indicated or approximating restricted range of motion if more aggressive techniques are indicated.
3. The clinician is at the patient's side facing the patient's hip.
4. The stabilizing hand grips the ankle and controls the amount of hip rotation.
5. The mobilizing/manipulating hand is positioned over the midpoint of the posterior surface of the ilium.

Procedure

1. The stabilizing hand holds the leg in position.
2. The mobilizing/manipulating hand glides the pelvis in an anteromedial direction, imparting a posterolateral force to the femur on the pelvis (see Fig. 6-6).

Particulars

1. It is important to screen for sacroiliac joint impairments before performing this technique.
2. This technique might be especially effective for increasing range of motion into hip joint medial rotation.

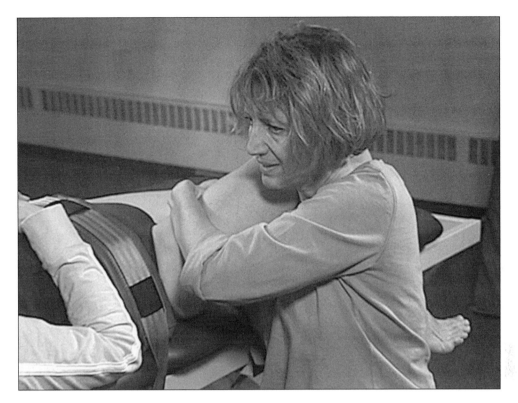

FIG. 6-7. Lateral glide.

LATERAL GLIDE (Fig. 6-7)

Purpose

- To examine for hip joint impairment
- To increase accessory motion into hip joint lateral glide
- To increase range of motion at the hip joint
- To decrease pain
- To improve periarticular muscle performance

Positioning

1. The patient is supine with the leg positioned over the clinician's shoulder.
2. The clinician can wrap a belt around the patient's pelvis and treatment table to help stabilize the pelvis.
3. The hip joint is placed as close to the resting position as possible if conservative techniques are indicated or approximating restricted range of motion if more aggressive techniques are indicated.
4. The clinician is at the patient's side facing the patient's hip.
5. Both hands are positioned on the medial surface of the proximal thigh.

Procedure

1. The clinician applies a grade I traction to the joint.
2. Both hands glide the femur in a lateral direction (see Fig. 6-7).

Particulars

1. This technique might be especially effective for increasing range of motion into hip joint adduction and medial rotation.

REFERENCES

1. Hoeksma HL, Dekker J, Ronday HK, et al: Comparison of manual therapy and exercise therapy in osteoarthritis of the hip: a randomized clinical trial. Arthritis Care Res 2004;51:722-729.
2. Kaltenborn FM: Manual Mobilization of the Joints: The Kaltenborn Method of Joint Examination and Treatment, Vol I: The Extremities, 6th ed. Oslo, Norway, Norli, 2002.
3. Cyriax J: Textbook of Orthopaedic Medicine, Vol 1: Diagnosis of Soft Tissue Lesions, 8th ed. London, Bailliere Tindall, 1982.

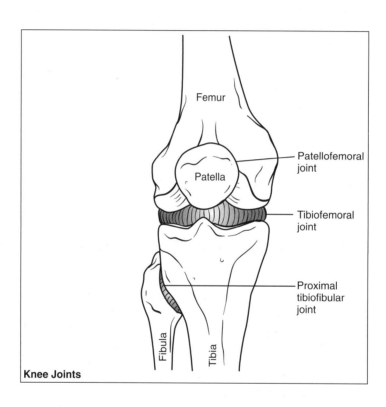

Femur

Patellofemoral joint

Patella

Tibiofemoral joint

Proximal tibiofibular joint

Fibula

Tibia

Knee Joints

The Knee

BASICS

The knee joint consists of two sets of articulating surfaces, the tibiofemoral joint and the patellofemoral joint. To perform most activities of daily living, these two joints must allow at least 110 degrees of knee flexion to occur.

Tibiofemoral Joint

Flexion at the knee is accompanied by medial rotation of the tibia, and extension is accompanied by lateral rotation. Lateral rotation occurs during the last 30 degrees of extension. This rotational motion is caused by tightening of ligamentous structures and the configuration of the two articular surfaces.

Patellofemoral Joint

The patellofemoral joint moves five to seven cm superiorly in the femoral groove as the knee extends. It also is believed to move from a lateral position to a more medial position and back to a more lateral position as the knee moves from full flexion to full extension.

SPECIFIC PATHOLOGY AND KNEE JOINT MOBILIZATION/MANIPULATION

Knee Osteoarthritis

In a study of 83 patients with knee osteoarthritis, subjects were randomly assigned to receive a combination of physical therapy interventions or subtherapeutic ultrasound to the knee. Physical therapy consisted of joint mobilization, soft tissue mobilization, and muscle stretching to the knee, lumbar spine, and ankle as indicated. The intervention group also performed a standardized knee exercise program. Outcomes were measured at four and six weeks and at one-year follow-up. The distance walked in six minutes was statistically and clinically higher in the group receiving physical therapy at all three time intervals. Similar improvements in function, pain, and stiffness were evident in the group receiving physical therapy by six weeks and at one-year follow-up. The investigators concluded that a combination of physical therapy interventions, including joint mobilization, was effective in reducing symptoms and improving function in subjects with knee osteoarthritis.[1]

Patellofemoral Joint Syndrome

In a randomized study of 19 patients with patellofemoral joint pain in which the efficacy of patellar mobilization was investigated, knee symptoms were not reduced significantly in subjects receiving mobilization compared with a placebo treatment.[2] A subsequent randomized trial was performed in which the investigators evaluated the effect of a combination of physical therapy interventions, which included joint mobilization and quadriceps muscle retraining, patellar taping, and home exercises, with a sham physical therapy treatment of taping and ultrasound. The study was performed on 67 subjects with patellofemoral pain. The group receiving combined physical therapy interventions showed a significant decrease in knee pain and improvement in function compared with the placebo group.[3] These two studies support the premise that joint mobilization, when performed in combination with other physical therapy interventions, can reduce pain and disability effectively.

TIBIOFEMORAL JOINT

Osteokinematic motions:
  Flexion/extension
  Medial/lateral rotation
Ligaments:
  Tibial collateral ligament
  Fibular collateral ligament
  Anterior cruciate ligament
  Posterior cruciate ligament
  Oblique ligament
  Arcuate popliteal ligament
Joint orientation:
  Femur: inferior
  Tibia: superior
Concave joint surface:
  Tibia
Type of joint:
  Synovial
Resting position:
  25 to 40 degrees of flexion[4]
Close-packed position:
  Full extension[4]
Capsular pattern of restriction:
  Gross limitations in flexion accompanied by slight limitations in extension[5]

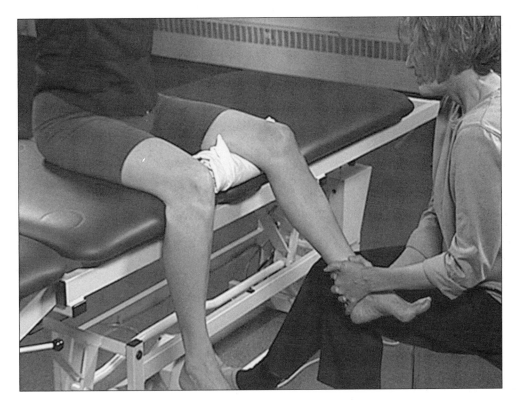

FIGURE 7-1. Distraction.

DISTRACTION (Fig. 7-1)

Purpose

- To examine for tibiofemoral joint impairment
- To increase accessory motion into tibiofemoral joint distraction
- To increase range of motion at the knee joint
- To decrease pain
- To improve periarticular muscle performance

Positioning

1. The patient is sitting with the knee off the edge of the treatment table.
2. The tibiofemoral joint is placed in the resting position if conservative techniques are indicated or approximating restricted range of motion if more aggressive techniques are indicated.
3. The clinician is at the patient's foot facing the patient's knee.
4. Both hands grip the distal tibia from the medial and lateral sides.
5. Alternatively, the clinician can use a specialized belt with a strap that wraps around the patient's tibia and a stirrup attachment for placement of the clinician's foot to perform this technique.

Procedure

1. Both hands move the tibia distally perpendicular to the tibial joint surface (see Fig. 7-1).

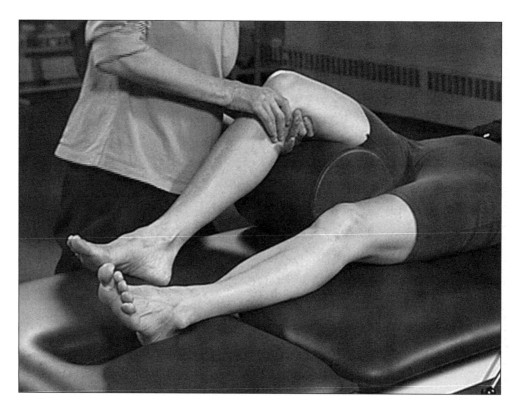

FIGURE 7-2. Posterior glide.

POSTERIOR GLIDE (Fig. 7-2)

Purpose

- To examine for tibiofemoral joint impairment
- To increase accessory motion into tibiofemoral joint posterior glide
- To increase range of motion at the tibiofemoral joint
- To decrease pain
- To improve periarticular muscle performance

Positioning

1. The patient is supine.
2. The tibiofemoral joint is placed in the resting position if conservative techniques are indicated or approximating restricted range of motion if more aggressive techniques are indicated.
3. The clinician is at the side of the patient's leg facing the patient's knee.
4. The stabilizing hand supports the femur from the posterior side.
5. The mobilizing/manipulating hand grips the proximal tibia from the anterior side.

Procedure

1. The clinician applies a grade I traction to the joint.
2. The stabilizing hand holds the femur in position.
3. The mobilizing/manipulating hand glides the tibia in a posterior direction (see Fig. 7-2).

Particulars

1. This technique might be especially effective for increasing range of motion into knee joint flexion.

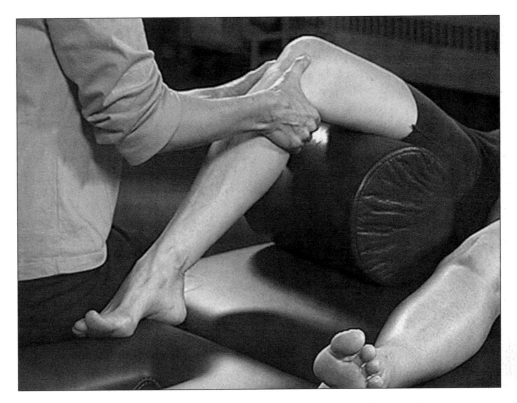

FIGURE 7-3. Anterior glide of the tibia on the femur: first technique.

ANTERIOR GLIDE OF THE TIBIA ON THE FEMUR: FIRST TECHNIQUE (Fig. 7-3)

Purpose
- To examine for tibiofemoral joint impairment
- To increase accessory motion into tibiofemoral joint anterior glide
- To increase range of motion at the tibiofemoral joint
- To decrease pain
- To improve periarticular muscle performance

Positioning
1. The patient is supine.
2. The tibiofemoral joint is placed in the resting position if conservative techniques are indicated or approximating restricted range of motion if more aggressive techniques are indicated.
3. The clinician is at the patient's foot facing the patient's knee.
4. Both hands grip the proximal tibia from the posterior side with the fingers while simultaneously positioning the thumbs over the anterior surface of the distal femur.

Procedure
1. Both hands glide the tibia in an anterior direction while stabilizing the femur with the thumbs (see Fig. 7-3).

Particulars
1. This technique might be especially effective for increasing range of motion into knee joint extension.

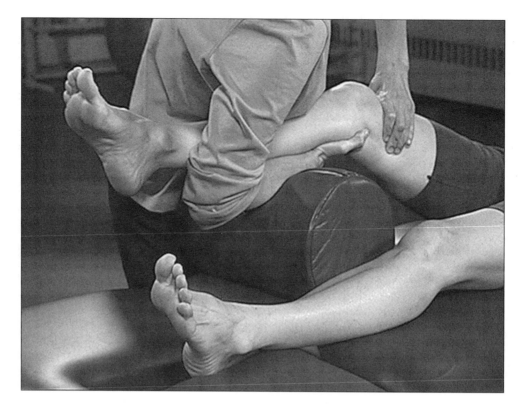

FIGURE 7-4. Anterior glide of the tibia on the femur: second technique.

ANTERIOR GLIDE OF THE TIBIA ON THE FEMUR: SECOND TECHNIQUE (Fig. 7-4)

Purpose

- To examine for tibiofemoral joint impairment
- To increase accessory motion into tibiofemoral joint anterior glide
- To increase range of motion at the tibiofemoral joint
- To decrease pain
- To improve periarticular muscle performance

Positioning

1. The patient is supine.
2. The tibiofemoral joint is placed in the resting position if conservative techniques are indicated or approximating restricted range of motion into extension if more aggressive techniques are indicated.
3. The clinician is at the side of the patient's leg facing the patient's knee.
4. The stabilizing hand grips the proximal tibia posteriorly.
5. The mobilizing/manipulating hand is positioned over the anterior surface of the distal femur.

Procedure

1. The clinician applies a grade I traction to the joint.
2. The stabilizing hand holds the tibia in position.
3. The mobilizing/manipulating hand glides the femur in a posterior direction, imparting an anterior force to the tibia on the femur (see Fig. 7-4).

Particulars

1. This technique might be especially effective for increasing range of motion into knee joint extension.

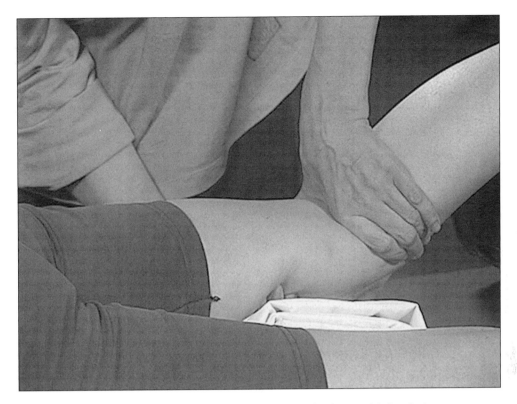

FIGURE 7-5. Anterior glide of the tibia on the femur: third technique.

ANTERIOR GLIDE OF THE TIBIA ON THE FEMUR: THIRD TECHNIQUE (Fig. 7-5)

Purpose

- To examine for tibiofemoral joint impairment
- To increase accessory motion into tibiofemoral joint anterior glide
- To increase range of motion at the tibiofemoral joint
- To decrease pain
- To improve periarticular muscle performance

Positioning

1. The patient is prone with a small pillow positioned under the distal femur to protect the patellofemoral joint.
2. The tibiofemoral joint is placed in the resting position if conservative techniques are indicated or approximating restricted range of motion into extension if more aggressive techniques are indicated.
3. The clinician is at the side of the patient's leg facing the patient's knee.
4. The stabilizing hand grips the distal femur from the anterior side.
5. The mobilizing/manipulating hand is positioned over the posterior surface of the proximal tibia.

Procedure

1. The clinician applies a grade I traction to the joint.
2. The stabilizing hand holds the femur in position.
3. The mobilizing/manipulating hand glides the tibia in an anterior direction (see Fig. 7-5).

Particulars

1. This technique might be especially effective for increasing range of motion into knee joint extension.

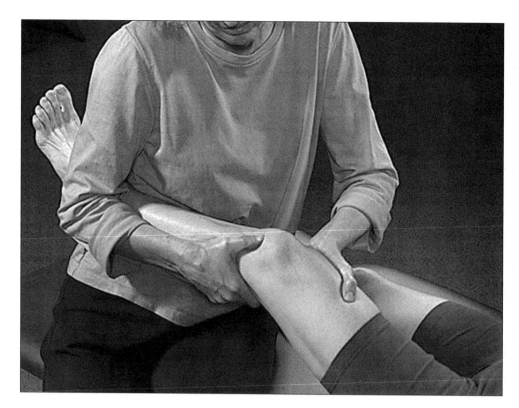

FIGURE 7-6. Medial glide.

MEDIAL GLIDE (Fig. 7-6)

Purpose

- To examine for tibiofemoral joint impairment
- To increase accessory motion into tibiofemoral joint medial glide
- To increase range of motion at the tibiofemoral joint
- To decrease pain
- To improve periarticular muscle performance

Positioning

1. The patient is supine.
2. The tibiofemoral joint is placed in the resting position if conservative techniques are indicated or approximating restricted range of motion if more aggressive techniques are indicated.
3. The clinician is between the patient's knees with the patient's lower leg between the clinician's arm and trunk.
4. The stabilizing hand grips the distal femur from the medial side.
5. The mobilizing/manipulating hand grips the proximal tibia and fibula from the lateral side and supports the lateral lower leg with the forearm.

Procedure

1. The clinician applies a grade I traction to the joint.
2. The stabilizing hand holds the femur in position.
3. The mobilizing/manipulating hand glides the proximal tibia in a medial direction indirectly through the fibula, while the trunk guides the motion (see Fig. 7-6).

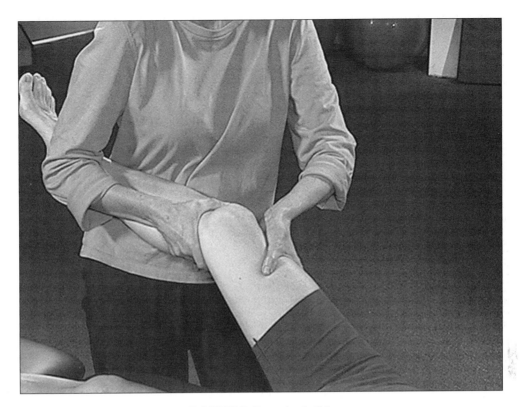

FIGURE 7-7. Lateral glide.

LATERAL GLIDE (Fig. 7-7)

Purpose
- To examine for tibiofemoral joint impairment
- To increase accessory motion into tibiofemoral joint lateral glide
- To increase range of motion at the tibiofemoral joint
- To decrease pain
- To improve periarticular muscle performance

Positioning
1. The patient is supine.
2. The tibiofemoral joint is placed in the resting position if conservative techniques are indicated or approximating restricted range of motion if more aggressive techniques are indicated.
3. The clinician is at the side of the treatment table facing the patient's knee with the patient's lower leg between the clinician's arm and trunk.
4. The stabilizing hand grips the distal femur from the lateral side.
5. The mobilizing/manipulating hand grips the proximal tibia from the medial side and supports the medial lower leg with the forearm.

Procedure
1. The clinician applies a grade I traction to the joint.
2. The stabilizing hand holds the femur in position.
3. The mobilizing/manipulating hand glides the proximal tibia in a lateral direction while the trunk guides the motion (see Fig. 7-7).

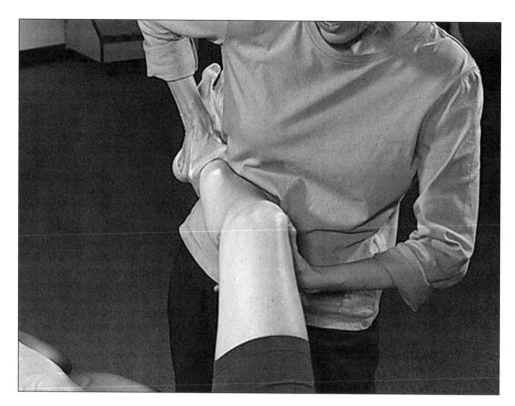

FIGURE 7-8. Medial gap.

MEDIAL GAP (Fig. 7-8)

Purpose

- To examine for tibiofemoral joint impairment
- To increase accessory motion into tibiofemoral joint medial gap
- To increase range of motion at the tibiofemoral joint
- To decrease pain
- To improve periarticular muscle performance

Positioning

1. The patient is supine.
2. The tibiofemoral joint is placed in the resting position if conservative techniques are indicated or approximating restricted range of motion if more aggressive techniques are indicated.
3. The clinician is at the side of the treatment table facing the patient's knee with the patient's lower leg between the clinician's arm and trunk.
4. The stabilizing hand supports the distal lower leg from the medial side and holds the lower leg against the clinician's trunk.
5. The mobilizing/manipulating hand grips the lateral side of the knee at the joint line.

Procedure

1. The stabilizing hand holds the lower leg in position.
2. The mobilizing/manipulating hand moves the knee at the lateral joint line in a medial direction, creating a gapping at the joint line medially (see Fig. 7-8).

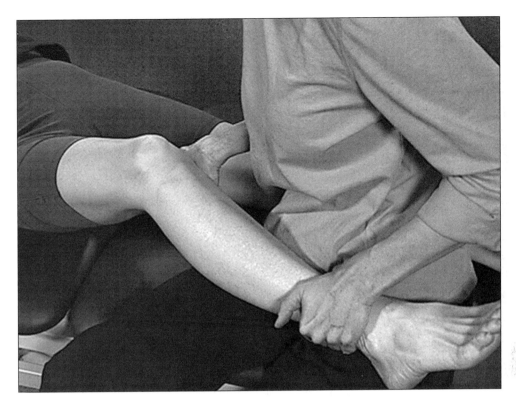

FIGURE 7-9. Lateral gap.

LATERAL GAP (Fig. 7-9)

Purpose
- To examine for tibiofemoral joint impairment
- To increase accessory motion into tibiofemoral joint lateral gap
- To increase range of motion at the tibiofemoral joint
- To decrease pain
- To improve periarticular muscle performance

Positioning
1. The patient is supine.
2. The tibiofemoral joint is placed in the resting position if conservative techniques are indicated or approximating restricted range of motion if more aggressive techniques are indicated.
3. The clinician is between the patient's knees with the patient's lower leg between the clinician's arm and trunk.
4. The stabilizing hand supports the distal lower leg from the lateral side and holds the lower leg against the clinician's trunk.
5. The mobilizing/manipulating hand grips the medial side of the knee at the joint line.

Procedure
1. The stabilizing hand holds the lower leg in position.
2. The mobilizing/manipulating hand moves the knee at the medial joint line in a lateral direction, creating a gapping at the joint line laterally (see Fig. 7-9).

PATELLOFEMORAL JOINT

Osteokinematic motion:
  Flexion/extension
Ligament:
  Patellofemoral ligament
Joint orientation:
  Patella: posterior
  Femur: anterior
Concave joint surface:
  Femur
Type of joint:
  Synovial
Resting position:
  25 to 40 degrees of flexion[4]
Close-packed position:
  Full extension[4]
Capsular pattern of restriction:
  Not described by Cyriax

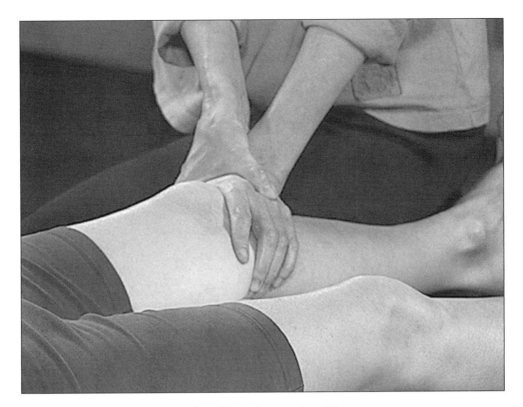

FIGURE 7-10. Superior glide.

SUPERIOR GLIDE (Fig. 7-10)

Purpose
- To examine for patellofemoral joint impairment
- To increase accessory motion into patellofemoral joint superior glide
- To increase range of motion at the patellofemoral joint
- To decrease pain
- To improve periarticular muscle performance

Positioning
1. The patient is supine.
2. The knee is placed in slight flexion by placing a rolled towel underneath the knee.
3. The clinician is at the patient's lower leg facing the patellofemoral joint.
4. The mobilizing/manipulating hand is positioned with either the web space or the heel of the hand on the inferior surface of the patella.
5. The guiding hand is positioned over the mobilizing/manipulating hand.

Procedure
1. The mobilizing/manipulating hand glides the patella in a superior direction, taking care to avoid compressing the patella into the femur.
2. The guiding hand controls the position of the mobilizing/manipulating hand (see Fig. 7-10).

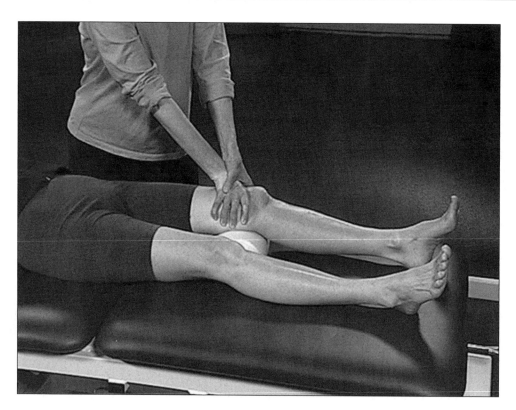

FIGURE 7-11. Inferior glide.

INFERIOR GLIDE (Fig. 7-11)

Purpose
- To examine for patellofemoral joint impairment
- To increase accessory motion into patellofemoral joint inferior glide
- To increase range of motion at the patellofemoral joint
- To decrease pain
- To improve periarticular muscle performance

Positioning
1. The patient is supine.
2. The knee is placed in slight flexion by placing a rolled towel underneath the knee.
3. The clinician is at the patient's hip facing the patellofemoral joint.
4. The mobilizing/manipulating hand is positioned with either the web space or the heel of the hand on the superior surface of the patella.
5. The guiding hand is positioned over the mobilizing/manipulating hand.

Procedure
1. The mobilizing/manipulating hand glides the patella in an inferior direction, taking care to avoid compressing the patella into the femur as much as possible by attempting to position the web space or the heel of the hand under the patella before initiating the technique.
2. The guiding hand controls the position of the mobilizing/manipulating hand (see Fig. 7-11).

Particulars
1. This technique might be especially effective for increasing range of motion into knee joint flexion.

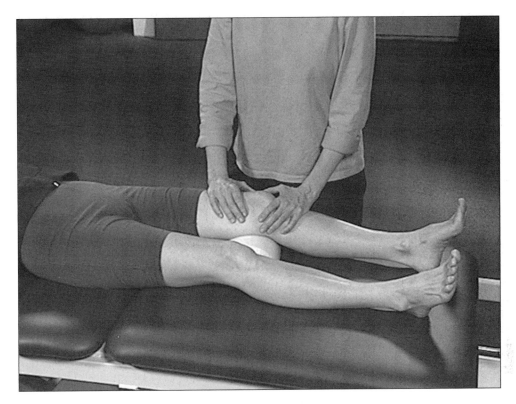

FIGURE 7-12. Medial glide.

MEDIAL GLIDE (Fig. 7-12)

Purpose
- To examine for patellofemoral joint impairment
- To increase accessory motion into patellofemoral joint medial glide
- To increase range of motion at the patellofemoral joint
- To decrease pain
- To improve periarticular muscle performance

Positioning
1. The patient is supine.
2. The knee is placed in slight flexion by placing a rolled towel underneath the knee.
3. The clinician is at the side of the patient's leg facing the patellofemoral joint.
4. The stabilizing hand is positioned with the fingers on the medial surface of the distal femur.
5. The mobilizing hand or hands are positioned with both thumbs or the heel of one hand on the lateral surface of the patella.

Procedure
1. The stabilizing hand holds the femur in position.
2. The mobilizing/manipulating hand or hands glide the patella in a medial direction, taking care to avoid compressing the patella into the femur (see Fig. 7-12).

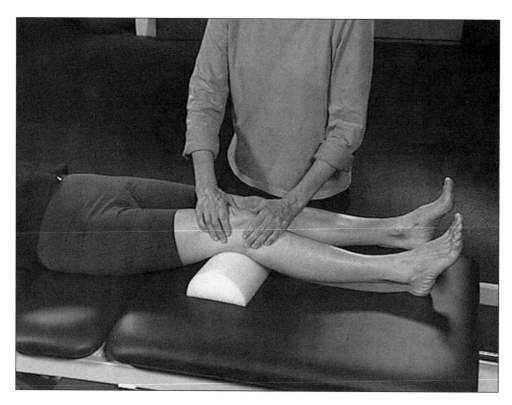

FIGURE 7-13. Lateral glide.

LATERAL GLIDE (Fig. 7-13)

Purpose

- To examine for patellofemoral joint impairment
- To increase accessory motion into patellofemoral joint lateral glide
- To increase range of motion at the patellofemoral joint
- To decrease pain
- To improve periarticular muscle performance

Positioning

1. The patient is supine.
2. The knee is placed in slight flexion by placing a rolled towel underneath the knee.
3. The clinician is at the side of the patient's unaffected leg facing the patellofemoral joint.
4. The stabilizing hand is positioned with the fingers on the lateral surface of the distal femur.
5. The mobilizing/manipulating hand or hands are positioned with both thumbs or the heel of one hand on the medial surface of the patella.

Procedure

1. The stabilizing hand holds the femur in position.
2. The mobilizing/manipulating hand or hands glide the patella in a lateral direction, taking care to avoid compressing the patella into the femur (see Fig. 7-13).

Particulars

1. The clinician should use caution in performing this technique because this motion might be hypermobile. If it is, performing a lateral glide mobilization/manipulation technique might cause the patella to dislocate.

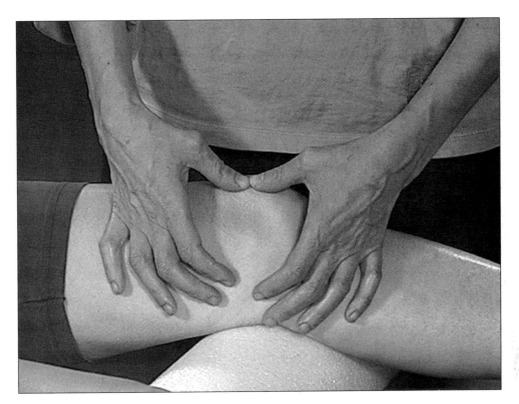

FIGURE 7-14. Medial tilt.

MEDIAL TILT (Fig. 7-14)

Purpose

- To examine for patellofemoral joint impairment
- To increase accessory motion into patellofemoral joint medial tilt
- To increase range of motion at the patellofemoral joint
- To decrease pain
- To improve periarticular muscle performance

Positioning

1. The patient is supine.
2. The knee is placed in slight flexion by placing a rolled towel underneath the knee.
3. The clinician is at the side of the patient's leg facing the patellofemoral joint.
4. The stabilizing hand is positioned with the fingers on the distal femur.
5. The mobilizing/manipulating hand or hands are positioned with both thumbs or the heel of one hand on the medial surface of the patella.

Procedure

1. The stabilizing hand holds the femur in position.
2. The mobilizing/manipulating hand or hands glide the medial surface of the patella in a posterior direction, tilting the anterior surface of the patella toward the midline of the body (see Fig. 7-14).

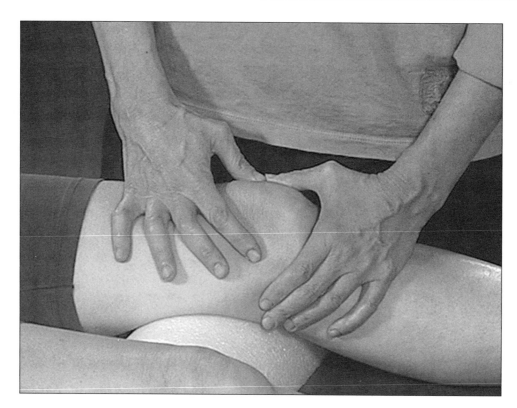

FIGURE 7-15. Lateral tilt.

LATERAL TILT (Fig. 7-15)

Purpose

- To examine for patellofemoral joint impairment
- To increase accessory motion into patellofemoral joint lateral tilt
- To increase range of motion at the patellofemoral joint
- To decrease pain
- To improve periarticular muscle performance

Positioning

1. The patient is supine.
2. The knee is placed in slight flexion by placing a rolled towel underneath the knee.
3. The clinician is at the side of the patient's leg facing the patellofemoral joint.
4. The stabilizing hand is positioned with the fingers on the distal femur.
5. The mobilizing/manipulating hand or hands are positioned with both thumbs or the heel of one hand on the lateral surface of the patella.

Procedure

1. The stabilizing hand holds the femur in position.
2. The mobilizing/manipulating hand or hands glide the lateral surface of the patella in a posterior direction, tilting the anterior surface of the patella away from the midline of the body (see Fig. 7-15).

REFERENCES

1. Deyle GD, Henderson NE, Matekel RL, et al: Effectiveness of manual physical therapy and exercise in osteoarthritis of the knee. Ann Intern Med 2000;132:173-181.
2. Rowlands BW, Brantigham JW: The efficacy of patellar mobilization in patients suffering from patellofemoral pain syndrome. J Neuromusculoskel Syst 1999;7:142-149.
3. Crossley K, Bennell K, Green S, et al: Physical therapy for patellofemoral pain: a randomized, double-blinded, placebo-controlled trial. Am J Sports Med 2002;30:857-865.
4. Kaltenborn FM: Manual Mobilization of the Joints: The Kaltenborn Method of Joint Examination and Treatment, Vol I: The Extremities, 6th ed. OPTP, 2002.
5. Cyriax J: Textbook of Orthopaedic Medicine, Vol I: Diagnosis of Soft Tissue Lesions, 8th ed. London, Bailliere Tindall, 1982.

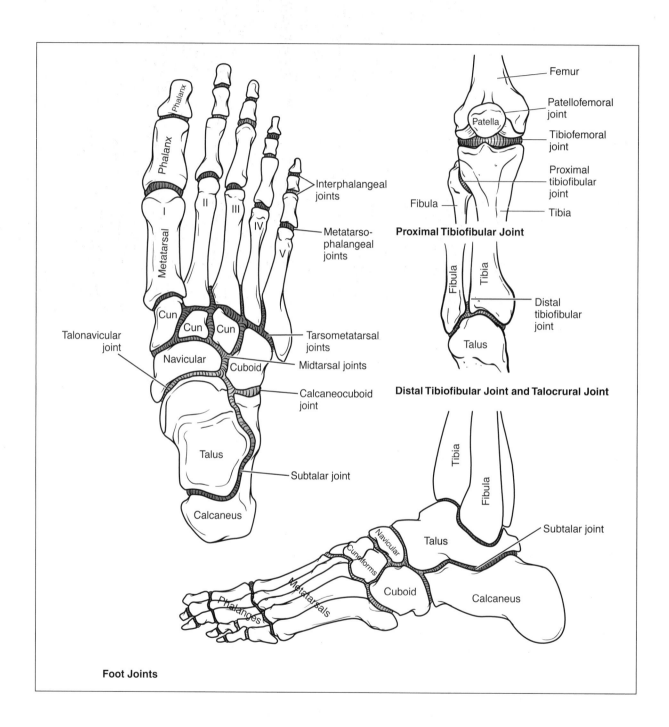

Proximal Tibiofibular Joint

Distal Tibiofibular Joint and Talocrural Joint

Foot Joints

CHAPTER 8

The Lower Leg, Ankle, and Foot

BASICS

Joints of the lower leg consist of the proximal and distal tibiofibular articulations. Motion at these articulations is minimal.

Ankle and foot motion is described as triplanar. The combined motions of dorsiflexion/abduction/eversion and plantar flexion/adduction/inversion occur together, but to a different extent at each of the following joints in the ankle and foot: talocrural joint, subtalar joint, midtarsal joints, and metatarsophalangeal joints. These composite motions are called *pronation* and *supination*. These movements at the ankle and foot allow for a flexible base of support that accommodates to changes in tibial rotation and produces a smooth transition from supination to pronation and back to supination during the stance phase of gait.

Range of motion is considered functional in the talocrural and subtalar joints if 10 to 20 degrees of dorsiflexion is present, 20 to 30 degrees of plantar flexion is present, and 6 to 10 degrees of motion is equally divided between inversion/adduction and eversion/abduction. Approximately 65 to 70 degrees of extension at the first metatarsophalangeal joint is necessary for push-off during the end of the stance phase of gait. Slightly less than 65 degrees of extension is necessary for normal gait at the other metatarsophalangeal joints.

Anatomical terminology in the ankle and the foot is often inconsistent. Thus far, in this text, *anterior* and *posterior* have referred to movement or positioning toward the front and back of the body (in the horizontal plane), and *medial* and *lateral* have indicated movement or positioning toward or away from the midline of the body, not the midline of the limb. *Superior* and *inferior* have referred to movement or positioning toward the head and foot respectively (in the vertical plane). The exception to these rules is at the foot, where *dorsal* indicates movement or positioning toward the top of the foot (or toward the head), and *plantar* indicates movement or positioning toward the bottom of the foot.

Proximal and Distal Tibiofibular Joints

The interosseous membrane connects the tibia and the fibula. Movement at the two joints is interrelated in a manner similar to that of the proximal and distal radioulnar joints of the forearm. Movement at these two joints probably influences ankle motion more than knee motion.

Talocrural Joint

The talocrural joint comprises the tibia and fibula and their articulation with the talus. Although triplanar motion occurs at this articulation, dorsiflexion and plantar flexion are the primary motions.

Subtalar Joint

Inversion and eversion are the primary motions occurring at the subtalar joint, which consists of the articulation between the talus and the calcaneus.

Midtarsal Joints

The midtarsal joint consists of the talonavicular and calcaneocuboid joints and the cuneiform articulations. Plantar flexion and dorsiflexion and inversion and eversion predominate at these joints.

Intermetatarsal Joints

The metatarsals move on one another, causing the transverse arch of the foot to increase and flatten. The axis for this motion is the second metatarsal.

Toe Joints

Toe flexion and extension occur at the metatarsophalangeal and interphalangeal joints. The metatarsophalangeal joints also are capable of moving into abduction and adduction, although these movements are not considered important for functional activities.

SPECIFIC PATHOLOGY AND LOWER LEG, ANKLE, AND FOOT JOINT MOBILIZATION/MANIPULATION

Lateral Ankle Sprains

Numerous studies in which the effectiveness of joint mobilization/manipulation was evaluated have been performed on subjects with ankle inversion injuries. One of these studies was performed on 15 subjects with acute ankle sprains. Subjects receiving a Maitland mobilization intervention to the ankle were compared with a control group that did not receive treatment. The treatment group experienced a significant decrease in swelling immediately after the mobilization compared with the control group.[1] In another study, 30 subjects were randomly assigned to receive talocrural traction or a placebo treatment consisting of detuned ultrasound. Subjects receiving the traction intervention experienced a significant reduction in pain, increase in ankle range of motion, and increase in function.[2]

In two studies involving subjects with ankle sprains, joint mobilization was administered as part of a comprehensive treatment. The first study compared talocrural posterior glide mobilization and a regimen of rest, ice, compression, and elevation (RICE) with the RICE regimen without mobilization. Forty-one subjects with acute ankle sprains were randomly assigned to one of these two interventions. Subjects receiving the mobilization required fewer physical therapy sessions and achieved greater increases in range of motion and stride speed.[3]

The second study was performed on 38 subjects with acute ankle sprains. The effect of RICE alone was compared with RICE with the addition of small-amplitude posterior glide joint mobilizations to the talocrural joint performed at a rate of three sets with each set lasting 60 seconds. Subjects receiving joint mobilization required fewer treatment sessions to achieve pain-free dorsiflexion range of motion. There was no difference between groups in relation to the mean number of days before returning to work, preinjury walking level, or participation in sports.[4]

Mulligan proposed that although ankle inversion injuries are believed to be a result of a sprain of the anterior talofibular ligament, in some cases the anterior talofibular ligament remains intact; instead the distal fibula moves in an anterior direction in relation to the tibia.[5] A study was performed to determine the validity of this theory. Both ankles of 25 subjects were tested for joint excursion into distal tibiofibular posterior glide. Of the 50 ankles, 6 had been diagnosed with an acute ankle sprain. Two ankles exhibited an increase in excursion, both of which had been sprained. This finding suggests that in approximately one third of diagnosed ankle sprains, the true pathology might be an anterior positional fault of the distal fibula on the tibia.[5]

A study addressing the effects of mobilization with movement on ankle sprains provided additional insight into Mulligan's theory. This study was performed on 14 subjects with grade II lateral ankle sprains. Subjects were assigned to receive mobilization to the distal tibiofibular joint into posterior glide performed simultaneously with repeated active inversion movements, a placebo treatment, and no treatment in random order. There was a significant improvement in range of motion, but no change in objective measures of pain after the mobilization compared with the other interventions.[6]

The results of these studies suggest that mobilization improves outcomes in subjects with lateral ankle sprains compared with standard treatment and placebo. Nevertheless, in a study of 30 subjects with acute ankle sprains in which manipulation of the talocrural and subtalar joints was compared with piroxicam, a medication that has been shown to be effective in the treatment of acute musculoskeletal injuries, there was no difference between groups in relation to pain, range of motion, or limitations in sports activities. Treatment consisted of ankle traction and subtalar eversion and gapping manipulations.[7] In this study, joint mobilization/manipulation might have shown greater effectiveness if it had been administered in combination with other interventions.

Decreased Ankle Joint Range of Motion

Several studies have investigated the effect of joint mobilization/manipulation on ankle joint range of motion. These studies are described in greater detail in Chapter 1. In one study, subjects who had been immobilized as a result of a fracture, and who received joint mobilization and exercise intervention to the ankle joint, had greater improvements in range of motion than similar subjects who were treated with exercise alone.[8] In the second study, subjects who received grade V manipulations to the proximal tibiofibular joint and the talocrural joint experienced greater range of motion improvements than a control group that received stretching exercises. The proximal tibiofibular joint manipulation consisted of anterior glides; the talocrural joint received distraction and posterior glide manipulations.[9]

First Metatarsophalangeal Hallux Rigidus

In a study of the effectiveness of physical therapy intervention for hallux rigidus, 20 subjects were randomly assigned to two groups: the first group received whirlpool, ultrasound, first metatarsophalangeal mobilization, calf and hamstring stretching, marble pick-up exercises, cold packs, and electrical stimulation; the second group received the same interventions with the addition of grade III glide sesamoid mobilization, flexor hallucis strengthening, and gait training. The group that received the additional interventions had greater improvements in strength and range of motion and a greater decrease in pain compared with the control group. Since subjects receiving sesamoid mobilization also received strengthening exercises and gait training, it is unclear what effect the addition of this mobilization technique had on the outcomes.[10]

PROXIMAL TIBIOFIBULAR JOINT

Osteokinematic motion:
    None
Ligaments:
    Posterior tibiofibular ligament
    Anterior tibiofibular ligament
Joint orientation:
    Tibia: lateral, posterior, inferior
    Fibula: medial, anterior, superior
Concave joint surface:
    Fibula
Type of joint:
    Synovial
Resting position:
    0 degrees of plantar flexion[11]
Close-packed position:
    Full dorsiflexion[11]
Capsular pattern:
    Pain with contracting the "biceps" (presumably, the biceps femoris) muscle[12]

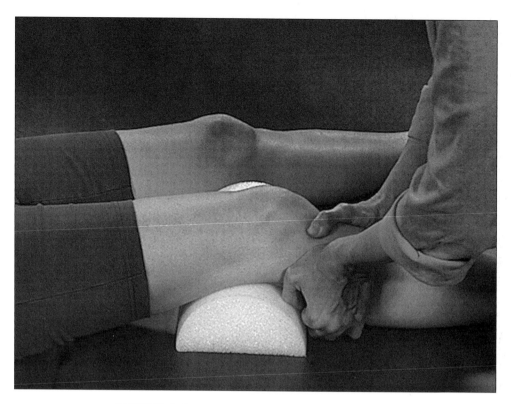

FIGURE 8-1. Posterior glide of the proximal fibula.

POSTERIOR GLIDE OF THE PROXIMAL FIBULA (Fig. 8-1)

Purpose

- To examine for proximal tibiofibular joint impairment
- To increase accessory motion into proximal tibiofibular joint posterior glide
- To decrease pain
- To improve periarticular muscle performance

Positioning

1. The patient is supine with the knee supported by a small pillow.
2. The proximal tibiofibular joint is placed in the resting position.
3. The clinician is at the side of the patient's leg facing the patient's knee.
4. The stabilizing hand grips the proximal tibia from the medial and posterior side.
5. The mobilizing/manipulating hand is positioned with the heel of the hand on the anterior surface of the fibular head, taking care to avoid contact with the common fibular nerve.

Procedure

1. The stabilizing hand holds the tibia in position.
2. The mobilizing/manipulating hand glides the proximal fibula in a posterior direction (see Fig. 8-1).

Particulars

1. The clinician should use caution in performing this technique because this motion might be hypermobile.
2. This technique might be effective in correcting a proximal tibiofibular joint positional fault.

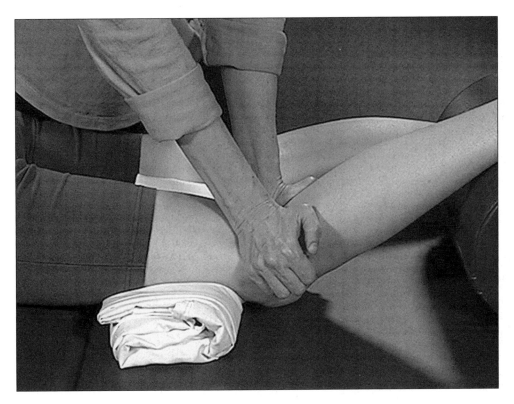

FIGURE 8-2. Anterior glide of the proximal fibula.

ANTERIOR GLIDE OF THE PROXIMAL FIBULA (Fig. 8-2)

Purpose

- To examine for proximal tibiofibular joint impairment
- To increase accessory motion into proximal tibiofibular joint anterior glide
- To decrease pain
- To improve periarticular muscle performance

Positioning

1. The patient is prone with the foot supported by a pillow and a towel roll under the distal thigh to protect the patellofemoral joint.
2. The proximal tibiofibular joint is placed in the resting position.
3. The clinician is at the side of the patient's unaffected leg facing the patient's knees.
4. The stabilizing hand grips the proximal tibia from the anterior and medial side.
5. The mobilizing/manipulating hand is positioned with the heel of the hand on the posterior surface of the fibular head, taking care to avoid contact with the common fibular nerve.

Procedure

1. The stabilizing hand holds the tibia in position.
2. The mobilizing/manipulating hand glides the proximal fibula in an anterior direction (see Fig. 8-2).

Particulars

1. The clinician should use caution in performing this technique because this motion might be hypermobile.
2. This technique, performed using grade V manipulations, has been shown to be effective in increasing ankle joint range of motion when performed along with talocrural joint manipulations.[9]
3. This technique might be effective in correcting a proximal tibiofibular joint positional fault.

DISTAL TIBIOFIBULAR JOINT

Osteokinematic motion:
    None
Ligaments:
    Anterior tibiofibular ligament
    Posterior tibiofibular ligament
    Inferior transverse ligament
    Interosseous membrane
Joint orientation:
    Tibia: lateral, posterior
    Fibula: medial, anterior
Concave joint surface:
    Tibia
Type of joint:
    Syndesmosis
Resting position:
    Not described by Kaltenborn
Close-packed position:
    Not described by Kaltenborn
Capsular pattern of restriction:
    Pain with performing a "springing" manipulation on the ankle[12]

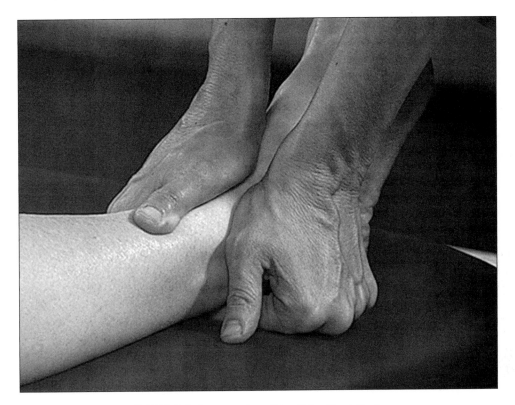

FIGURE 8-3. Posterior glide of the distal fibula.

POSTERIOR GLIDE OF THE DISTAL FIBULA (Fig. 8-3)

Purpose
- To examine for distal tibiofibular joint impairment
- To increase accessory motion into distal tibiofibular joint posterior glide
- To decrease pain
- To improve periarticular muscle performance

Positioning
1. The patient is supine.
2. The distal tibiofibular joint is placed in a neutral position.
3. The clinician is at the foot of the treatment table facing the patient's lower leg.
4. The stabilizing hand grips the distal tibia.
5. The mobilizing/manipulating hand is positioned with the heel of the hand over the anterior surface of the lateral malleolus (distal fibula).

Procedure
1. The stabilizing hand holds the tibia in position.
2. The mobilizing/manipulating hand glides the lateral malleolus (distal fibula) in a posterior direction (see Fig. 8-3).

Particulars
1. The clinician should use caution in performing this technique because this motion might be hypermobile.
2. A variation of this technique, using mobilization with movement, has been shown to be effective in increasing ankle range of motion in subjects with lateral ankle sprains. In the study, a posterior glide was performed while the subject performed active ankle inversion range of motion.[6]
3. This technique might be effective in correcting a distal tibiofibular joint positional fault.[5]

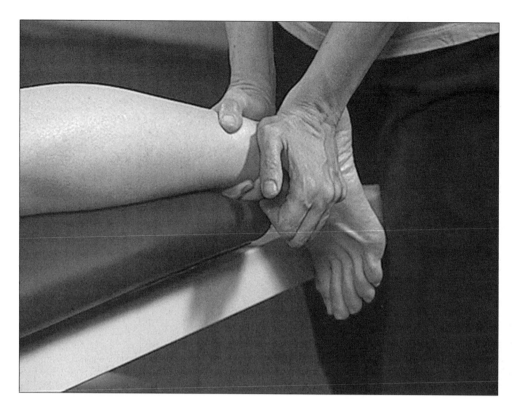

FIGURE 8-4. Anterior glide of the distal fibula.

ANTERIOR GLIDE OF THE DISTAL FIBULA (Fig. 8-4)

Purpose

- To examine for distal tibiofibular joint impairment
- To increase accessory motion into distal tibiofibular joint anterior glide
- To decrease pain
- To improve periarticular muscle performance

Positioning

1. The patient is prone.
2. The distal tibiofibular joint is placed in a neutral position.
3. The clinician is at the foot of the treatment table facing the patient's lower leg.
4. The stabilizing hand grips the distal tibia.
5. The mobilizing/manipulating hand is positioned with the heel of the hand over the posterior surface of the lateral malleolus (distal fibula).

Procedure

1. The stabilizing hand holds the tibia in position.
2. The mobilizing/manipulating hand glides the lateral malleolus (distal fibula) in an anterior direction (see Fig. 8-4).

Particulars

1. The clinician should use caution in performing this technique because this motion might be hypermobile.
2. This technique might be effective in correcting a distal tibiofibular joint positional fault.

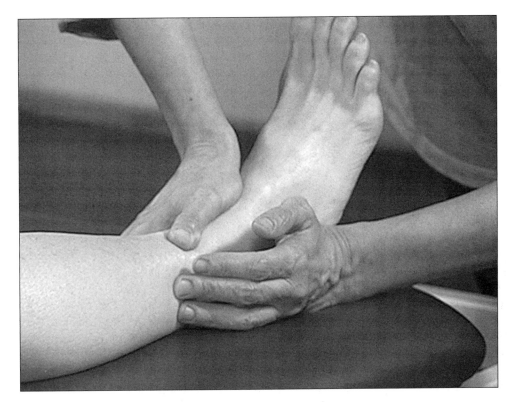

FIGURE 8-5. Superior glide of the fibula.

SUPERIOR GLIDE OF THE FIBULA (Fig. 8-5)

Purpose
- To examine for impairment at the tibiofibular joints
- To increase accessory motion into tibiofibular joint superior glide
- To decrease pain
- To improve periarticular muscle performance

Positioning
1. The patient is supine.
2. The tibiofibular joints are placed in a neutral position.
3. The clinician is at the foot of the treatment table facing the patient's lower leg.
4. The stabilizing hand grips the distal tibia.
5. The mobilizing/manipulating hand is positioned with the heel of the hand on the inferior surface of the lateral malleolus (distal fibula).

Procedure
1. The stabilizing hand holds the tibia in position.
2. The mobilizing/manipulating hand glides the fibula in a superior direction (see Fig. 8-5).

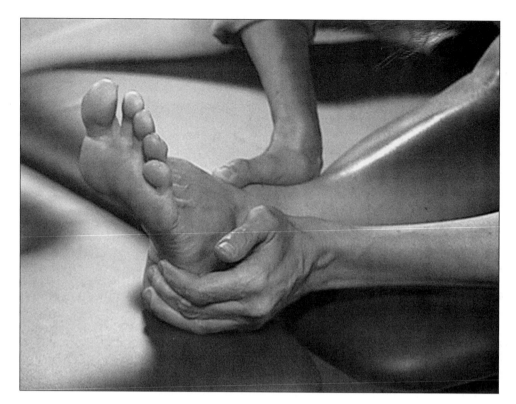

FIGURE 8-6. Inferior glide of the fibula.

INFERIOR GLIDE OF THE FIBULA (Fig. 8-6)

Purpose

- To examine for impairment at the tibiofibular joints
- To increase accessory motion into tibiofibular joint inferior glide
- To decrease pain
- To improve periarticular muscle performance

Positioning

1. The patient is supine.
2. The tibiofibular joints are placed in a neutral position.
3. The clinician is at the side of the patient's leg facing the patient's foot.
4. The stabilizing hand grips the distal tibia.
5. The mobilizing/manipulating hand is positioned with the heel of the hand on the superior surface of the lateral malleolus (distal fibula).

Procedure

1. The stabilizing hand holds the tibia in position.
2. The mobilizing/manipulating hand glides the fibula in an inferior direction (see Fig. 8-6).

TALOCRURAL JOINT

Osteokinematic motions:
Dorsiflexion/plantar flexion
Inversion/eversion
Abduction/adduction

Ligaments:
Medial collateral ligament/deltoid ligament (anterior tibiotalar, posterior tibiotalar, tibiocalcaneal, tibionavicular)
Lateral collateral ligament (anterior talofibular, posterior talofibular, calcaneofibular)

Joint orientation:
Tibia: inferior, lateral
Fibula: medial
Talus: superior, medial, lateral

Concave joint surface:
Tibia and fibula

Type of joint:
Synovial

Resting position:
10 degrees plantar flexion and midway between inversion and eversion[11]

Close-packed position:
Full dorsiflexion[11]

Capsular pattern of restriction:
If the calf muscles are not tight, plantar flexion is more limited than dorsiflexion, whereas if the calf muscles are tight, the capsular pattern is simply limitation into plantar flexion[12]

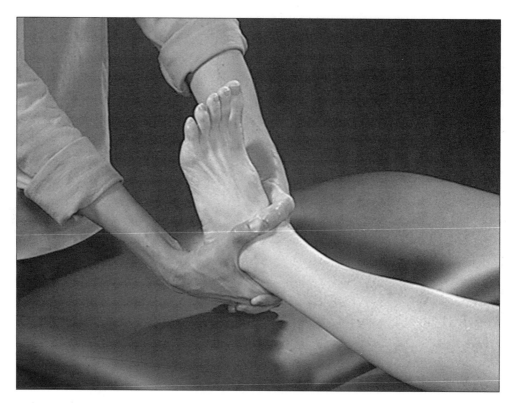

FIGURE 8-7. Distraction.

DISTRACTION (Fig. 8-7)

Purpose

- To examine for talocrural joint impairment
- To increase accessory motion into talocrural joint distraction
- To increase range of motion at the talocrural joint
- To decrease pain
- To improve periarticular muscle performance

Positioning

1. The patient is supine with the knee in extension.
2. The talocrural joint is placed in the resting position if conservative techniques are indicated or approximating restricted range of motion if more aggressive techniques are indicated.
3. The clinician is at the foot of the treatment table facing the patient's foot.
4. Both hands grip the proximal talus with fingers intertwined.
5. The clinician's arms are lined up parallel to the patient's leg.

Procedure

1. Both hands move the talus in a direction perpendicular to the tibia and fibula joint surfaces as the clinician leans away from the joint (see Fig. 8-7).

Particulars

1. It is important to screen for tibiofemoral joint impairments before performing this technique.
2. This technique is commonly performed using a grade V manipulation.

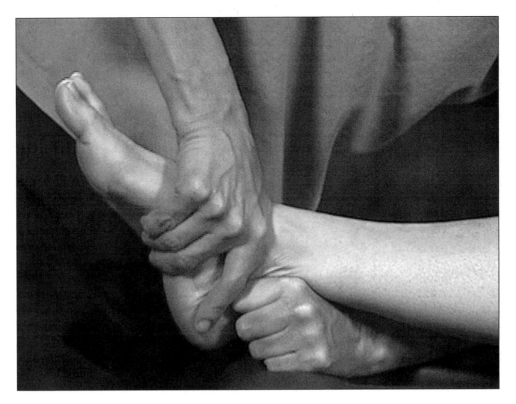

FIGURE 8-8. Posterior glide.

POSTERIOR GLIDE (Fig. 8-8)

Purpose

- To examine for talocrural joint impairment
- To increase accessory motion into talocrural joint posterior glide
- To increase range of motion at the talocrural joint
- To decrease pain
- To improve periarticular muscle performance

Positioning

1. The patient is supine with the foot positioned over the edge of the treatment table.
2. The talocrural joint is placed in the resting position if more conservative techniques are indicated or approximating restricted range of motion if more aggressive techniques are indicated.
3. The clinician is at the foot of the treatment table facing the patient's foot.
4. The stabilizing hand grips the posterior surface of the distal lower leg.
5. The mobilizing/manipulating hand grips the talus at the anterior surface.

Procedure

1. The clinician applies a grade I traction to the joint.
2. The stabilizing hand holds the distal lower leg in position.
3. The mobilizing/manipulating hand glides the talus in a posterior direction (see Fig. 8-8).

Particulars

1. This technique might be especially effective for increasing range of motion into ankle joint dorsiflexion.

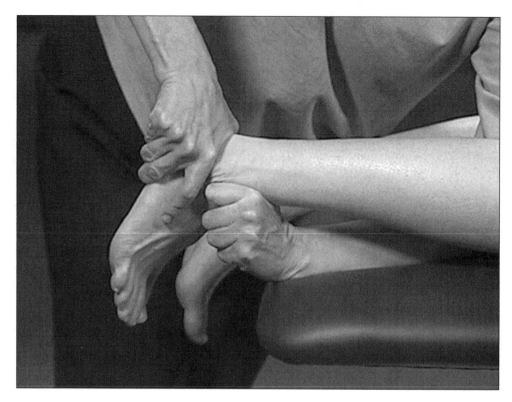

FIGURE 8-9. Anterior glide of the talus on the tibia and fibula: first technique.

ANTERIOR GLIDE OF THE TALUS ON THE TIBIA AND FIBULA: FIRST TECHNIQUE (Fig. 8-9)

Purpose

- To examine for talocrural joint impairment
- To increase accessory motion into talocrural joint anterior glide
- To increase range of motion at the talocrural joint
- To decrease pain
- To improve periarticular muscle performance

Positioning

1. The patient is prone with the foot positioned off the edge of the treatment table.
2. The talocrural joint is placed in the resting position if conservative techniques are indicated or approximating restricted range of motion if more aggressive techniques are indicated.
3. The clinician is at the foot of the treatment table facing the patient's foot.
4. The stabilizing hand grips the anterior surface of the distal lower leg.
5. The mobilizing/manipulating hand grips the talus at the posterior surface if the ankle is in the resting position or the calcaneus at the posterior surface if the foot is in too much plantar flexion to allow contact with the talus.

Procedure

1. The clinician applies a grade I traction to the joint.
2. The stabilizing hand holds the distal lower leg in position.
3. The mobilizing/manipulating hand glides the talus in an anterior direction, either directly or through the calcaneus (see Fig. 8-9).

Particulars

1. This technique might be especially effective for increasing range of motion into ankle joint plantar flexion.

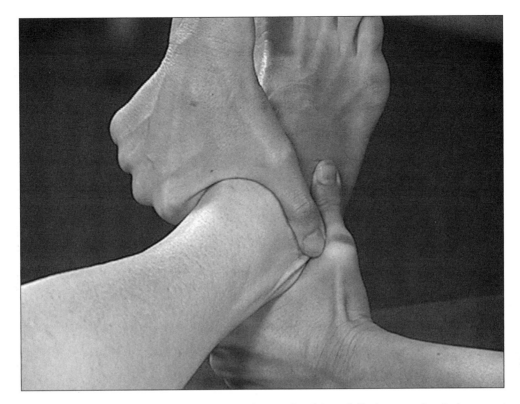

FIGURE 8-10. Anterior glide of the talus on the tibia and fibula: second technique.

ANTERIOR GLIDE OF THE TALUS ON THE TIBIA AND FIBULA: SECOND TECHNIQUE (Fig. 8-10)

Purpose

- To examine for talocrural joint impairment
- To increase accessory motion into talocrural joint anterior glide
- To increase range of motion at the talocrural joint
- To decrease pain
- To improve periarticular muscle performance

Positioning

1. The patient is supine.
2. The talocrural joint is placed in the resting position if more conservative techniques are indicated or approximating restricted range of motion if more aggressive techniques are indicated.
3. The clinician is at the foot of the treatment table facing the patient's foot.
4. The stabilizing hand grips the talus at the posterior surface.
5. The mobilizing/manipulating hand grips the anterior surface of the distal lower leg.

Procedure

1. The clinician applies a grade I traction to the joint.
2. The stabilizing hand holds the talus in position.
3. The mobilizing/manipulating hand glides the tibia and fibula in a posterior direction, imparting an anterior force to the talus on the tibia and fibula (see Fig. 8-10).

Particulars

1. This technique might be especially effective for increasing range of motion into ankle joint plantar flexion.

SUBTALAR JOINT

Osteokinematic motion:
   Inversion/eversion
Ligaments:
   Interosseous talocalcaneal ligament
   Cervical ligament
   Lateral talocalcaneal ligament
   Medial talocalcaneal ligament
Joint orientation:
   Talus: inferior, posterior, lateral
   Calcaneus: superior, anterior, medial
Concave joint surface:
   None, this is a plane joint
Type of joint:
   Synovial
Resting position:
   10 degrees of plantar flexion and midway between inversion and eversion[11]
Close-packed position:
   Full inversion[11]
Capsular pattern of restriction:
   Limitation in inversion[12]

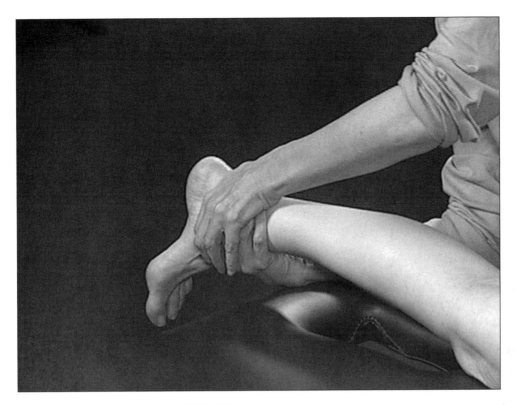

FIGURE 8-11. Distraction.

DISTRACTION (Fig. 8-11)

Purpose

- To examine for subtalar joint impairment
- To increase accessory motion into subtalar joint distraction
- To increase range of motion at the subtalar joint
- To decrease pain
- To improve periarticular muscle performance

Positioning

1. The patient is prone with the foot off the treatment table.
2. The subtalar joint is placed in the resting position if conservative techniques are indicated or approximating restricted range of motion if more aggressive techniques are indicated.
3. The clinician is at the side of the treatment table facing the patient's foot.
4. The stabilizing hand grips the talus at the anterior surface with the web space.
5. The mobilizing/manipulating hand is positioned with the web space on the posterior and superior surface of the calcaneus and the thumb and index finger on the medial and lateral surface of the calcaneus.

Procedure

1. The stabilizing hand holds the talus in position.
2. The mobilizing/manipulating hand moves the calcaneus inferiorly in a direction perpendicular to the talocalcaneal joint surface (see Fig. 8-11).

Particulars

1. This technique is commonly performed using a grade V manipulation.

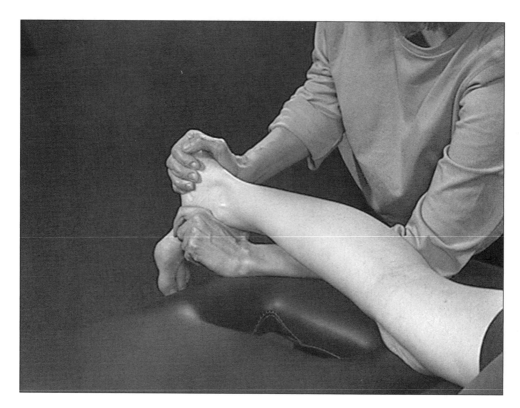

FIGURE 8-12. Medial glide.

MEDIAL GLIDE (Fig. 8-12)

Purpose

- To examine for subtalar joint impairment
- To increase accessory motion into subtalar joint medial glide
- To increase range of motion at the subtalar joint
- To decrease pain
- To improve periarticular muscle performance

Positioning

1. The patient is prone with the foot off the treatment table.
2. The subtalar joint is placed in the resting position if conservative techniques are indicated or approximating restricted range of motion if more aggressive techniques are indicated.
3. The clinician is at the side of the treatment table facing the patient's foot.
4. The stabilizing hand grips the talus at the anterior and medial surface with the web space.
5. The mobilizing/manipulating hand grips the calcaneus with the heel of the hand on the lateral surface.

Procedure

1. The clinician applies a grade I traction to the joint.
2. The stabilizing hand holds the talus in position.
3. The mobilizing/manipulating hand glides the calcaneus in a medial direction (see Fig. 8-12).

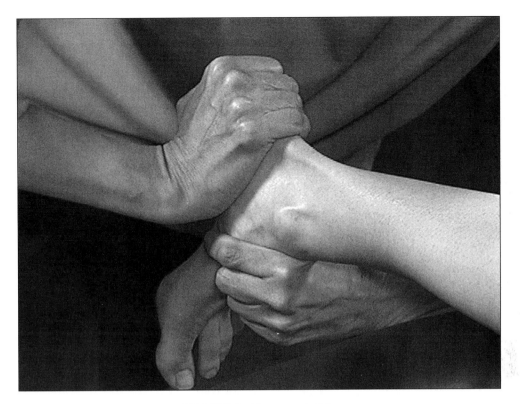

FIGURE 8-13. Lateral glide.

LATERAL GLIDE (Fig. 8-13)

Purpose

- To examine for subtalar joint impairment
- To increase accessory motion into subtalar joint lateral glide
- To increase range of motion at the subtalar joint
- To decrease pain
- To improve periarticular muscle performance

Positioning

1. The patient is prone with the foot off the treatment table.
2. The subtalar joint is placed in the resting position if conservative techniques are indicated or approximating restricted range of motion if more aggressive techniques are indicated.
3. The clinician is at the side of the treatment table facing the patient's foot.
4. The stabilizing hand grips the talus at the anterior and lateral surface with the web space.
5. The mobilizing/manipulating hand grips the calcaneus with the heel of the hand on the medial surface.

Procedure

1. The clinician applies a grade I traction to the joint.
2. The stabilizing hand holds the talus in position.
3. The mobilizing/manipulating hand glides the calcaneus in a lateral direction (see Fig. 8-13).

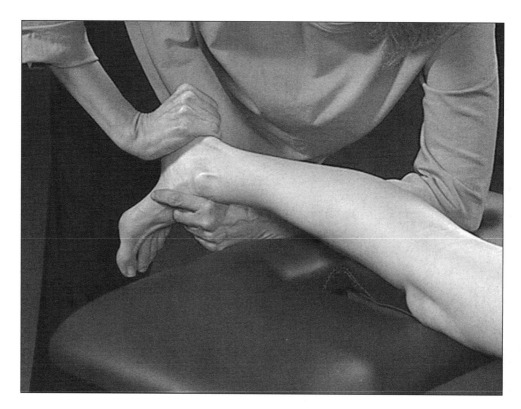

FIGURE 8-14. Medial gap.

MEDIAL GAP (Fig. 8-14)

Purpose

- To examine for subtalar joint impairment
- To increase accessory motion into subtalar joint medial gap
- To increase range of motion at the subtalar joint
- To decrease pain
- To improve periarticular muscle performance

Positioning

1. The patient is prone with the foot off the treatment table.
2. The subtalar joint is placed in the resting position.
3. The clinician is at the side of the treatment table facing the patient's foot.
4. The stabilizing hand grips the talus at the anterior and lateral surface with the web space.
5. The mobilizing/manipulating hand grips the calcaneus with the heel of the hand on the medial surface.

Procedure

1. The stabilizing hand holds the talus in position.
2. The mobilizing/manipulating hand tilts the calcaneus in a valgus direction (see Fig. 8-14).

Particulars

1. This technique might be especially effective for increasing range of motion into subtalar joint eversion.

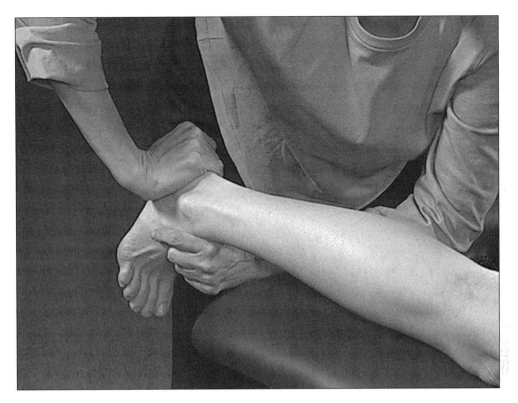

FIGURE 8-15. Lateral gap.

LATERAL GAP (Fig. 8-15)

Purpose

- To examine for subtalar joint impairment
- To increase accessory motion into subtalar joint lateral gap
- To increase range of motion at the subtalar joint
- To decrease pain
- To improve periarticular muscle performance

Positioning

1. The patient is prone with the foot off the treatment table.
2. The subtalar joint is placed in the resting position.
3. The clinician is at the side of the treatment table facing the patient's foot.
4. The stabilizing hand grips the talus at the anterior and medial surface with the web space.
5. The mobilizing/manipulating hand grips the calcaneus with the heel of the hand on the lateral surface.

Procedure

1. The stabilizing hand holds the talus in position.
2. The mobilizing/manipulating hand tilts the calcaneus in a varus direction (see Fig. 8-15).

Particulars

1. This technique might be especially effective for increasing range of motion into subtalar joint inversion.

MIDTARSAL JOINTS

This section discusses the talonavicular and calcaneocuboid joints.

Osteokinematic motions:
   Dorsiflexion/plantar flexion
   Inversion/eversion

Ligaments:
   Long plantar ligament
   Plantar calcaneonavicular ligament
   Bifurcate ligament

Joint orientation: Talonavicular joint
   Talus: anterior, lateral
   Navicular: posterior, medial

Joint orientation: Calcaneocuboid joint
   Calcaneus: anterior, medial
   Cuboid: posterior, lateral

Concave joint surface:
   None, these are plane joints

Type of joint:
   Synovial

Resting position:
   10 degrees plantar flexion and midway between inversion and eversion[11]

Close-packed position:
   Full inversion[11]

Capsular pattern of restriction:
   Limitations in dorsiflexion, plantar flexion, adduction, and inversion[12]

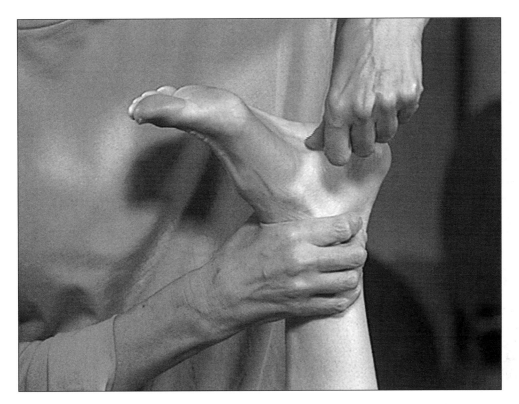

FIGURE 8-16. Dorsal glide of the navicular.

DORSAL GLIDE OF THE NAVICULAR (Fig. 8-16)

Purpose

- To examine for talonavicular joint impairment
- To increase accessory motion into talonavicular dorsal glide
- To increase range of motion at the midtarsal joint
- To decrease pain
- To improve periarticular muscle performance

Positioning

1. The patient is prone with the knee flexed to 90 degrees.
2. The talonavicular joint is placed in the resting position.
3. The clinician is facing the plantar surface of the patient's foot.
4. The stabilizing hand grips the talus at the dorsal surface with the web space or with the thumb on the plantar surface and the index finger on the dorsal surface.
5. The mobilizing/manipulating hand grips the navicular with the thumb on the plantar surface and the index finger on the dorsal surface.

Procedure

1. The clinician applies a grade I traction to the joint.
2. The stabilizing hand holds the talus in position.
3. The mobilizing/manipulating hand glides the navicular in a dorsal direction (see Fig. 8-16).

Particulars

1. The clinician should use caution in performing this technique because this motion might be hypermobile.

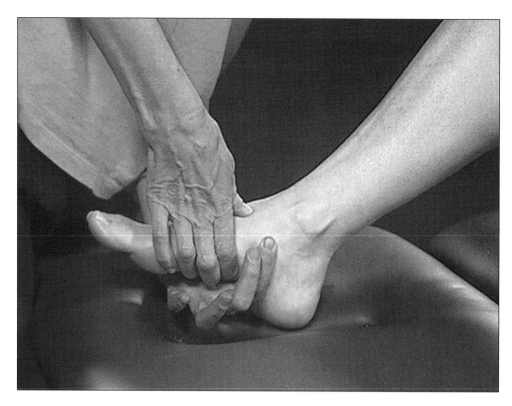

FIGURE 8-17. Plantar glide of the navicular.

PLANTAR GLIDE OF THE NAVICULAR (Fig. 8-17)

Purpose

- To examine for talonavicular joint impairment
- To increase accessory motion into talonavicular plantar glide
- To increase range of motion at the midtarsal joint
- To decrease pain
- To improve periarticular muscle performance

Positioning

1. The patient is supine.
2. The talonavicular joint is placed in the resting position.
3. The clinician is facing the dorsal surface of the patient's foot.
4. The stabilizing hand grips the talus at the plantar surface with the web space or with the thumb on the dorsal surface and the index finger on the plantar surface.
5. The mobilizing/manipulating hand grips the navicular with the thumb on the dorsal surface and the index finger on the plantar surface.

Procedure

1. The clinician applies a grade I traction to the joint.
2. The stabilizing hand holds the talus in position.
3. The mobilizing/manipulating hand glides the navicular in a plantar direction (see Fig. 8-17).

Particulars

1. The clinician should use caution in performing this technique because this motion might be hypermobile.

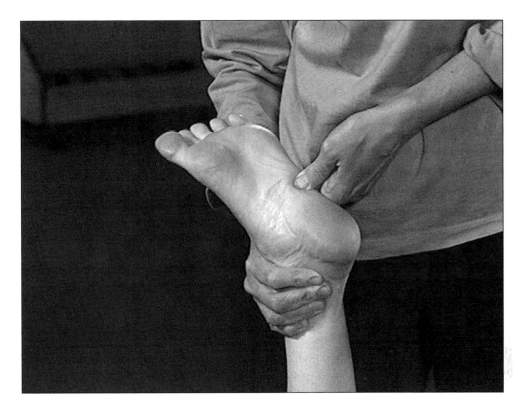

FIGURE 8-18. Dorsal glide of the cuboid.

DORSAL GLIDE OF THE CUBOID (Fig. 8-18)

Purpose

- To examine for calcaneocuboid joint impairment
- To increase accessory motion into calcaneocuboid dorsal glide
- To increase range of motion at the midtarsal joint
- To decrease pain
- To improve periarticular muscle performance

Positioning

1. The patient is prone with the knee flexed to 90 degrees.
2. The calcaneocuboid joint is placed in the resting position.
3. The clinician is facing the plantar surface of the patient's foot.
4. The stabilizing hand grips the talus at the dorsal surface with the web space, indirectly stabilizing the calcaneus.
5. The mobilizing/manipulating hand grips the cuboid with the thumb on the plantar surface and the index finger on the dorsal surface.

Procedure

1. The clinician applies a grade I traction to the joint.
2. The stabilizing hand holds the calcaneus in position.
3. The mobilizing/manipulating hand glides the cuboid in a dorsal direction (see Fig. 8-18).

Particulars

1. The clinician should use caution in performing this technique because this motion might be hypermobile.
2. This technique might be effective in correcting a calcaneocuboid joint positional fault.

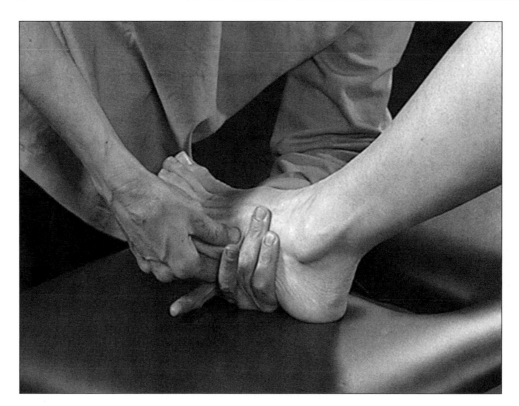

FIGURE 8-19. Plantar glide of the cuboid.

PLANTAR GLIDE OF THE CUBOID (Fig. 8-19)

Purpose

- To examine for calcaneocuboid joint impairment
- To increase accessory motion into calcaneocuboid plantar glide
- To increase range of motion at the midtarsal joint
- To decrease pain
- To improve periarticular muscle performance

Positioning

1. The patient is supine.
2. The calcaneocuboid joint is placed in the resting position.
3. The clinician is facing the dorsal surface of the patient's foot.
4. The stabilizing hand grips the calcaneus at the plantar surface with the web space.
5. The mobilizing/manipulating hand grips the cuboid with the thumb on the dorsal surface and the index finger on the plantar surface.

Procedure

1. The clinician applies a grade I traction to the joint.
2. The stabilizing hand holds the calcaneus in position.
3. The mobilizing/manipulating hand glides the cuboid in a plantar direction (see Fig. 8-19).

Particulars

1. The clinician should use caution in performing this technique because this motion might be hypermobile.

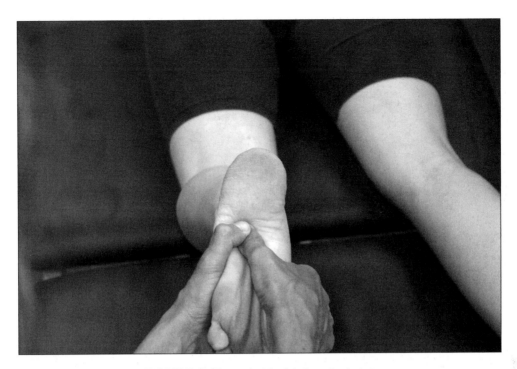

FIGURE 8-20. Cuboid whip/manipulation.

CUBOID WHIP/MANIPULATION (Fig. 8-20)

Purpose

- To increase accessory motion into calcaneocuboid dorsal glide
- To increase range of motion at the midtarsal joint
- To decrease pain
- To improve periarticular muscle performance

Positioning

1. The patient is prone with the knee flexed to about 75 degrees and the ankle in slight plantar flexion.
2. The clinician is facing the plantar surface of the patient's foot.
3. The manipulating hand is positioned with the thumb over the thumb of the guiding hand and the fingers on the dorsal surface of the foot distal to the cuboid.
4. The guiding hand is positioned with the thumb over the plantar surface of the cuboid and the fingers interlacing the fingers of the manipulating hand on the dorsal surface of the foot.

Procedure

1. The manipulating hand glides the cuboid in a dorsal direction, while moving the ankle slightly into plantar flexion and the knee slightly into extension.
2. The guiding hand supports the manipulating hand (see Fig. 8-20).

Particulars

1. The clinician should use caution in performing this technique because this motion might be hypermobile.
2. This technique should be performed using grade V manipulations.
3. This technique might be effective in correcting a calcaneocuboid joint positional fault.

INTERMETATARSAL JOINTS ONE THROUGH FIVE

Osteokinematic motion:
   Increasing/flattening the transverse arch of the foot
Ligaments:
   Transverse metatarsal ligaments
Joint orientation:
   Medial metatarsal: lateral
   Lateral metatarsal: medial
Concave joint surface:
   None, this is a plane joint
Type of joint:
   Synarthrosis
Resting position:
   Unknown[11]
Close-packed position:
   Unknown[11]
Capsular pattern of restriction:
   None, not a synovial joint

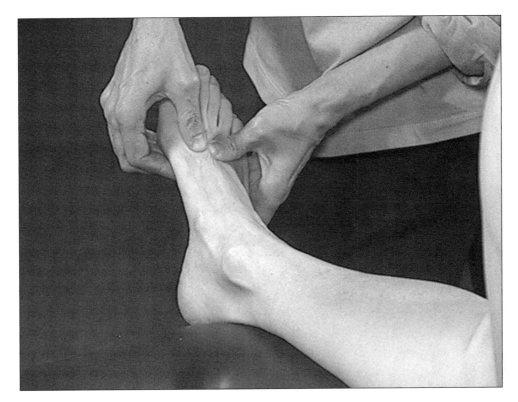

FIGURE 8-21. Dorsal glide.

DORSAL GLIDE (Fig. 8-21)

Purpose
- To examine for intermetatarsal joint impairment
- To increase accessory motion into intermetatarsal joint dorsal glide, using the second metatarsal as a reference point
- To increase range of motion at the intermetatarsal joints
- To decrease pain
- To improve periarticular muscle performance

Positioning
1. The patient is supine.
2. The foot is placed in a neutral position.
3. The clinician is facing the dorsal surface of the patient's foot.
4. The stabilizing hand grips the midshaft of one metatarsal with the thumb on the dorsal surface and the index finger on the plantar surface.
5. The mobilizing/manipulating hand grips the midshaft of the other metatarsal with the thumb on the dorsal surface and the index finger on the plantar surface.

Procedure
1. The clinician applies a grade I traction to the joint.
2. The stabilizing hand holds one metatarsal in position.
3. The mobilizing/manipulating hand glides the first metatarsal in a dorsal direction on the second metatarsal, the third metatarsal in a dorsal direction on the second metatarsal, the fourth metatarsal in a dorsal direction on the third metatarsal, and the fifth metatarsal in a dorsal direction on the fourth metatarsal (see Fig. 8-21).

Particulars
1. This technique might be especially effective for increasing range of motion into flattening the transverse arch of the foot.

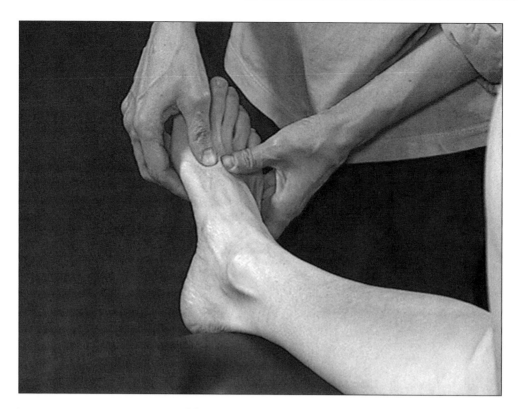

FIGURE 8-22. Plantar glide.

PLANTAR GLIDE (Fig. 8-22)

Purpose

- To examine for intermetatarsal joint impairment
- To increase accessory motion into intermetatarsal joint plantar glide, using the second metatarsal as a reference point
- To increase range of motion at the intermetatarsal joints
- To decrease pain
- To improve periarticular muscle performance

Positioning

1. The patient is supine.
2. The foot is placed in a neutral position.
3. The clinician is facing the dorsal surface of the patient's foot.
4. The stabilizing hand grips the midshaft of one metatarsal with the thumb on the dorsal surface and the index finger on the plantar surface.
5. The mobilizing/manipulating hand grips the midshaft of the other metatarsal with the thumb on the dorsal surface and the index finger on the plantar surface.

Procedure

1. The clinician applies a grade I traction to the joint.
2. The stabilizing hand holds one metatarsal in position.
3. The mobilizing/manipulating hand glides the first metatarsal in a plantar direction on the second metatarsal, the third metatarsal in a plantar direction on the second metatarsal, the fourth metatarsal in a plantar direction on the third metatarsal, and the fifth metatarsal in a plantar direction on the fourth metatarsal (see Fig. 8-22).

Particulars

1. This technique might be especially effective for increasing range of motion into increasing the transverse arch of the foot.

METATARSOPHALANGEAL JOINTS

Osteokinematic motions:
Flexion/extension
Abduction/adduction

Ligaments:
Plantar ligaments
Collateral ligaments

Joint orientation:
Metatarsals: anterior
Phalanges: posterior

Concave joint surface:
Proximal phalanx

Type of joint:
Synovial

Resting position:
10 degrees of extension[11]

Close-packed position:
First metatarsophalangeal joint: full extension
Second through fifth metatarsophalangeal joints: full flexion[11]

Capsular pattern of restriction:
First metatarsophalangeal joint: marked limitation in extension and slight limitation in flexion
Second through fifth metatarsophalangeal joints: variable, but flexion is generally more limited than extension[12]

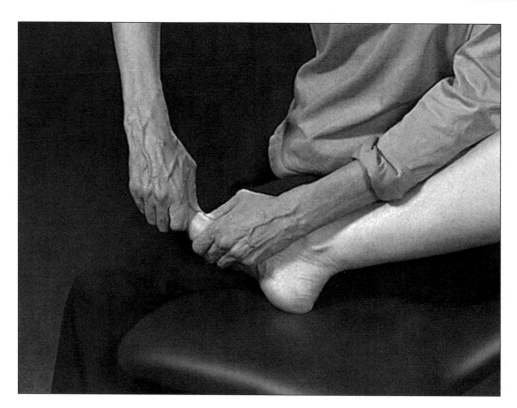

FIGURE 8-23. Distraction.

DISTRACTION (Fig. 8-23)

Purpose

- To examine for metatarsophalangeal joint impairment
- To increase accessory motion into metatarsophalangeal joint distraction
- To increase range of motion at the metatarsophalangeal joints
- To decrease pain
- To improve periarticular muscle performance

Positioning

1. The patient is supine.
2. The metatarsophalangeal joint is placed in the resting position if conservative techniques are indicated or approximating restricted range of motion if more aggressive techniques are indicated.
3. The clinician is facing the lateral surface of the patient's foot.
4. The stabilizing hand grips the head of the metatarsal with the thumb on the dorsal surface and the index finger on the plantar surface.
5. The mobilizing/manipulating hand grips the proximal end of the proximal phalanx with the thumb on the dorsal surface and the index finger on the plantar surface.

Procedure

1. The stabilizing hand holds the metatarsal in position.
2. The mobilizing/manipulating hand moves the proximal phalanx distally in a direction perpendicular to the joint surface of the proximal phalanx (see Fig. 8-23).
3. The clinician could grip the patient's digit with a padded tongue depressor to assist in directing a more precise mobilization/manipulation.
4. The clinician could wear surgical gloves to reduce slippage against the patient's skin.

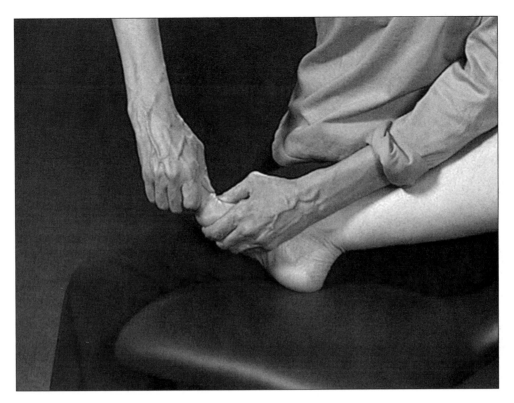

FIGURE 8-24. Dorsal glide.

DORSAL GLIDE (Fig. 8-24)

Purpose

- To examine for metatarsophalangeal joint impairment
- To increase accessory motion into metatarsophalangeal joint dorsal glide
- To increase range of motion at the metatarsophalangeal joint
- To decrease pain
- To improve periarticular muscle performance

Positioning

1. The patient is supine.
2. The metatarsophalangeal joint is placed in the resting position if conservative techniques are indicated or approximating restricted range of motion if more aggressive techniques are indicated.
3. The clinician is facing the lateral surface of the patient's foot.
4. The stabilizing hand grips the head of the metatarsal with the thumb on the dorsal surface and the index finger on the plantar surface.
5. The mobilizing/manipulating hand grips the proximal end of the proximal phalanx with the thumb on the dorsal surface and the index finger on the plantar surface.

Procedure

1. The clinician applies a grade I traction to the joint.
2. The stabilizing hand holds the metatarsal in position.
3. The mobilizing/manipulating hand glides the proximal phalanx in a dorsal direction (see Fig. 8-24).
4. The clinician could grip the patient's digit with a padded tongue depressor to assist in directing a more precise mobilization/manipulation.
5. The clinician could wear surgical gloves to reduce slippage against the patient's skin.

Particulars

1. This technique might be especially effective for increasing range of motion into metatarsophalangeal joint extension.

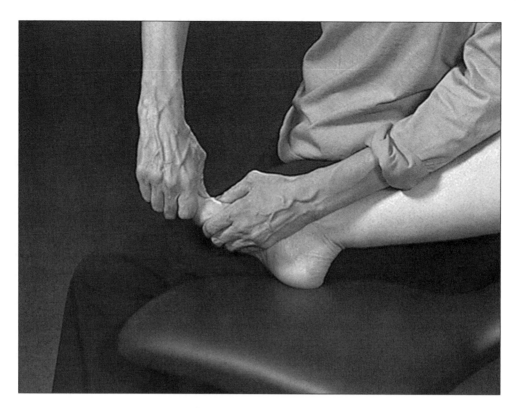

FIGURE 8-25. Plantar glide.

PLANTAR GLIDE (Fig. 8-25)

Purpose

- To examine for metatarsophalangeal joint impairment
- To increase accessory motion into metatarsophalangeal joint plantar glide
- To increase range of motion at the metatarsophalangeal joint
- To decrease pain
- To improve periarticular muscle performance

Positioning

1. The patient is supine.
2. The metatarsophalangeal joint is placed in the resting position if conservative techniques are indicated or approximating restricted range of motion if more aggressive techniques are indicated.
3. The clinician is facing the lateral surface of the patient's foot.
4. The stabilizing hand grips the head of the metatarsal with the thumb on the dorsal surface and the index finger on the plantar surface.
5. The mobilizing/manipulating hand grips the proximal end of the proximal phalanx with the thumb on the dorsal surface and the index finger on the plantar surface.

Procedure

1. The clinician applies a grade I traction to the joint.
2. The stabilizing hand holds the metatarsal in position.
3. The mobilizing/manipulating hand glides the proximal phalanx in a plantar direction (see Fig. 8-25).
4. The clinician could grip the patient's digit with a padded tongue depressor to assist in directing a more precise mobilization/manipulation.
5. The clinician could wear surgical gloves to reduce slippage against the patient's skin.

Particulars

1. This technique might be especially effective for increasing range of motion into metatarsophalangeal joint flexion.

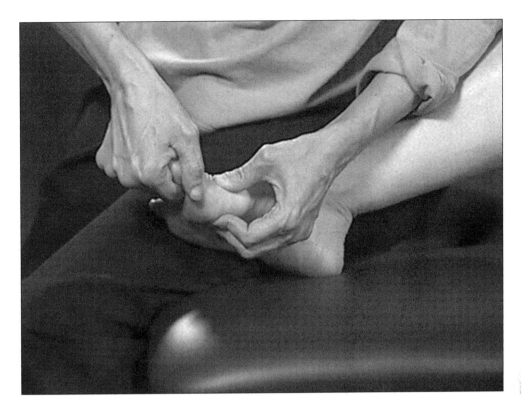

FIGURE 8-26. Medial glide.

MEDIAL GLIDE (Fig. 8-26)

Purpose

- To examine for metatarsophalangeal joint impairment
- To increase accessory motion into metatarsophalangeal joint medial glide
- To increase range of motion at the metatarsophalangeal joint
- To decrease pain
- To improve periarticular muscle performance

Positioning

1. The patient is supine.
2. The metatarsophalangeal joint is placed in the resting position if conservative techniques are indicated or approximating restricted range of motion if more aggressive techniques are indicated.
3. The clinician is facing the lateral surface of the patient's foot.
4. The stabilizing hand grips the head of the metatarsal with the thumb on the dorsal and medial surfaces and the index finger on the plantar and medial surfaces.
5. The mobilizing/manipulating hand grips the proximal end of the proximal phalanx on the lateral and medial surfaces.

Procedure

1. The clinician applies a grade I traction to the joint.
2. The stabilizing hand holds the metatarsal in position.
3. The mobilizing/manipulating hand glides the proximal phalanx in a medial direction (see Fig. 8-26).
4. The clinician could grip the patient's digit with a padded tongue depressor to assist in directing a more precise mobilization/manipulation.
5. The clinician could wear surgical gloves to reduce slippage against the patient's skin.

Particulars

1. This technique might be especially effective for increasing range of motion into metatarsophalangeal joint movement toward the midline of the body.

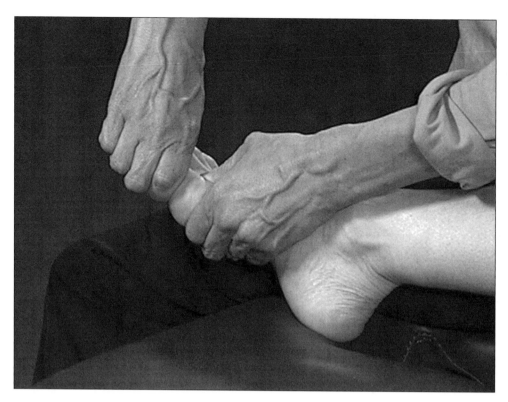

FIGURE 8-27. Lateral glide.

LATERAL GLIDE (Fig. 8-27)

Purpose

- To examine for metatarsophalangeal joint impairment
- To increase accessory motion into metatarsophalangeal joint lateral glide
- To increase range of motion at the metatarsophalangeal joint
- To decrease pain
- To improve periarticular muscle performance

Positioning

1. The patient is supine.
2. The metatarsophalangeal joint is placed in the resting position if conservative techniques are indicated or approximating restricted range of motion if more aggressive techniques are indicated.
3. The clinician is facing the lateral surface of the patient's foot.
4. The stabilizing hand grips the head of the metatarsal with the thumb on the dorsal and lateral surfaces and the index finger on the plantar and lateral surfaces.
5. The mobilizing/manipulating hand grips the proximal end of the proximal phalanx on the lateral and medial surfaces.

Procedure

1. The clinician applies a grade I traction to the joint.
2. The stabilizing hand holds the metatarsal in position.
3. The mobilizing/manipulating hand glides the proximal phalanx in a lateral direction (see Fig. 8-27).
4. The clinician could grip the patient's digit with a padded tongue depressor to assist in directing a more precise mobilization/manipulation.
5. The clinician could wear surgical gloves to reduce slippage against the patient's skin.

Particulars

1. This technique might be especially effective for increasing range of motion into metatarsophalangeal joint movement away from the midline of the body.

INTERPHALANGEAL JOINTS OF TOES ONE THROUGH FIVE

Osteokinematic motion:
Flexion/extension
Ligaments:
Medial collateral
Lateral collateral
Joint orientation:
Proximal phalanx: anterior (distal)
Distal phalanx: posterior (proximal)
Concave joint surface:
Distal phalanx
Type of joint:
Synovial
Resting position:
Slight flexion[11]
Close-packed position:
Full extension[11]
Capsular pattern of restriction:
Not described by Cyriax

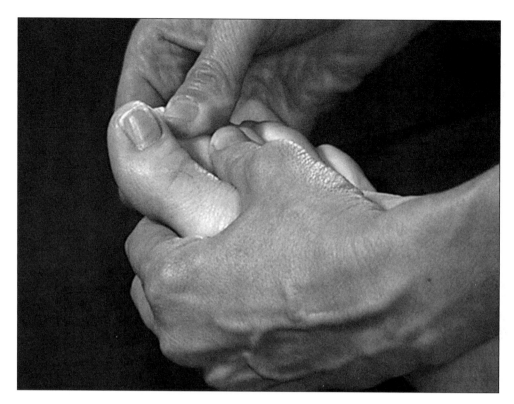

FIGURE 8-28. Distraction.

DISTRACTION (Fig. 8-28)

Purpose

- To examine for toe interphalangeal joint impairment
- To increase accessory motion into toe interphalangeal joint distraction
- To increase range of motion at the toe interphalangeal joints
- To decrease pain
- To improve periarticular muscle performance

Positioning

1. The patient is supine.
2. The interphalangeal joint is placed in the resting position if conservative techniques are indicated or approximating restricted range of motion if more aggressive techniques are indicated.
3. The clinician is facing the lateral of the patient's foot.
4. The stabilizing hand grips the distal end of the more proximal phalanx with the thumb on the dorsal surface and the index finger on the plantar surface.
5. The mobilizing/manipulating hand grips the proximal end of the more distal phalanx with the thumb on the dorsal surface and the index finger on the plantar surface.

Procedure

1. The stabilizing hand holds the more proximal phalanx in position.
2. The mobilizing/manipulating hand moves the more distal phalanx distally in a direction perpendicular to the joint surface of the distal phalanx (see Fig. 8-28).
3. The clinician could grip the patient's digit with a padded tongue depressor to assist in directing a more precise mobilization/manipulation.
4. The clinician could wear surgical gloves to reduce slippage against the patient's skin.

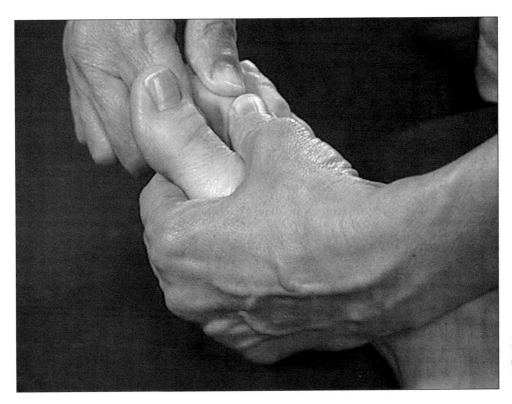

FIGURE 8-29. Dorsal glide.

DORSAL GLIDE (Fig. 8-29)

Purpose

- To examine for toe interphalangeal joint impairment
- To increase accessory motion into toe interphalangeal joint dorsal glide
- To increase range of motion at the interphalangeal joints
- To decrease pain
- To improve periarticular muscle performance

Positioning

1. The patient is supine.
2. The interphalangeal joint is placed in the resting position if conservative techniques are indicated or approximating restricted range of motion if more aggressive techniques are indicated.
3. The clinician is facing the lateral surface of the patient's foot.
4. The stabilizing hand grips the distal end of the more proximal phalanx with the thumb on the dorsal surface and the index finger on the plantar surface.
5. The mobilizing/manipulating hand grips the proximal end of the more distal phalanx with the thumb on the dorsal surface and the index finger on the plantar surface.

Procedure

1. The clinician applies a grade I traction to the joint.
2. The stabilizing hand holds the more proximal phalanx in position.
3. The mobilizing/manipulating hand glides the more distal phalanx in a dorsal direction (see Fig. 8-29).
4. The clinician could grip the patient's digit with a padded tongue depressor to assist in directing a more precise mobilization/manipulation.
5. The clinician could wear surgical gloves to reduce slippage against the patient's skin.

Particulars

1. This technique might be especially effective for increasing range of motion into interphalangeal joint extension.

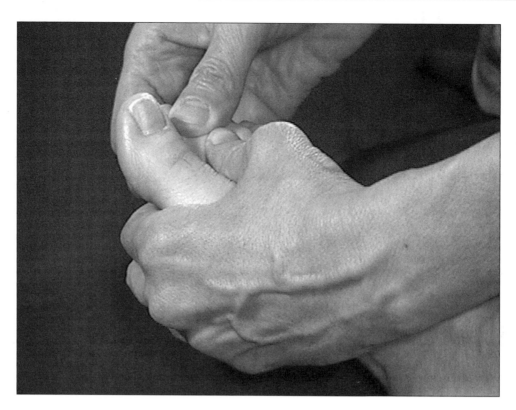

FIGURE 8-30. Plantar glide.

PLANTAR GLIDE (Fig. 8-30)

Purpose

- To examine for toe interphalangeal joint impairment
- To increase accessory motion into toe interphalangeal joint plantar glide
- To increase range of motion at the interphalangeal joints
- To decrease pain
- To improve periarticular muscle performance

Positioning

1. The patient is supine.
2. The interphalangeal joint is placed in the resting position if conservative techniques are indicated or approximating restricted range of motion if more aggressive techniques are indicated.
3. The clinician is facing the lateral surface of the patient's foot.
4. The stabilizing hand grips the distal end of the more proximal phalanx with the thumb on the dorsal surface and the index finger on the plantar surface.
5. The mobilizing/manipulating hand grips the proximal end of the more distal phalanx with the thumb on the dorsal surface and the index finger on the plantar surface.

Procedure

1. The clinician applies a grade I traction to the joint.
2. The stabilizing hand holds the more proximal phalanx in position.
3. The mobilizing/manipulating hand glides the more distal phalanx in a plantar direction (see Fig. 8-30).
4. The clinician could grip the patient's digit with a padded tongue depressor to assist in directing a more precise mobilization/manipulation.
5. The clinician could wear surgical gloves to reduce slippage against the patient's skin.

Particulars

1. This technique might be especially effective for increasing range of motion into interphalangeal joint flexion.

REFERENCES

1. Fay F, Egerod S: The effects of joint mobilizations on swelling in the acutely sprained ankle joint: a pilot study. Aust J Physiother 1985;31:168.
2. Pellow JE, Brantigham JW: The efficacy of adjusting the ankle in the treatment of subacute and chronic grade I and grade II ankle inversion sprains. J Manip Physiol Therap 2001;24:17-24.
3. Green T, Refshauge K, Crosbie J, et al: A randomized controlled trial of a passive accessory joint mobilization on acute ankle inversion sprains. Phys Ther 2001;81:984-994.
4. Hart LE, Macintyre J: Passive joint mobilization for acute ankle inversion sprains. Clin J Sport Med 2002;12:54-56.
5. Kavanagh J: Is there a positional fault at the inferior tibiofibular joint in patients with acute or chronic ankle sprains compared to normals? Manual Ther 1999;4:19-24.
6. Collins N, Teys P, Vicenzino B: The initial effects of a Mulligan's mobilization with movement technique on dorsiflexion and pain in subacute ankle sprains. Manual Ther 2004;9:77-82.
7. Coetzer D, Brantigham J, Nook B: The relative effectiveness of Piroxicam compared to manipulation in the treatment of acute grades 1 and 2 inversion ankle sprains. J Neuromusculoskel Syst 2001;9:1-12.
8. Wilson F: Manual therapy versus traditional exercises in mobilization of the ankle post-ankle fracture: a pilot study. N Z J Physiother 1991;19:11-16.
9. Dananberg HJ, Shearstone J, Guiliano M: Manipulation method for the treatment of ankle equinus. J Am Podiatr Med Assoc 2000;90:385-389.
10. Shamus J, Shamus E, Gugel RN, et al: The effect of sesamoid mobilization, flexor hallucis strengthening, and gait training on reducing pain and restoring function in individuals with hallux limitus: a clinical trial. J Orthop Sports Phys Ther 2004;34:368-376.
11. Kaltenborn FM: Manual Mobilization of the Joints: The Kaltenborn Method of Joint Examination and Treatment, Vol I: The Extremities, 6th ed. OPTP, 2002.
12. Cyriax J: Textbook of Orthopaedic Medicine, Vol 1: Diagnosis of Soft Tissue Lesions, 8th ed. London, Bailliere Tindall, 1982.

Section **III**

The Axillary Skeletal System

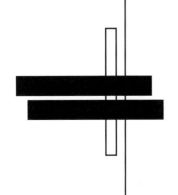

Introduction to the Axillary Skeletal System

The axial skeletal system differs from the appendicular skeletal system in several important ways. One major difference is that movement in one joint is mechanically linked to movement at the same joint on the opposite side of the body. For example, with normal lower cervical forward bending, the facet joint surfaces on the left side and the right side of C2 glide up and forward simultaneously on the facet joint surfaces of C3. Additionally, most of the axial skeletal system shelters the spinal cord and spinal nerve roots and contains multiple small muscles and joints that are located in close proximity to one another. These considerations render the axial skeletal system far more complex and more difficult to evaluate and treat than the appendicular skeletal system. Accessory motion examination and joint mobilization/manipulation intervention also differ in the axial skeletal system in several important ways and are described subsequently.

TERMINOLOGY

Vertebral motion at C2-3 through L5-S1 involves movement of the vertebral bodies and the paired facet joints. To differentiate movement of a vertebra from that of the articulation between two vertebrae, the latter is commonly referred to as a *motion segment*. By convention, movement at a motion segment is defined by the movement of the more superior vertebral body on the more inferior vertebral body; this is the case regardless of which vertebra is actually moving. For example, if a patient is lying prone and lifts the left shoulder off the treatment table, T8 is rotating left on T9. Some clinicians simply would state that T8 is rotating left. If the prone patient lifts the right pelvis off the treatment table, motion is still described as T8 rotating left on T9, even though the actual movement is that of T9 rotating right on T8. The reference point for motion is the vertebral body and not the spinous processes, even though the clinician evaluating spinal movement from behind the patient observes or palpates the T8 spinous process moving to the right of midline when the patient moves into left rotation at T8 on T9.

In this description of joint movement, the assumption is made that vertebral motion occurs sequentially from the structure initiating the motion. In the case of the prone patient lifting the left shoulder off the treatment table, the assumption is that motion starts around T2 or T3, and when this motion segment has moved to end range, rotation begins at the adjacent motion segment below, then sequentially moves down the spine one motion segment at a time.

PRECAUTIONS AND CONTRAINDICATIONS TO JOINT MOBILIZATION AND MANIPULATION RELATED SPECIFICALLY TO THE SPINE

Since spinal joints differ from peripheral joints, many additional concerns need to be considered when determining whether and how to perform spinal mobilization/manipulation techniques. These concerns are listed subsequently. The potential adverse effects of mobilization/manipulation are more severe in the spine than in the extremities. All of the conditions listed should therefore be viewed more as contraindications than as precautions.

Precautions and Contraindications to Spinal Mobilization and Manipulation Interventions

1. Spinal cord involvement in the area being treated
2. Spondylolisthesis in the area being treated
3. Severe scoliosis in the area being treated

4. Suspected aneurysm in the area being treated
5. Positive neurologic signs if the spine or pelvis is being treated with grade V techniques

Precautions and Contraindications Specifically to Cervical Spine Mobilization and Manipulation Interventions

1. Any indication of vertebrobasilar insufficiency in the upper cervical spine, such as reports of dizziness with extension or rotation movements, because cervical spine joint manipulation has been shown to produce cerebrovascular accidents
2. Any indication of ligamentous instability in the upper cervical spine because cervical spine joint manipulation has been shown to cause injury to the spinal cord
3. Rheumatoid arthritis in the cervical spine because joint mobilization/manipulation might produce subluxation or dislocation of cervical spine joints
4. Traumatized upper cervical ligaments, if there is any evidence that the trauma might have caused the upper cervical joints to become unstable
5. Genetic disorders affecting joint laxity in the spine, such as Down syndrome

Precautions and Contraindications Specifically to Lumbar Spine and Pelvic Joint Mobilization and Manipulation Interventions

1. Cauda equina syndrome because mobilization/manipulation might exacerbate the condition
2. Pregnancy because there is speculation (but no evidence) that mobilization/manipulation techniques might induce labor

PASSIVE ACCESSORY VERTEBRAL MOTION VERSUS PASSIVE PHYSIOLOGIC VERTEBRAL MOTION

In Section II of this book (The Appendicular Skeletal System), most of the techniques described are performed without physiologic (passive or active) movement. Regardless of whether the technique is performed with or without passive or active movement, in the peripheral joints, the motion that accompanies joint mobilization/ manipulation techniques is called *joint accessory motion*. In the spine, the term commonly used to describe joint accessory motion is *passive intervertebral motion*. Spinal techniques performed without physiologic motion are called *passive accessory vertebral motion* or *passive accessory intervertebral motion*; the corresponding mobilization/ manipulation technique used sometimes is called passive accessory mobilization/manipulation. Joint mobilization/ manipulation in the spine also commonly is performed such that the clinician or the patient moves the joint being treated at the same time that the joint mobilization/manipulation procedure is being performed. This type of motion is called *passive physiologic vertebral motion,* and the corresponding joint mobilization/manipulation technique sometimes is called passive physiologic mobilization/manipulation.

Most likely, these two types of mobilization/manipulation techniques evaluate different types of joint accessory motion and have different clinical effects; however, no research has been performed that addresses the nature or the clinical relevance of the differences. Some clinicians believe that passive physiologic techniques are more therapeutic because they incorporate physiologic movements in the mobilization/manipulation technique. Often, the determination of which type of technique to perform is made based on the nature of the patient's pain. Although passive physiologic techniques often are less traumatic to capsular and periarticular tissue, they can involve physiologic motions that cause the patient to experience an increase in pain.

JOINT LOCKING

Since spinal joints are positioned in relatively close proximity to one another, one issue that arises specifically with spinal joint mobilization/manipulation interventions is that of preventing unintended motion from occurring at joints located in close proximity to the motion segment being treated. In some cases, judicious and accurate hand placement can prevent this unintended motion from occurring. In other cases, it is advantageous to *lock* joints located close to the motion segment being mobilized/manipulated, using principles of ligamentous or bony locking. With both locking techniques, adjacent joints are positioned at the end of the available range of motion for forward/backward bending, side bending, or rotation. This positioning prevents further movement (and stretching) at these joints because either the ligaments are taut or the articular surfaces are contacting one another, and any further motion induced by the mobilization/manipulation technique is likely to occur at the motion segment with the most slack, which is also the motion segment targeted for treatment.

EVALUATION VERSUS INTERVENTION

Since it is unnecessary to lock joints located close to the motion segment being treated when examining passive intervertebral motion, the process of evaluating passive intervertebral motion is sometimes performed using a different examination procedure than the one used to treat. In this text, when the examination and corresponding treatment procedure differ, the examination procedure also is described along with the description of the treatment mobilization/manipulation.

SPRINGING

One technique, sometimes called *springing*, is commonly performed on spinal structures. With this technique, a vertebra is glided in an anterior direction without any attempt to stabilize adjacent vertebrae. The motion resulting from this technique is believed to occur at the motion segments superior and inferior to the vertebra being mobilized/manipulated. In two studies investigating the motion effects of this technique on lumbar spinous processes, investigators concluded that the motion that occurred was not a pure gliding motion, but rather one of extension[1] and translation.[1,2] A greater amount of the motion occurred at the motion segment inferior to the vertebra being mobilized than at the superior motion segment.[1] Furthermore, there was a sagging of the entire lumbar spine during this technique.[1,2] This sagging effect generally is considered to be an unintended consequence. These findings suggest that the spinal movements occurring during this springing technique, and most likely with other spinal mobilization/manipulation techniques, are more complex than our assumptions about passive accessory vertebral motion would suggest.

Many clinicians use springing as a method of determining the location of the spinal lesion causing the patient's neck or back pain. If springing on T4 reproduced the patient's symptoms, the clinician would be more likely to conclude that the pathology causing pain was located at either the T3-4 or T4-5 motion segment. This assumption should be re-evaluated, at least in relation to the lumbar spine, given the evidence that suggests that springing produces sagging at all lumbar joints.

COUPLED MOTION

Articular surfaces are not entirely congruent, and they are not consistently located in cardinal planes. Motion in one plane should therefore be accompanied by a specific pattern of motion in at least one other plane. This phenomenon is called *coupled motion,* and although it is most likely present in peripheral joints, principles of coupled motion are applied primarily in relation to the spine.

Many clinicians use information about specific patterns of spinal coupled motion to evaluate for joint hypomobility and to determine patient positioning and direction of glide mobilization/manipulation interventions. For example, assuming that side bending and rotation are coupled toward the same side in the lower cervical spine, when a person side bends to the left at C5-6, that person also would rotate simultaneously to the left at that motion segment. Based on knowledge of the pattern of coupled motion, the clinician might assume that if left side bending were hypomobile at C5-6, left rotation also would be hypomobile at that motion segment, and treatment directed at restoring motion into left rotation at C5-6 also would also treat the hypomobility into left side bending at C5-6.

In the lumbar and thoracic spine, some clinicians have suggested that abnormal patterns of coupled motion indicate facet joint impairment at that level. For example, assuming that side bending and rotation are coupled to the same side, a clinician might conclude that there is impairment at a motion segment if the clinician palpated motion into side bending right when he or she rotated the patient's thoracic or lumbar spine to the left.

No studies specifically address upper cervical spine coupled motion. In one study investigating coupled motion in the lower cervical spine, the investigators concluded that side bending and rotation are coupled to the same side.[3] This finding is consistent with what would be expected to occur, given that the lower cervical facet joints are angulated 45 degrees anteriorly and superiorly.

Normal and abnormal coupling in the lumbar spine has been studied extensively. Some form of coupled motion is most likely present in these spinal joints; however, there is a great deal of disagreement in the literature regarding the nature of this coupled motion. Results from numerous studies are inconsistent regarding the specific spinal motions that are coupled with one another.[4,5] Additionally, this coupling has been shown to entail movements in the range of less than three degrees. Such small values cannot be measured without three-dimensional computer-aided equipment[5] and therefore cannot be determined with manual palpation techniques. Although coupled motion in the thoracic spine has been less well studied, conclusions similar to those for the lumbar spine regarding the nature and extent of movement have been drawn.[4]

Concepts related to coupled motion are not likely to be helpful in evaluating and treating spinal conditions in the thoracic and lumbar spine. First, coupled patterns are likely not detectable using manual techniques. Second, there is no evidence to show that even if coupled motion can be detected, there is any therapeutic value in doing so. Clinicians should consider eliminating the use of coupled motion patterns in their evaluation and intervention of patients with thoracic and lumbar spine conditions using joint mobilization/manipulation techniques. Since the evidence suggests that there is a pattern of coupled motion in the lower cervical spine, concepts related to lower cervical spine coupled motion might be more clinically useful.

REFERENCES

1. Kulig K, Landel R, Powers C: Assessment of lumbar spine kinematics using dynamic MRI: a proposed mechanism of sagittal plane motion induced by manual posterior-to-anterior mobilization. J Orthop Sports Phys Ther 2004;34:57-61.
2. Lee R, Evans J: Toward a better understanding of spinal posteroanterior mobilization. Physiotherapy 1994;80:68-73.
3. Mimura M, Moriya H, Watanabe T, et al: Three dimensional motion analysis of the cervical spine with special reference to the axial rotation. Spine 1989;14:1135-1139.
4. Gibbons P, Tehan P: Muscle energy concepts and coupled motion of the spine. Manual Ther 1998;3:95-101.
5. Harrison DE, Harrison DD, Troyanovich SJ: Three-dimensional spinal coupling mechanics: Part I. a review of the literature. J Manip Physiol Therap 1998;21:101-113.

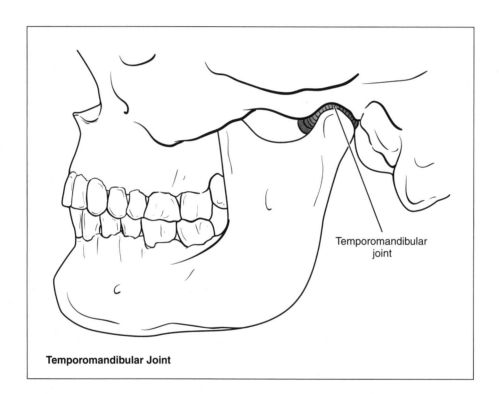

Temporomandibular
joint

Temporomandibular Joint

CHAPTER 10

The Temporomandibular Joint

BASICS

The temporomandibular joints are an integral component of basic functional activities including eating and talking. For most activities, an individual should be able to open the mouth wide enough at both temporomandibular joints to allow placement of two of the individual's knuckles or three of the individual's fingers between the teeth.

Temporomandibular Joints

Anatomically, the temporomandibular joints consist of the paired convex articular surface of the mandible, which articulates with the paired concave articular surface of the temporal bone. An intra-articular disc separates these joint surfaces. Motion at the temporomandibular joint includes opening and closing, protraction and retraction, and side gliding.

Jaw opening occurs as a result of a combination of temporomandibular rotation and gliding. Protraction and retraction occur via a gliding motion, with minimal, if any, rotation. Limitations in retraction are uncommon. With side gliding, the temporomandibular joint on the side to which the chin is moving rotates and shifts slightly laterally, and the temporomandibular joint on the opposite side glides forward, medially, and downward.

SPECIFIC PATHOLOGY AND TEMPOROMANDIBULAR JOINT MOBILIZATION/ MANIPULATION

Temporomandibular Pain Syndrome

Only a few studies have addressed the role of joint mobilization/manipulation in the treatment of temporomandibular pain. In an early study of patients with myofascial pain syndrome, which was defined as unilateral facial pain, masticatory muscle tenderness, joint crepitus, and limitation of mandibular movement, 34 subjects were alternately assigned to receive physical therapy or relaxation therapy with biofeedback. Physical therapy consisted of ultrasound and joint mobilization. Subjects receiving relaxation therapy experienced a significant decrease in pain compared with the group receiving a physical therapy program that included joint mobilization.[1]

Conversely, in a more recent study, 15 subjects with chronic temporomandibular pain and limited jaw movement were randomly assigned to receive grade IV distraction mobilization to the temporomandibular joint and sham treatment consisting of superficial massage. When subjects received joint mobilization, they had a significant increase in range of motion and decrease in masseter muscle electromyogram activity compared with the sham intervention. The increase in range of motion disappeared after 15 minutes.[2] In these two studies, joint mobilization/manipulation might have produced a more positive effect if it had been administered in conjunction with other interventions, such as exercise.

Temporomandibular Disc Derangement

Numerous studies have investigated the effect of joint mobilization/manipulation on internal derangement of the temporomandibular joint disc. Results generally do not support using joint mobilization/manipulation techniques to correct disc derangements. Studies that did show improvement with interventions that included joint mobilization/manipulation did not incorporate a comparison group in the study.[3-5] It is therefore difficult to conclude that these subjects improved as a result of treatment, and not as a result of time or placebo effects. In studies in which the actual position of the disc was compared via radiography before and after the subject received joint mobilization/manipulation intervention, only a small percentage of subjects showed disc reduction.[4,6]

In the only randomized controlled trial in which joint mobilization was compared with another intervention, 69 subjects with disc derangements without reduction were assigned to receive advice only; advice and nonsteroidal anti-inflammatory drugs (NSAIDs); or advice, NSAIDs, an occlusal appliance, and joint mobilization. Outcome measures included pain, range of motion, and activity level. At the end of treatment, there was a difference among groups for activity level only, and this difference was in favor of the group receiving self-care instruction and NSAIDs.[7]

TEMPOROMANDIBULAR JOINTS

Osteokinematic motions:
    Opening/closing
    Protraction/retraction
    Side gliding left and right
Ligaments:
    Temporomandibular ligament
    Sphenomandibular ligament
    Stylomandibular ligament
Joint orientation:
    Temporalis: inferior, anterior, lateral
    Mandible: superior, posterior, medial
Type of joint:
    Synovial
Concave joint surface:
    Temporalis
Resting position:
    Mouth slightly open[8]
Close-packed position:
    Mouth closed[8]
Capsular pattern of restriction:
    Limitation in mouth opening[9]

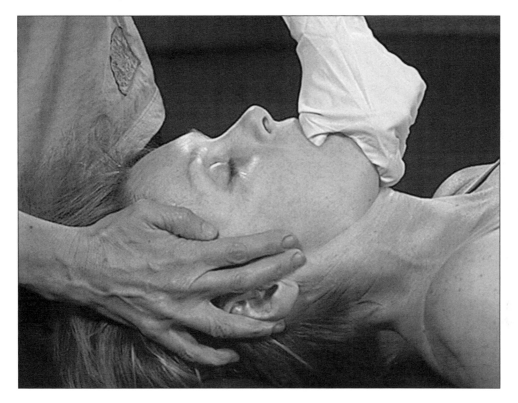

FIGURE 10-1. Distraction.

DISTRACTION (Fig. 10-1)

Purpose

- To examine for temporomandibular joint impairment
- To increase accessory motion into temporomandibular joint distraction
- To increase range of motion at the temporomandibular joint
- To decrease pain
- To improve periarticular muscle performance

Positioning

1. The patient is supine.
2. The temporomandibular joint is placed in the resting position if conservative techniques are indicated or approximating restricted range of motion if more aggressive techniques are indicated.
3. The clinician is at the head of the treatment table facing the temporomandibular joint.
4. The clinician should wear surgical gloves to protect the clinician and patient from transmission of infection.
5. The stabilizing hand supports the head laterally on the same side as the joint being mobilized/manipulated.
6. The mobilizing/manipulating hand is positioned with the thumb over the lower molars and the fingers wrapped around the lateral lower jaw on the side to be mobilized/manipulated.

Procedure

1. The stabilizing hand holds the head in position.
2. The mobilizing/manipulating hand moves the mandible inferiorly in a direction perpendicular to the joint surface of the temporalis and guides this movement with the fingers (see Fig. 10-1).

Particulars

1. In the case of bilateral temporomandibular joint impairment, this technique can be performed on both temporomandibular joints simultaneously by positioning and moving both hands as if they were both "mobilizing/manipulating" hands.

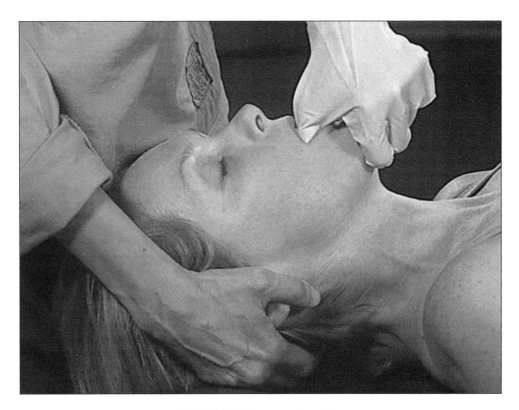

FIGURE 10-2. Anterior glide.

ANTERIOR GLIDE (Fig. 10-2)

Purpose

- To examine for temporomandibular joint impairment
- To increase accessory motion into temporomandibular joint anterior glide
- To increase range of motion at the temporomandibular joint
- To decrease pain
- To improve periarticular muscle performance

Positioning

1. The patient is supine.
2. The temporomandibular joint is placed in the resting position if conservative techniques are indicated or approximating restricted range of motion if more aggressive techniques are indicated.
3. The clinician is at the head of the treatment table facing the temporomandibular joint.
4. The clinician should wear surgical gloves to protect the clinician and patient from transmission of infection.
5. The stabilizing hand supports the head laterally and anteriorly on the same side as the joint being mobilized/manipulated.
6. The mobilizing/manipulating hand is positioned with the thumb over the lower molars and the fingers wrapped around the lateral lower jaw on the side to be mobilized/manipulated.

Procedure

1. The clinician applies a grade I traction to the joint.
2. The stabilizing hand holds the head in position.
3. The mobilizing/manipulating hand glides the mandible in an anterior direction with the thumb and guides the movement with the fingers (see Fig. 10-2).

Particulars

1. This technique might be especially effective for increasing range of motion into temporomandibular joint protraction.

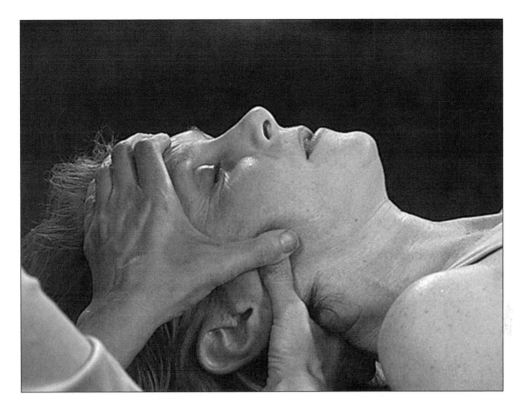

FIGURE 10-3. Medial glide.

MEDIAL GLIDE (Fig. 10-3)

Purpose
- To examine for temporomandibular joint impairment
- To increase accessory motion into temporomandibular joint medial glide
- To increase range of motion at the temporomandibular joint
- To decrease pain
- To improve periarticular muscle performance

Positioning
1. The patient is supine.
2. The temporomandibular joint is placed in the resting position if conservative techniques are indicated or approximating restricted range of motion if more aggressive techniques are indicated.
3. The clinician is at the side of the patient's head facing the temporomandibular joint.
4. The mobilizing/manipulating hand is positioned with the thumb over the guiding hand.
5. The guiding hand is positioned with the thumb on the mandibular condyle.

Procedure
1. The mobilizing/manipulating hand glides the mandible in a medial direction with the thumb.
2. The guiding hand controls the position of the mobilizing/manipulating hand (see Fig. 10-3).

Particulars
1. This technique might be especially effective for increasing range of motion into temporomandibular joint side gliding to the side away from the side of the joint being treated.

REFERENCES

1. Trott PH, Goss AN: Physiotherapy in diagnosis and treatment of the myofascial pain dysfunction syndrome. Int J Oral Surg 1978;7:360-365.

2. Taylor M, Suvinen T, Reade P: The effect of grade IV distraction mobilization on patients with temporomandibular pain-dysfunction disorder. Physiother Theory Pract 1994;10:129-136.

3. Kirk WS, Calabrese DK: Clinical evaluation of physical therapy in the management of internal derangement of the temporomandibular joint. J Oral Maxillofac Surg 1989;47:113-119.

4. Segami N, Murakami K, Iizuka T, et al: Arthrographic evaluation of disk position following mandibular manipulation technique for internal derangement with closed lock of the temporomandibular joint. J Craniomandib Disord Facial Oral Pain 1990;4:99-108.

5. Minagi S, Nozaki S, Sato T, et al: A manipulation technique for treatment of anterior disk displacement without reduction. J Prosthet Dent 1991;65:686-691.

6. Kurita H, Kurashina K, Ohtsuka A: Efficacy of a mandibular manipulation technique in reducing the permanently displaced temporomandibular joint disc. J Oral Maxillofac Surg 1999;57:784-787.

7. Minakuchi H, Kuboki T, Matsuka Y, et al: Randomized controlled evaluation of non-surgical treatments for temporomandibular joint anterior disk displacement without reduction. J Dent Res 2001;80:924-928.

8. Kaltenborn FM: Manual Mobilization of the Joints: The Kaltenborn Method of Joint Examination and Treatment, Vol II: The Spine, 4th ed. OPTP, 2003.

9. Cyriax J: Textbook of Orthopaedic Medicine, Vol 1: Diagnosis of Soft Tissue Lesions, 8th ed. London, Bailliere Tindall, 1982.

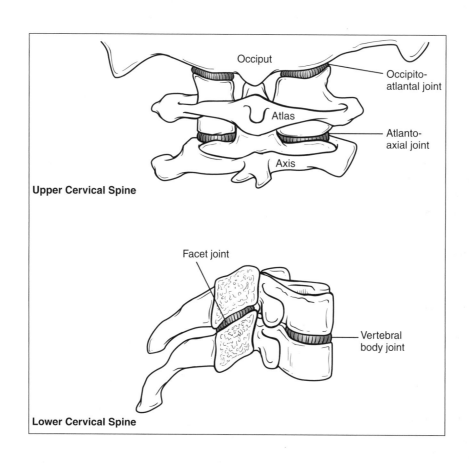

Occiput

Occipito-
atlantal joint

Atlas

Atlanto-
axial joint

Axis

Upper Cervical Spine

Facet joint

Vertebral
body joint

Lower Cervical Spine

CHAPTER 11

Cervical Spine

BASICS

The cervical spine is commonly divided into upper (occiput through C1-2) and lower (C2-3 and below) components. Most clinicians categorize the upper thoracic motion segments (T1-2 and T2-3) as if they were part of the lower cervical spine.

Upper Cervical Joints

Forward bending and backward bending are the primary motions occurring at the occipitoatlantal joint. This joint accounts for 15 degrees of motion in the sagittal plane. Rotation occurs primarily at the atlantoaxial joint, accounting for 45 degrees of rotation in each direction.

Movement at the occipitoatlantoaxial joint has the potential to restrict blood flow in the vertebral arteries. If there is ligamentous instability in the upper cervical area, upper cervical motion could cause impingement by the dens on the spinal cord. It is therefore crucial that the clinician evaluate for signs and symptoms of potential adverse responses to upper cervical movement before proceeding with any of the techniques described for the upper cervical spine or any of the lower cervical spine techniques involving neck passive or active physiological movement.

Lower Cervical and Upper Thoracic Joints

Motion into forward and backward bending is completed by the lower cervical spine. More movement occurs at the C5-6 motion segment than at any other lower cervical spine motion segment. Lower cervical spine motion is guided by the facet joints, which are angulated 45 degrees anteriorly from the frontal plane. Forward bending occurs as the inferior facets of the more superior vertebra glide up and forward on the superior facets of the more inferior vertebra. Backward bending is associated with a downward and backward gliding of the facets of the more superior vertebra on the facets of the more inferior vertebra.

The lower cervical spine is responsible for approximately 45 degrees of rotation in either direction, accounting for about 50% of total movement into rotation. More movement into lower cervical side bending and rotation occurs at the C5-6 motion segment than at any other lower cervical spine motion segment. As with forward bending, lower cervical side bending and rotation are guided by the angulation of the facet joints. Movement into side bending and rotation to the left is accompanied by an upward and forward glide of the right facet joints and a downward and backward glide of the left facet joints of the more superior vertebra, and vice versa for movement into right side bending and rotation. Most clinicians assume that lower cervical side bending and rotation are coupled to the same side.

A limitation in facet joint movement in a superior and anterior direction is sometimes called an *opening restriction*. Conversely, a limitation in facet joint inferior and posterior movement is sometimes called a *closing restriction*. An opening restriction on the right could result in decreased motion into forward bending, side bending left, and rotation left, whereas a right closing restriction could result in decreased motion into backward bending, side bending right, and rotation right.

RISKS AND BENEFITS OF MOBILIZATION VERSUS MANIPULATION

Numerous serious complications have been reported as a result of grade V manipulations performed on the cervical spine. Most of the more serious complications involved vertebrobasilar accidents resulting in a brainstem or cerebellar infarct, obstruction of the posterior inferior cerebellar artery (Wallenberg syndrome), or occlusion of the basilar artery. Also reported were spinal cord compression, vertebral fracture, tracheal rupture, diaphragm paralysis, internal carotid hematoma, and cardiac arrest.[1-3] If one of the aforementioned complications does occur, immediate medical attention is necessary.

Several investigators have attempted to calculate the incidence of a serious complication from cervical spine grade V manipulations. Estimates range from 1 to 100 incidents per one million manipulations.[1-4] Manipulations involving movement into rotation[1,5,6] or extension[6] are considered to be the most dangerous, although the movement or movements that increase risk of an adverse effect have not been determined with any certainty.[6] To date, no serious adverse effects have been reported in the medical literature from mobilization techniques, including techniques involving movement into rotation or extension.

In a review of the literature addressing the identification of patients at risk for experiencing these complications, the authors concluded that there is no indication that trauma history, neck movement, type of manipulation, or examination procedure can be used to identify increased risk.[6] Nevertheless, the Manipulation Association of Chartered Physiotherapists and the Society of Orthopaedic Medicine have provided guidelines for testing to determine if the patient is at risk for an adverse effect from cervical spine grade V manipulations. These guidelines include performing a thorough examination, including identification of a history of symptoms related to vertebrobasilar artery insufficiency and a recognized premanipulation vertebrobasilar artery test. The authors also recommend obtaining informed consent from the patient before performing any cervical spine grade V manipulation.[7]

Several studies have addressed the relative benefits of mobilization versus grade V manipulation. In a small study comparing the effects of cervical spine mobilization with manipulation on subjects with chronic neck pain, there was a greater increase in pain threshold with manipulation.[8] In a second publication, in which 100 subjects with neck pain were studied, there was no difference in relation to range of motion or pain between subjects receiving mobilization using muscle energy techniques and subjects receiving manipulation.[9,10] In a third study, 336 subjects with neck pain were randomly assigned to receive manipulation or mobilization in various combinations with heat and electrical stimulation. Cervical spine manipulation and mobilization interventions resulted in comparable reductions in pain and disability.[11]

Grade V manipulations seem to be only slightly more effective than mobilization techniques in treating patients with mechanical neck pain. In a review of the risks and benefits of cervical manipulation, one investigator concluded that the risks of cervical manipulation outweigh the benefits, and cervical manipulation should not be used to treat musculoskeletal cervical spine conditions.[12]

The relative benefits of two different grade V manipulations also were studied in a randomized clinical trial of 30 subjects. The investigators concluded that both manipulations produced equal amounts of subjective improvement.[13] In a different randomized trial, the relative effect of two manipulation procedures on 40 asymptomatic subjects with evidence of atlantoaxial rotation asymmetry was studied.[14] Results showed that the direction of the grade V manipulation had no effect on range of motion improvements. These studies suggest that in relation to cervical spine manipulations, there is insufficient evidence to suggest that the specific type of the grade V manipulation has an effect on outcome.

SPECIFIC PATHOLOGY AND CERVICAL SPINE JOINT MOBILIZATION/MANIPULATION

Mechanical Neck Pain

In recent years, numerous systematic reviews addressing the efficacy of mobilization/manipulation of the cervical spine for treatment of neck pain have been published. One set of reviews was performed by many of the same investigators. The authors' conclusions were similar across articles and can be summarized as follows:
- Mobilization produces short-term benefits for patients with acute neck pain when performed alone[1] or in combination with other interventions.[1,4,15,16]
- Mobilization and manipulation in combination with other interventions that include exercise produce short-term benefits for patients with subacute and chronic neck pain.[1,4,15,16,17]
- Manipulation is slightly more beneficial than mobilization in patients with subacute and chronic neck pain.[1,15]

These conclusions are consistent with results from several other critical reviews and from a recent clinical trial. Two of these critical reviews were published by the same author. This author concluded that cervical mobilization and manipulation produce at least short-term benefit to some patients with acute and subacute/chronic neck pain.[2,3] In the final critical review, the authors supported the use of spinal manipulation for reduction in pain, and improvement in range of motion and activities of daily living.[18]

In the clinical trial, 183 subjects with nonspecific neck pain were randomly assigned to receive mobilization combined with other manual therapy techniques; exercise therapy; or analgesics, counseling, and education. Subjects receiving mobilization experienced a significant reduction in pain and improvement in most functional activities compared with the other two groups for up to 28 weeks follow-up.[19]

The research supports the use of mobilization and manipulation for the treatment of mechanical neck pain. Issues related to the implementation of mobilization/manipulation techniques, such as the identification of specific patients who would benefit most from cervical spine mobilization/manipulation and the inclusion of other interventions with mobilization/manipulation techniques, need further exploration.

Whiplash

In a critical review of the literature specifically addressing acute neck pain after whiplash injuries, the author concluded that within the first 8 weeks after a whiplash injury, pain might decrease more rapidly with mobilization compared with a placebo. The short-term benefits were the same as with exercise, however, and with exercise patients had a greater chance of being pain-free at 2-year follow-up.[20] Possibly, long-term outcomes would have improved if mobilization had been combined with exercise.

Headache

In several critical reviews, outcomes from mobilization/manipulation for the treatment of headaches were reported. In two of the reviews, the authors concluded that manipulation or mobilization or both might provide short-term relief for some patients with cervicogenic headaches.[1,3] Conversely, in two different critical reviews, the authors stated that there was insufficient evidence to draw a conclusion regarding the efficacy of mobilization/manipulation for cervicogenic headaches.[21,22]

A subsequent study was performed in which 200 subjects with cervicogenic headaches were randomly assigned to receive grade V manipulation, exercise, grade V manipulation and exercise, or a control intervention. At 12-month follow-up, the manipulation and the exercise groups experienced a significant decrease in headache pain and frequency compared with the control group. The group receiving a combination of manipulation and exercise experienced an even greater decrease in symptoms, but this finding did not reach statistical significance.[23]

Lateral Epicondylalgia

In a study of 15 subjects with lateral epicondylalgia, subjects received a grade III lateral glide mobilization to C5-6, a sham intervention consisting of manual contact, and a control condition consisting of no manual contact in random order. The mobilization intervention resulted in a significant increase in pressure pain threshold and pain-free grip strength and a reduction in pain compared with the other two groups.[24]

A second study was performed on 24 subjects with lateral epicondylalgia using the same study design. There was evidence of greater hypoalgesia after mobilization compared with the other two conditions.[25]

UPPER CERVICAL JOINTS (OCCIPUT THROUGH C2)

Osteokinematic motions: Occipitoatlantal joint:
   Forward/backward bending
   Side bending
   Rotation
Osteokinematic motions: Atlantoaxial joint:
   Rotation
   Forward/backward bending
   Side bending
Ligaments:
   Tectorial membrane
   Ligamentum nuchae
   Alar ligaments
   Transverse ligaments
   Apical ligament

Interspinous ligament
Supraspinous ligament
Anterior longitudinal ligament
Posterior longitudinal ligament
Joint orientation:
Occiput: inferior
Atlas superior surface: superior
Atlas inferior facet: inferior, medial
Axis superior facet: superior, lateral
Atlas also encircles the odontoid process of the axis
Type of joint:
Synovial
Concave joint surface:
None, these are plane joints
Resting position:
Not described by Kaltenborn
Close-packed position:
Not described by Kaltenborn
Capsular pattern of restriction:
For the entire cervical spine, side bending and rotation are equally limited, and extension is more limited than flexion[26]

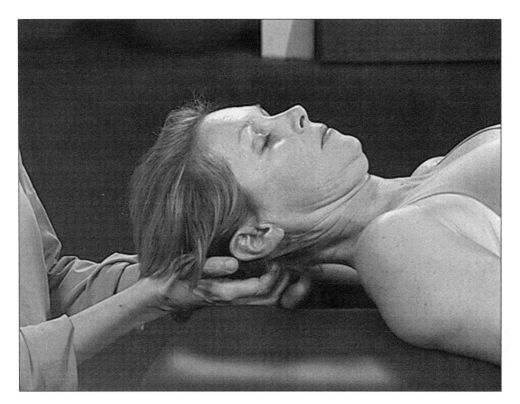

FIGURE 11-1. Distraction/passive accessory vertebral motion.

DISTRACTION/PASSIVE ACCESSORY VERTEBRAL MOTION (Fig. 11-1)

Purpose

- To examine for upper cervical spine joint impairment
- To increase accessory motion into upper cervical joint distraction
- To increase range of motion at the upper cervical spine
- To decrease pain
- To improve periarticular muscle performance

Positioning

1. The patient is supine.
2. The cervical spine is placed in midrange in relation to forward/ backward bending, side bending, and rotation.
3. The clinician is at the patient's head facing the patient.
4. Both hands are positioned with the fingertips inferior to the base of the occiput and the hands on the posterior surface of the skull.

Procedure

1. Testing for signs and symptoms of a potential adverse response to upper cervical movement should be done before performing this or any other mobilization/manipulation technique on the upper cervical spine.
2. Both fingers move the occiput superiorly in a direction perpendicular to the joint surface of the suboccipital joint by lifting the skull away from the clinician's palms and allowing the weight of the head to distract the occiput from the cervical spine.
3. This position can be maintained for several minutes to stretch suboccipital tissue maximally (see Fig. 11-1).

Particulars

1. This is not a grade V manipulation technique.
2. This technique also stretches the suboccipital musculature.

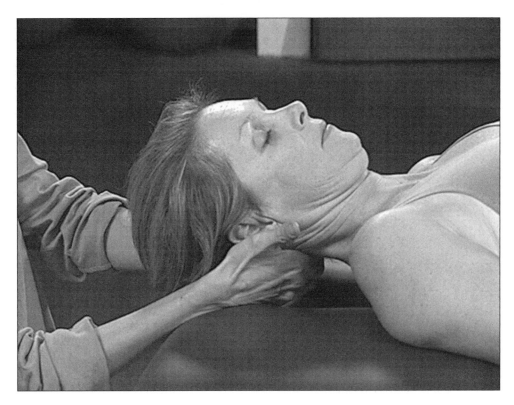

FIGURE 11-2. Forward bending glide/passive physiological vertebral motion.

FORWARD BENDING GLIDE/PASSIVE PHYSIOLOGICAL VERTEBRAL MOTION
(Fig. 11-2)

Purpose
- To examine for upper cervical spine joint impairment
- To increase accessory motion into upper cervical spine forward bending
- To increase range of motion at the upper cervical spine
- To decrease pain
- To improve periarticular muscle performance

Positioning
1. The patient is supine.
2. The cervical spine is placed in midrange in relation to forward/backward bending, side bending, and rotation.
3. The clinician is at the patient's head facing the patient.
4. The stabilizing hand holds the axis in position by placing the lateral (radial) border of the index finger on the superior surface of the spinous process of the axis.
5. The mobilizing hand grips the occiput posteriorly with the web space.

Procedure
1. Testing for signs and symptoms of a potential adverse response to upper cervical movement should be done before performing this or any other mobilization/manipulation technique on the upper cervical spine.
2. The stabilizing hand holds the axis in position.
3. The mobilizing hand glides the occiput superiorly, allowing the head to move into forward bending (see Fig. 11-2).

Particulars
1. This is not a grade V manipulation technique.
2. This technique might be especially effective for increasing range of motion into upper cervical spine forward bending.

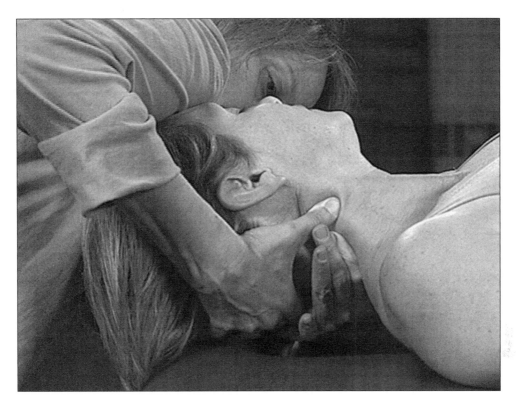

FIGURE 11-3. Rotation glide/passive physiological vertebral motion.

ROTATION GLIDE/PASSIVE PHYSIOLOGICAL VERTEBRAL MOTION (Fig. 11-3)

Purpose

- To examine for upper cervical spine joint impairment
- To increase accessory motion into upper cervical spine rotation
- To increase range of motion at the upper cervical spine
- To decrease pain
- To improve periarticular muscle performance

Positioning

1. The patient is supine.
2. The cervical spine is placed in midrange in relation to forward/backward bending, side bending, and rotation.
3. The clinician is at the patient's head facing the patient with the clinician's anterior shoulder (the shoulder on the same side as the mobilizing/manipulating hand) positioned on the patient's forehead.
4. The stabilizing hand grips the axis posteriorly with the web space and laterally with the fingers and thumb.
5. The mobilizing/manipulating hand grips the occiput posteriorly.

Procedure

1. Testing for signs and symptoms of a potential adverse response to upper cervical movement should be done before performing this or any other mobilization/manipulation technique on the upper cervical spine.
2. The clinician applies a grade I traction to the joints.
3. The stabilizing hand holds the axis.
4. The mobilizing/manipulating hand glides the occiput into rotation as the shoulder guides the motion (see Fig. 11-3).

Particulars

1. This technique might be especially effective for increasing range of motion into upper cervical spine rotation in the direction of vertebral body movement.
2. This technique might be effective in correcting an upper cervical rotational positional fault.

LOWER CERVICAL JOINTS (C3-4 THROUGH T2-3)

Osteokinematic motions:
   Forward/backward bending
   Side bending
   Rotation
Ligaments:
   Anterior longitudinal ligament
   Posterior longitudinal ligament
   Supraspinous ligament
   Interspinous ligament
   Ligamentum flavum
   Intertransverse ligaments
Joint orientation:
   Inferior facet of superior vertebra: inferior, anterior, lateral
   Superior facet of inferior vertebra: superior, posterior, medial
   Superior vertebral body: inferior
   Inferior vertebral body: superior
Type of joint:
   Facets: synovial
   Disc: amphiarthrodial
Concave joint surface:
   None, these are plane joints
Resting position:
   Not described by Kaltenborn
Close-packed position:
   Not described by Kaltenborn
Capsular pattern of restriction:
   For the entire cervical spine, side bending and rotation are equally limited, and extension is more limited than
      flexion[26]

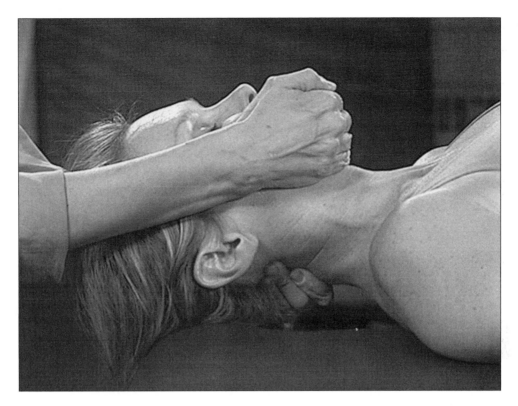

FIGURE 11-4. Distraction/passive accessory vertebral motion.

DISTRACTION/PASSIVE ACCESSORY VERTEBRAL MOTION (Fig. 11-4)

Purpose
- To examine for cervical spine joint impairment
- To increase accessory motion into cervical vertebral body distraction
- To increase range of motion at the cervical spine
- To decrease pain
- To improve periarticular muscle performance

Positioning
1. The patient is supine.
2. The cervical spine is placed in midrange in relation to forward/backward bending, side bending, and rotation.
3. The clinician is at the patient's head facing the patient.
4. The mobilizing/manipulating hand grips the occiput posteriorly with the web space.
5. The guiding hand gently grips the chin.

Procedure
1. Testing for signs and symptoms of a potential adverse response to upper cervical movement should be done before performing this technique.
2. The clinician leans backward, moving the head in a superior direction and distracting the vertebral bodies from one another.
3. Most of the force exerted by the clinician should be directed to the occiput because excessive pressure on the chin might cause the patient to develop temporomandibular joint problems (see Fig. 11-4).

Particulars
1. It is important to screen for temporomandibular joint impairments before performing this technique.

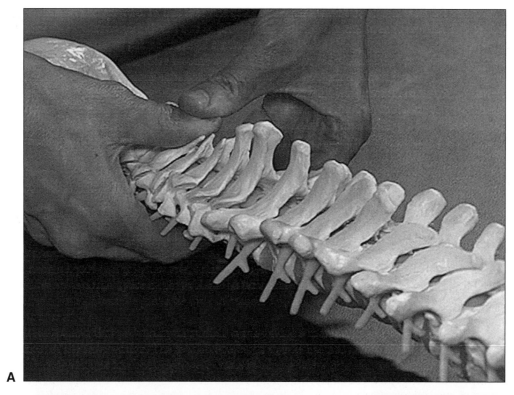

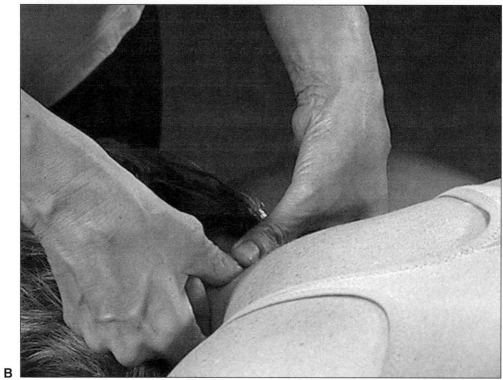

FIGURE 11-5. Anterior glide using the spinous processes/passive accessory vertebral motion.

ANTERIOR GLIDE USING THE SPINOUS PROCESSES/PASSIVE ACCESSORY VERTEBRAL MOTION (Fig. 11-5)

Purpose

- To examine for lower cervical spine joint impairment
- To increase accessory motion into lower cervical joint anterior glide
- To increase range of motion at the lower cervical spine
- To decrease pain
- To improve periarticular muscle performance

Positioning

1. The patient is supine or prone.
2. The cervical spine is placed in midrange in relation to forward/backward bending, side bending, and rotation.
3. The clinician is at the patient's head facing the lower cervical spine.
4. The mobilizing/manipulating hand is positioned with the thumb over the thumb of the guiding hand.
5. The guiding hand is positioned with the thumb over the spinous process being mobilized/manipulated.

Procedure

1. The mobilizing/manipulating hand glides the spinous process anteriorly.
2. The guiding hand controls the position of the mobilizing/manipulating hand (see Fig. 11-5).

Particulars

1. When performed with the patient prone, this technique also is called *springing*. If it is being performed as an examination technique, the term *spring testing* is used.
2. This technique is commonly performed using a grade V manipulation.

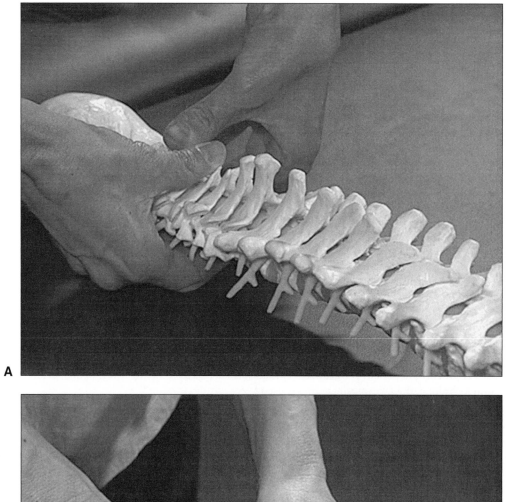

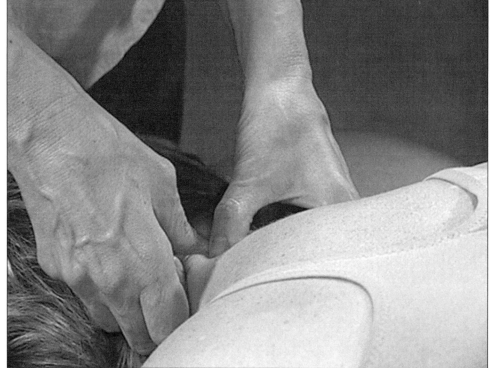

FIGURE 11-6. Anterior/superior glide using the spinous processes/passive accessory vertebral motion: first technique.

ANTERIOR/SUPERIOR GLIDE USING THE SPINOUS PROCESSES/PASSIVE ACCESSORY VERTEBRAL MOTION: FIRST TECHNIQUE (Fig. 11-6)

Purpose

- To examine for lower cervical spine joint impairment
- To increase accessory motion into lower cervical joint anterior/superior glide
- To increase range of motion at the lower cervical spine
- To decrease pain
- To improve periarticular muscle performance

Positioning

1. The patient is supine or prone.
2. The cervical spine is placed in midrange in relation to forward/backward bending, side bending, and rotation.
3. The clinician is at the patient's head facing the lower cervical spine.
4. The stabilizing hand is positioned with the middle finger or the thumb on the spinous process of the more inferior vertebra.
5. The mobilizing/manipulating hand is positioned with the middle finger or the thumb over the most inferior surface of the spinous process of the more superior vertebra.

Procedure

1. The stabilizing hand holds the more inferior vertebra in position.
2. The mobilizing/manipulating hand glides the spinous process of the more superior vertebra anteriorly and superiorly (see Fig. 11-6).

Particulars

1. This technique might be especially effective for increasing range of motion into lower cervical spine forward bending.
2. This technique might be effective in correcting a lower cervical joint forward/backward bending positional fault.

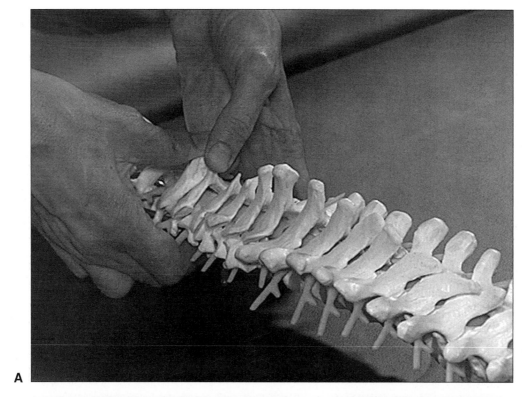

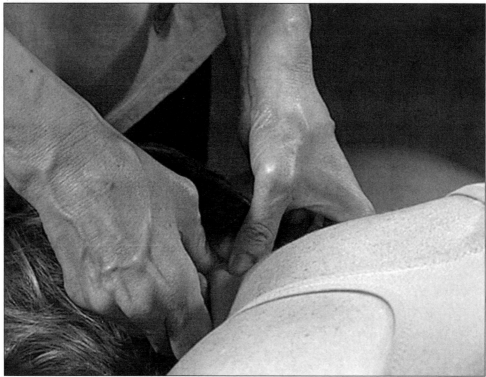

FIGURE 11-7. Anterior/superior glide using the spinous processes/passive accessory vertebral motion: second technique.

ANTERIOR/SUPERIOR GLIDE USING THE SPINOUS PROCESSES/PASSIVE ACCESSORY VERTEBRAL MOTION: SECOND TECHNIQUE (Fig. 11-7)

Purpose

- To examine for lower cervical spine joint impairment
- To increase accessory motion into lower cervical joint anterior/superior glide
- To increase range of motion at the lower cervical spine
- To decrease pain
- To improve periarticular muscle performance

Positioning

1. The patient is supine or prone.
2. The cervical spine is placed in midrange in relation to forward/backward bending, side bending, and rotation.
3. The clinician is at the patient's head facing the lower cervical spine.
4. The stabilizing hand is positioned with the middle finger or the thumb on the spinous process of the more superior vertebra.
5. The mobilizing/manipulating hand is positioned with the middle finger or the thumb over the most inferior surface of the spinous process of the more inferior vertebra.

Procedure

1. The stabilizing hand holds the more superior vertebra in position.
2. The mobilizing/manipulating hand glides the spinous process of the more inferior vertebra anteriorly and superiorly (see Fig. 11-7).

Particulars

1. This technique might be especially effective for increasing range of motion into lower cervical spine backward bending.
2. This technique might be effective in correcting a lower cervical joint forward/backward bending positional fault.

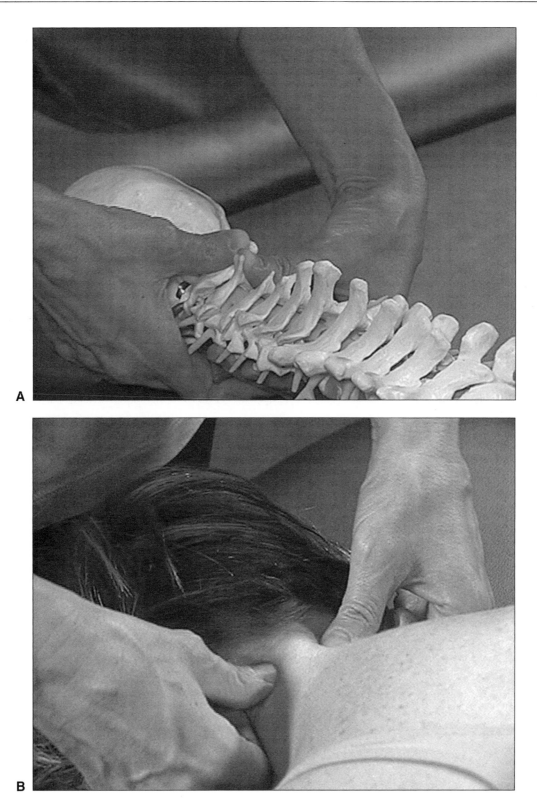

FIGURE 11-8. Lateral glide using the spinous processes/passive accessory vertebral motion.

LATERAL GLIDE USING THE SPINOUS PROCESSES/PASSIVE ACCESSORY VERTEBRAL MOTION (Fig. 11-8)

Purpose

- To examine for lower cervical spine joint impairment
- To increase accessory motion into lower cervical vertebral body rotation and into facet joint distraction on the side toward which the vertebral body is rotating
- To increase range of motion at the lower cervical spine
- To decrease pain
- To improve periarticular muscle performance

Positioning

1. The patient is supine or prone.
2. The cervical spine is placed in midrange in relation to forward/backward bending, side bending, and rotation.
3. The clinician is at the patient's head facing the lower cervical spine.
4. The stabilizing hand is positioned with the tip of the middle finger or the thumb on the lateral surface of the spinous process of the more inferior vertebra.
5. The mobilizing/manipulating hand is positioned with the tip of the middle finger or the thumb on the lateral surface of the spinous process of the more superior vertebra opposite the side of the stabilizing hand.

Procedure

1. The stabilizing hand holds the more inferior vertebra in position.
2. The mobilizing/manipulating hand glides the more superior spinous process toward the contralateral side (see Fig. 11-8).

Particulars

1. This technique might be especially effective for increasing range of motion into lower cervical spine rotation in the direction of vertebral body movement (in the direction opposite the movement of the spinous processes).
2. This technique might be effective in correcting a lower cervical joint rotation positional fault.

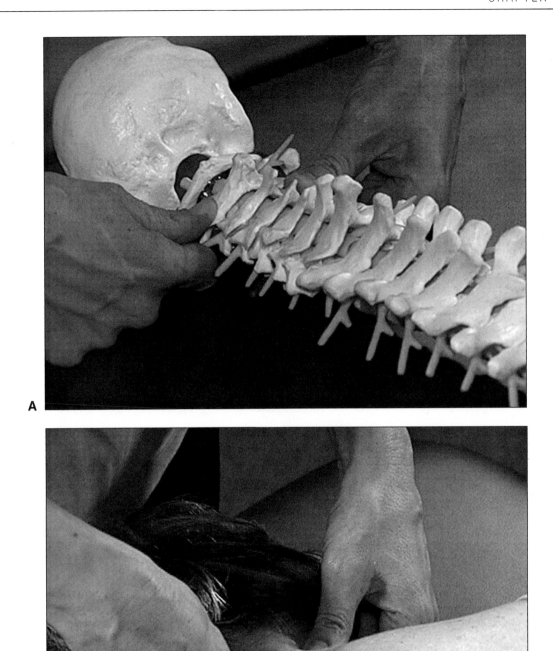

FIGURE 11-9. Anterior glide using the facet joints/passive accessory vertebral motion.

ANTERIOR GLIDE USING THE FACET JOINTS/PASSIVE ACCESSORY VERTEBRAL MOTION (Fig. 11-9)

Purpose
- To examine for lower cervical spine joint impairment
- To increase accessory motion into lower cervical vertebral body rotation and into facet joint distraction on the side toward which the vertebral body is rotating
- To increase range of motion at the lower cervical spine
- To decrease pain
- To improve periarticular muscle performance

Positioning
1. The patient is supine or prone.
2. The cervical spine is placed in midrange in relation to forward/backward bending, side bending, and rotation.
3. The clinician is at the patient's head facing the lower cervical spine.
4. The stabilizing hand is positioned with the tip of the middle finger or the thumb on the facet articular pillars of the more inferior vertebra.
5. The mobilizing/manipulating hand is positioned with the tip of the middle finger or the thumb on the facet articular pillars of the more superior vertebra opposite the side of the stabilizing hand.

Procedure
1. The stabilizing hand holds the more inferior vertebra in position.
2. The mobilizing/manipulating hand glides the more superior facet in an anterior and superior direction (see Fig. 11-9).

Particulars
1. This technique might be especially effective for increasing range of motion into lower cervical spine rotation in the direction of vertebral body movement.
2. This technique might be effective in correcting a lower cervical joint rotation positional fault.
3. This technique is commonly performed using a grade V manipulation.

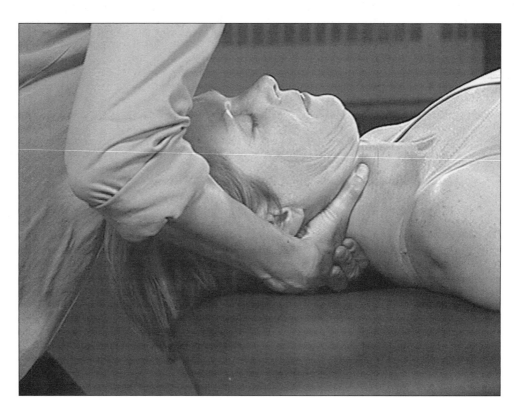

FIGURE 11-10. Side glide/passive accessory vertebral motion.

SIDE GLIDE/PASSIVE ACCESSORY VERTEBRAL MOTION (Fig. 11-10)

Purpose

- To examine for lower cervical spine joint impairment
- To increase accessory motion into lower cervical joint side glide
- To increase range of motion at the lower cervical spine
- To decrease pain
- To improve periarticular muscle performance

Position

1. The patient is supine.
2. The cervical spine is placed in midrange in relation to forward/backward bending, side bending and rotation.
3. The clinician is at the patient's head facing the lower cervical spine.
4. The clinician locks the more superior vertebra of the motion segment being mobilized/manipulated by side bending the patient's neck away from the mobilizing hand to the extent that the motion segment above the one being mobilized/manipulated is fully side bent, but the motion segment being mobilized/manipulated has not yet moved.
5. The stabilizing hand is positioned with the second metacarpophalangeal joint over the facet joint of the more inferior vertebra of the motion segment being mobilized/manipulated on the side to which the patient is side bent.
6. The mobilizing/manipulating hand is positioned with the second metacarpophalangeal joint over the facet joint of the more superior vertebra of the motion segment being mobilized/manipulated on the opposite side as the stabilizing hand and supports the patient's head and neck with the palm of the mobilizing/manipulating hand.

Procedure

1. Testing for signs and symptoms of a potential adverse response to upper cervical movement should be done before performing this or any other lower cervical mobilization/manipulation technique involving cervical spine movement.
2. The stabilizing hand supports the more inferior vertebra.
3. The mobilizing/manipulating hand glides the more superior vertebra toward the contralateral side (see Fig. 11-10).

Particulars

1. This technique is commonly performed using a grade V manipulation.

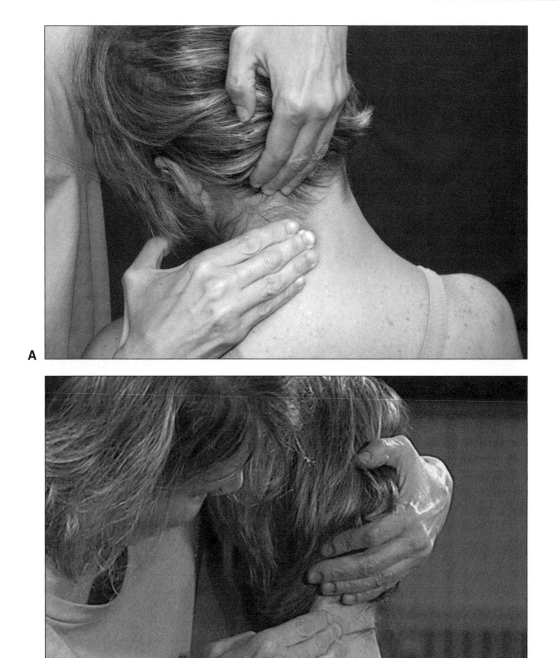

FIGURE 11-11. Rotation glide/passive physiological vertebral motion.

ROTATION GLIDE/PASSIVE PHYSIOLOGICAL VERTEBRAL MOTION (Fig. 11-11)

Purpose

- To increase accessory motion into lower cervical vertebral body rotation, and into facet joint distraction on the side toward which the patient is rotating
- To increase range of motion at the lower cervical spine
- To decrease pain
- To improve periarticular muscle performance

Positioning

1. The patient is sitting.
2. The cervical spine is placed in midrange in relation to forward/backward bending, side bending, and rotation.
3. The clinician is at the patient's side facing the patient with the clinician's arm supporting the patient's head.
4. The clinician locks the more superior vertebrae by rotating the neck toward the clinician (and to the same side as the direction of intended vertebral body motion) to the extent that the motion segment above the one being mobilized/manipulated is fully rotated, but the motion segment being mobilized/manipulated has not yet moved.
5. The stabilizing hand is positioned with the middle finger on the lateral surface of the more inferior spinous process on the opposite side of the direction of the intended vertebral body motion.

Procedure

1. Testing for signs and symptoms of a potential adverse response to upper cervical movement should be done before performing this or any other lower cervical mobilization/manipulation technique involving cervical spine movement.
2. The clinician applies a grade I traction to the vertebral body by lifting the head slightly.
3. The stabilizing hand holds the inferior vertebra in position.
4. The mobilizing/manipulating hand rotates the patient's neck toward the clinician (see Fig. 11-11B).

Particulars

1. The examination procedure for this technique differs from the intervention procedure. To examine for joint mobility, the patient is positioned sitting. The clinician is facing the side of the patient's trunk with one arm supporting the patient's head. The clinician palpates the C2-3 motion segment by placing the palpating finger between the C2 and C3 spinous processes, rotates the patient's neck toward himself or herself until the he or she feels motion between C2 and C3, and grades the amount of motion into rotation that occurred. After grading the motion, the clinician restores slack to the C2-3 motion segment by moving the head slightly back toward neutral and moves the palpating finger to the C3-4 motion segment. This process is repeated until motion into rotation at all lower cervical vertebral motion segments is graded. Mobility into left and right rotation is graded (see Fig. 11-11A).
2. The intervention technique might be especially effective for increasing range of motion into lower cervical spine rotation in the direction of vertebral body movement.
3. The intervention technique might be effective in correcting a lower cervical joint rotation positional fault.
4. The intervention technique is commonly performed using a grade V manipulation.

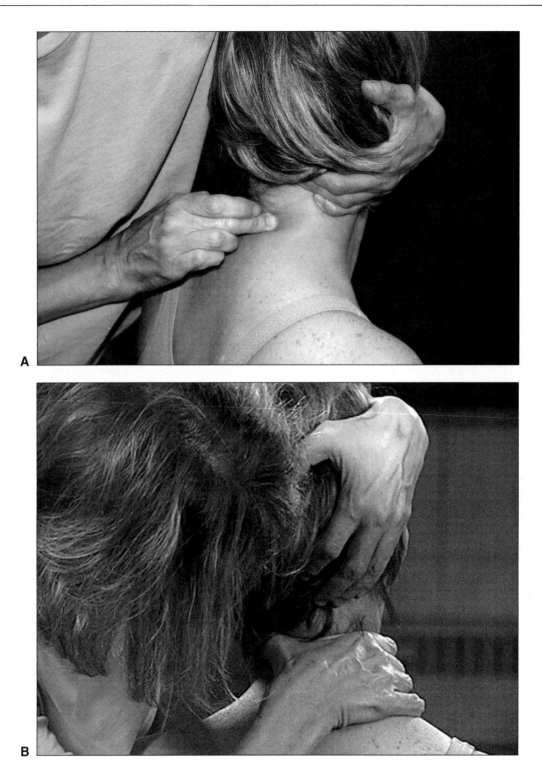

A

B

FIGURE 11-12. Side bending glide/passive physiological vertebral motion.

SIDE BENDING GLIDE/PASSIVE PHYSIOLOGICAL VERTEBRAL MOTION
(Fig. 11-12)

Purpose

- To increase accessory motion into lower cervical joint side bending
- To increase range of motion at the lower cervical spine
- To decrease pain
- To improve periarticular muscle performance

Positioning

1. The patient is sitting.
2. The cervical spine is placed in midrange in relation to forward/backward bending, side bending, and rotation.
3. The clinician is at the patient's side facing the patient with the clinician's arm supporting the patient's head.
4. The clinician locks the more superior vertebrae by side bending the neck toward the clinician (and to the same side as the direction of intended vertebral body motion) to the extent that the motion segment above the one being mobilized/manipulated is fully side bent, but the motion segment being mobilized/manipulated has not yet moved.
5. The stabilizing hand is positioned with the web space gripping the more inferior vertebra.

Procedure

1. Testing for signs and symptoms of a potential adverse response to upper cervical movement should be done before performing this or any other lower cervical mobilization/manipulation technique involving cervical spine movement.
2. The clinician applies a grade I traction to the vertebral body by lifting the head slightly.
3. The stabilizing hand holds the inferior vertebra in position.
4. The mobilizing/manipulating hand side bends the patient's neck toward the clinician (see Fig. 11-12B).

Particulars

1. The examination procedure for this technique differs from the intervention procedure. To examine for joint mobility, the patient is positioned sitting. The clinician is facing the side of the patient's trunk with one arm supporting the patient's head. The clinician palpates the C2-3 motion segment by placing the palpating finger between the C2 and C3 spinous processes, side bends the patient's neck toward himself or herself until he or she feels motion between C2 and C3, and grades the amount of motion into side bending that occurred. After grading the motion, the clinician restores slack to the C2-3 motion segment by moving the head slightly back toward neutral and moves the palpating finger to the C3-4 motion segment. This process is repeated until motion into side bending at all lower cervical vertebral motion segments is graded. Mobility into left and right side bending is graded (see Fig. 11-12A).
2. The intervention technique might be especially effective for increasing range of motion into lower cervical spine side bending in the direction of vertebral body movement.
3. The intervention technique is commonly performed using a grade V manipulation.

REFERENCES

1. Hurwitz EL, Aker PD, Adams AH, et al: Manipulation and mobilization of the cervical spine: a systematic review of the literature. Spine 1996;21:1746-1760.
2. Coulter I: Manipulation and mobilization of the cervical spine: the results of a literature survey and consensus panel. J Musculoskel Pain 1996;4:113-123.
3. Coulter I: Efficacy and risks of chiropractic manipulation: what does the evidence suggest? Integr Med 1998;1:61-66.
4. Gross AR, Aker PD, Goldsmith CH, et al: Conservative management of mechanical neck disorders: a systematic overview and meta-analysis. Online J Curr Clin Trials 1994;3.
5. Assendelft WJJ, Bouter LM, Knipschild PG: Complications of spinal manipulation: a comprehensive review of the literature. J Fam Pract 1996;42:475-480.
6. Haldeman S, Kohlbeck FJ, McGregor M: Risk factors and precipitating neck movements causing vertebrobasilar artery dissection after cervical trauma and spinal manipulation. Spine 1999;24:785-794.
7. Barker S, Kesson M, Ashmore J, et al: Guidance for pre-manipulative testing of the cervical spine. Physiotherapy 2001;87:318-322.
8. Vernon HT, Aker P, Burns S, et al: Pressure pain threshold evaluation of the effect of spinal manipulation in the treatment of chronic neck pain: a pilot study. J Manip Physiol Therap 1990;13:13-16.
9. Cassidy JD, Lopes AA, Yong-Hing K: The immediate effect of manipulation versus mobilization on pain and range of motion in the cervical spine: a randomized controlled trial. J Manip Physiol Therap 1992;15:570-587.
10. Cassidy JD, Lopes AA, Yong-Hing K: The immediate effect of manipulation versus mobilization on pain and range of motion in the cervical spine: a randomized controlled trial (letter to the editor). J Manip Physiol Therap 1993;16:279-280.
11. Hurwitz EL, Morgenstern H, Harber P, et al: A randomized trial of chiropractic manipulation and mobilization for patients with neck pain: clinical outcomes from the UCLA Neck-Pain Study. Am J Public Health 2002;92:1634-1641.
12. DiFabio RP: Manipulation of the cervical spine: risks and benefits. Phys Ther 1999;79:50-65.
13. van Schalkwyk R, Parkin-Smith GF: A clinical trial investigating the possible effect of the supine cervical rotatory manipulation and the supine lateral break manipulation in the treatment of mechanical neck pain: a pilot study. J Manip Physiol Therap 2000;23:324-331.
14. Clements B, Gibbons P, McLaughlin P: The amelioration of atlanto-axial rotation asymmetry using high velocity low amplitude manipulations: is the direction of thrust important? J Osteopath Med 2001;4:8-14.
15. Gross AR, Aker PD, Quartly C: Manual therapy in the treatment of neck pain. Rheum Dis Clin North Am 1996;22:579-598.
16. Aker PD, Gross AR, Goldsmith CH, et al: Conservative management of mechanical neck pain: systematic overview and meta-analysis. BMJ 1996;313:1291-1296.
17. Gross AR, Hoving JL, Haines TA, et al. Manipulation and Mobilization for Mechanical neck disorders: The Cochrane Database of Systematic Reviews 2005 (4).
18. Kjellman GV, Skargren EI, Oberg BE: A critical analysis of randomized clinical trials on neck pain and treatment efficacy: a review of the literature. Scand J Rehabil Med 1999;31:139-152.
19. Korthals-de Bos IB, Hoving JL, van Tulder MW, et al. Cost effectiveness of physiotherapy, manual therapy, and general practitioner care for neck pain: Economic evaluation alongside a randomized controlled trial. BMJ 2003;326:911.
20. Bogduk N: Whiplash. "Why pay for what does not work?" J Musculoskel Pain 2000;8:29-53.
21. Vernon H, McDermaid CS, Hagino C: Systematic review of randomized clinical trials of complementary/alternative therapies in the treatment of tension-type and cervicogenic headache. Complement Ther Med 1999;7:142-155.
22. Astin JA, Ernst E: The effectiveness of spinal manipulation for the treatment of headache disorders: a systematic review of randomized clinical trials. Cephalalgia 2002;22:617-623.
23. Jull G, Trott P, Potter H, et al: A randomized controlled trial of exercise and manipulative therapy for cervicogenic headache. Spine 2002;27:1835-1843.
24. Vicenzino B, Collins D, Wright A: The initial effects of a cervical spine manipulative physiotherapy treatment on the pain and dysfunction of lateral epicondylalgia. Pain 1996;68:69-74.
25. Vicenzino B, Collins D, Benson H, et al: An investigation of the interrelationship between manipulative therapy-induced hypoalgesia and sympathetoexcitation. J Manip Physiol Therap 1998;21:448-453.
26. Cyriax J: Textbook of Orthopaedic Medicine, Vol 1: Diagnosis of Soft Tissue Lesions, 8th ed. London, Bailliere Tindall, 1982.

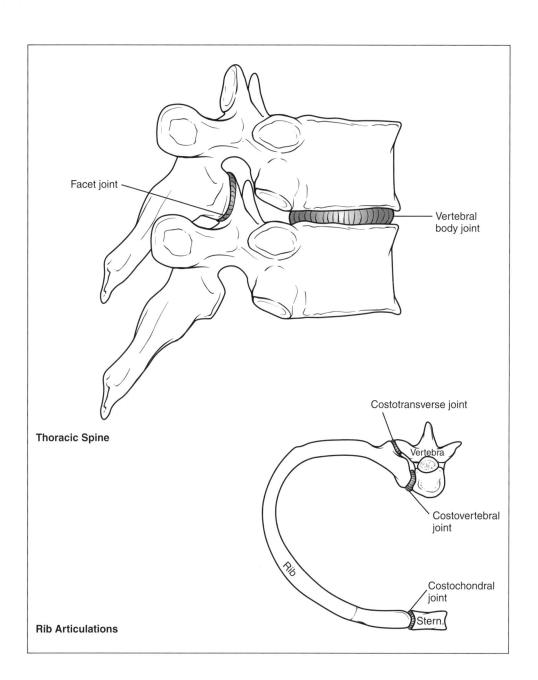

Thoracic Spine

Facet joint

Vertebral body joint

Rib Articulations

Costotransverse joint

Vertebra

Costovertebral joint

Rib

Costochondral joint

Stern.

CHAPTER 12

The Thoracic Spine and Ribs

BASICS

One major role related specifically to the thoracic spine and ribs is the protection of vital organs. The thoracic spine also provides stability in the upright position. The ribs assist in this role by blocking thoracic spine motion. Despite its function as a supporting structure, the thoracic spine contributes to 25% of the total movement in the spine.

Thoracic Joints

The spinous processes in the thoracic spine are positioned inferior to the motion segment. They can be used as a lever to move the vertebral body, resulting in a gliding of the facet articulations that corresponds to the physiological movement that occurs with forward and backward bending in the thoracic spine.

The facet joints in the thoracic spine are oriented in a similar manner to the facet joints of the cervical spine except that they are aligned more vertically, almost parallel with the frontal plane. Similar to the lower cervical spine, forward and backward bending is accompanied by a gliding motion between the two facet articulations, although with less movement in an anterior direction.

Rib Joints

Thoracic spine motion is restricted primarily by the ribs. The ribs attach to the vertebral bodies and to the vertebral transverse processes of the thoracic spine. Rib movement is guided in part by thoracic spine motion and in part by the act of breathing.

The first rib is capable of only a small amount of motion because it is fused anteriorly to the sternum. Ribs two through five move primarily in an anterior and superior direction with inspiration and in a posterior and inferior direction with expiration; this is called *pump-handle motion*. Ribs seven through ten move primarily laterally and superiorly with inspiration and medially and inferiorly with expiration; this is called *bucket-handle motion*. Ribs five through seven are transitional ribs and exhibit characteristics of both types of movements. All of these motions are accompanied by rotation of the ribs around their longitudinal axes. Ribs 11 and 12 are capable of movement, but generally are held in a relative position of expiration posteriorly by the quadratus lumborum muscle. When they do move, it is in a lateral direction with inspiration and in a medial direction with expiration; this is called *caliper motion*.

SPECIFIC PATHOLOGY AND THORACIC SPINE AND RIB JOINT MOBILIZATION/MANIPULATION

Mechanical Mid Back Pain

Only one major study has been performed investigating the efficacy of mobilization/manipulation on patients with thoracic spine pain,[1] and no studies specifically have addressed the ribs. In the study of thoracic spine pain, 30 subjects with mechanical mid back pain were randomly assigned to receive grade V manipulation to hypomobile thoracic segments or detuned ultrasound for a maximum of six treatment sessions. Subjects receiving manipulation showed a significant reduction in pain at follow-up compared with the placebo group. These changes were maintained at one-month follow-up.

THORACIC JOINTS (T3-4 THROUGH T12-L1)

Osteokinematic motions:
   Forward/backward bending
   Side bending
   Rotation
Ligaments:
   Anterior longitudinal ligament
   Posterior longitudinal ligament
   Supraspinous ligament
   Interspinous ligament
   Ligamentum flavum
   Intertransverse ligaments

Joint orientation:
   Inferior facet of superior vertebra: anterior, inferior, medial
   Superior facet of inferior vertebra: posterior, superior, lateral
   Superior vertebral body: inferior
   Inferior vertebral body: superior
Type of joint:
   Facets: synovial
   Disc: amphiarthrodial
Concave joint surface:
   None, these are plane joints
Resting position:
   Not described by Kaltenborn
Close-packed position:
   Not described by Kaltenborn
Capsular pattern of restriction:
   Difficult to determine[2]

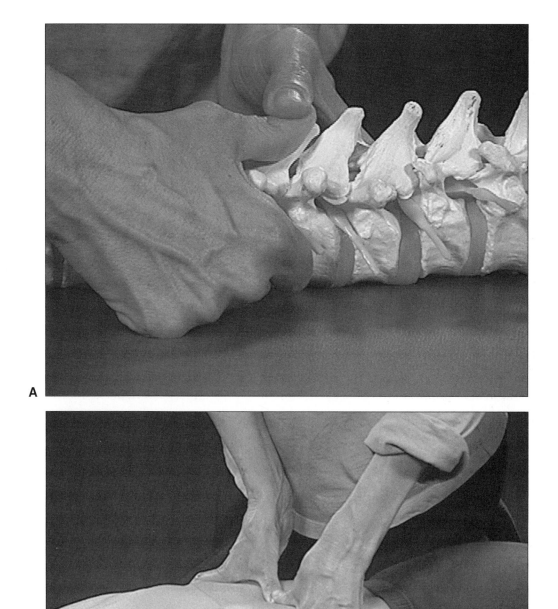

A

B

FIGURE 12-1. Anterior glide using the spinous processes/passive accessory vertebral motion: first technique.

ANTERIOR GLIDE USING THE SPINOUS PROCESSES/PASSIVE ACCESSORY VERTEBRAL MOTION: FIRST TECHNIQUE (Fig. 12-1)

Purpose

- To examine for thoracic spine joint impairment
- To increase accessory motion into thoracic joint anterior glide
- To increase range of motion at the thoracic spine
- To decrease pain
- To improve periarticular muscle performance

Positioning

1. The patient is prone.
2. The thoracic spine is placed in midrange in relation to forward/backward bending, side bending, and rotation.
3. The clinician is at the patient's side facing the thoracic spine.
4. The mobilizing/manipulating hand is positioned with the heel of the hand or the thumb over the guiding hand.
5. The guiding hand is positioned with the thumb over the spinous process being mobilized/manipulated.

Procedure

1. The mobilizing/manipulating hand glides the spinous process anteriorly as the patient exhales.
2. The guiding hand controls the position of the mobilizing/manipulating hand (see Fig. 12-1).

Particulars

1. This technique also is called *springing*. If it is being performed as an examination technique, the term *spring testing* is used.
2. This technique is commonly performed using a grade V manipulation.

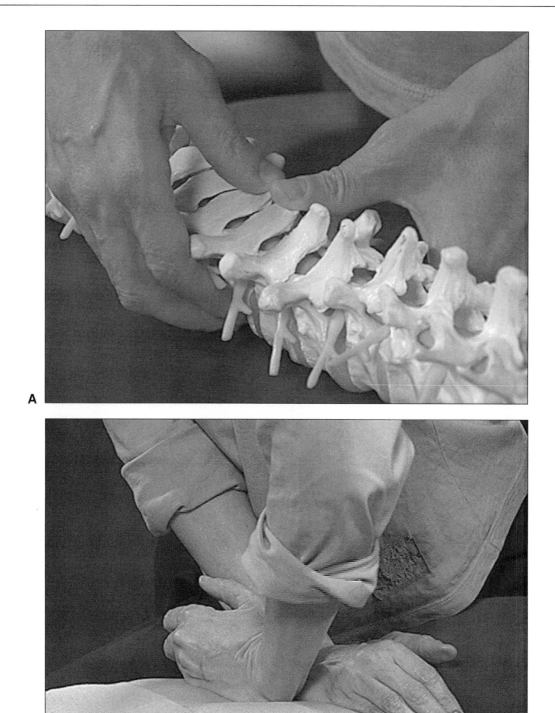

FIGURE 12-2. Anterior glide using the spinous processes/passive accessory vertebral motion: second technique.

ANTERIOR GLIDE USING THE SPINOUS PROCESSES/PASSIVE ACCESSORY VERTEBRAL MOTION: SECOND TECHNIQUE (Fig. 12-2)

Purpose

- To examine for thoracic spine joint impairment
- To increase accessory motion into thoracic joint anterior glide
- To increase range of motion at the thoracic spine
- To decrease pain
- To improve periarticular muscle performance

Positioning

1. The patient is prone.
2. The thoracic spine is placed in midrange in relation to forward/backward bending, side bending, and rotation.
3. The clinician is at the patient's side facing the thoracic spine.
4. The stabilizing hand is positioned with the thumb or the anterior surface of the pisiform on the spinous process of the more inferior vertebra.
5. The mobilizing/manipulating hand is positioned with the thumb or the medial (ulnar) surface of the pisiform over the spinous process of the more superior vertebra.

Procedure

1. The stabilizing hand holds the vertebra in position.
2. The mobilizing/manipulating hand glides the spinous process anteriorly as the patient exhales (see Fig. 12-2).

Particulars

1. This technique might be especially effective for increasing range of motion into thoracic spine backward bending.
2. This technique might be effective in correcting a thoracic joint forward/backward bending positional fault.
3. This technique is commonly performed using a grade V manipulation.

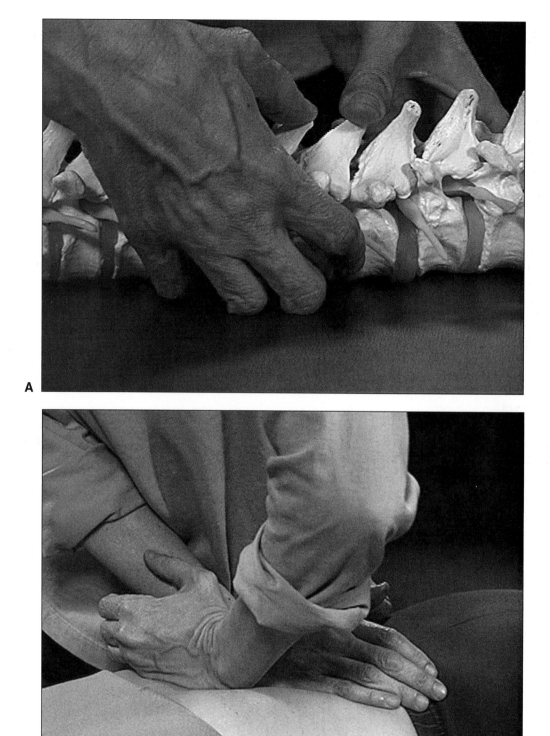

FIGURE 12-3. Anterior glide using the spinous processes/passive accessory vertebral motion: third technique.

ANTERIOR GLIDE USING THE SPINOUS PROCESSES/PASSIVE ACCESSORY VERTEBRAL MOTION: THIRD TECHNIQUE (Fig. 12-3)

Purpose
- To examine for thoracic spine joint impairment
- To increase accessory motion into thoracic joint anterior glide
- To increase range of motion at the thoracic spine
- To decrease pain
- To improve periarticular muscle performance

Positioning
1. The patient is prone.
2. The thoracic spine is placed in midrange in relation to forward/backward bending, side bending, and rotation.
3. The clinician is at the patient's side facing the thoracic spine.
4. The stabilizing hand is positioned with the thumb or the medial (ulnar) surface of the pisiform on the spinous process of the more superior vertebra.
5. The mobilizing/manipulating hand is positioned with the thumb or the anterior surface of the pisiform over the spinous process of the more inferior vertebra.

Procedure
1. The stabilizing hand holds the vertebra in position.
2. The mobilizing/manipulating hand glides the spinous process anteriorly as the patient exhales (see Fig. 12-3).

Particulars
1. This technique might be especially effective for increasing range of motion into thoracic spine forward bending.
2. This technique might be effective in correcting a thoracic joint forward/backward bending positional fault.
3. This technique is commonly performed using a grade V manipulation.

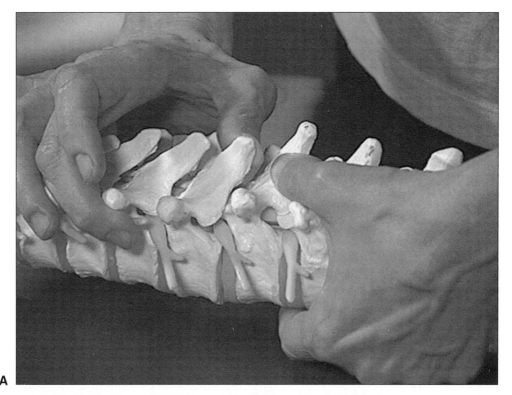

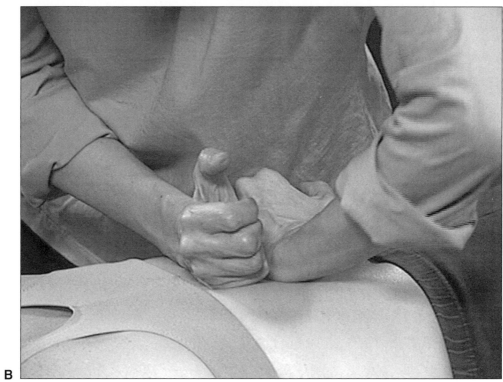

FIGURE 12-4. Lateral glide using the spinous processes/passive accessory vertebral motion.

LATERAL GLIDE USING THE SPINOUS PROCESSES/PASSIVE ACCESSORY VERTEBRAL MOTION (Fig. 12-4)

Purpose

- To examine for thoracic spine joint impairment
- To increase accessory motion into thoracic vertebral body rotation and into facet joint distraction on the side toward which the vertebral body is rotating
- To increase range of motion at the thoracic spine
- To decrease pain
- To improve periarticular muscle performance

Positioning

1. The patient is prone.
2. The thoracic spine is placed in midrange in relation to forward/backward bending, side bending, and rotation.
3. The clinician is at the patient's side facing the thoracic spine.
4. The stabilizing hand is positioned with the thumb or the anterior surface of the pisiform on the lateral surface of the spinous process of the more inferior vertebra.
5. The mobilizing/manipulating hand is positioned with the thumb or the anterior surface of the pisiform on the lateral surface of the spinous process of the more superior vertebra opposite the side of the stabilizing hand.

Procedure

1. The stabilizing hand holds the more inferior vertebra in position.
2. The mobilizing/manipulating hand glides the more superior spinous process toward the contralateral side as the patient exhales (see Fig. 12-4).

Particulars

1. This technique might be especially effective for increasing range of motion into thoracic spine rotation in the direction of vertebral body movement (in the direction opposite the movement of the spinous processes).
2. This technique might be effective in correcting a thoracic joint rotation positional fault.
3. This technique is commonly performed using a grade V manipulation.

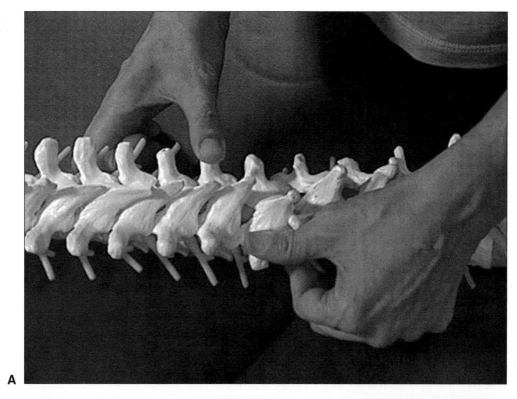

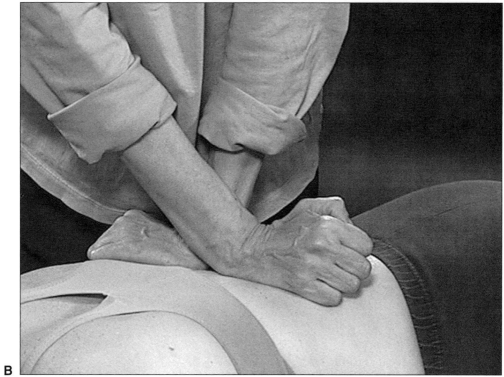

FIGURE 12-5. Anterior glide using the transverse processes/passive accessory vertebral motion.

ANTERIOR GLIDE USING THE TRANSVERSE PROCESSES/PASSIVE ACCESSORY VERTEBRAL MOTION (Fig. 12-5)

Purpose

- To examine for thoracic spine joint impairment
- To increase accessory motion into thoracic vertebral body rotation and into facet joint distraction on the side toward which the vertebral body is rotating
- To increase range of motion at the thoracic spine
- To decrease pain
- To improve periarticular muscle performance

Positioning

1. The patient is prone.
2. The thoracic spine is placed in midrange in relation to forward/backward bending, side bending, and rotation.
3. The clinician is at the patient's side facing the thoracic spine.
4. The stabilizing hand is positioned with the thumb or the anterior surface of the pisiform on the transverse process of the more inferior vertebra.
5. The mobilizing/manipulating hand is positioned with the thumb or the anterior surface of the pisiform on the transverse process of the more superior vertebra opposite the side of the stabilizing hand.

Procedure

1. The stabilizing hand holds the more inferior vertebra in position.
2. The mobilizing/manipulating hand glides the more superior transverse process in an anterior direction as the patient exhales (see Fig. 12-5).

Particulars

1. This technique might be especially effective for increasing range of motion into thoracic spine rotation in the direction of vertebral body movement.
2. This technique might be effective in correcting a thoracic joint rotation positional fault.
3. This technique is commonly performed using a grade V manipulation.

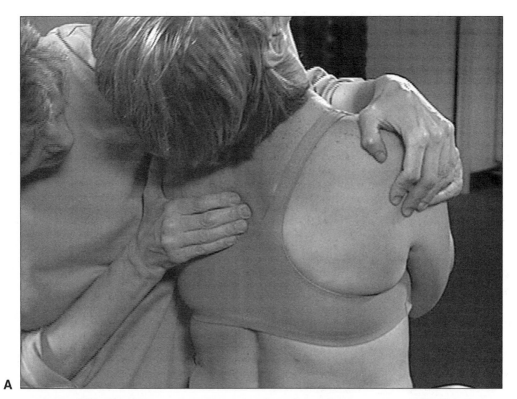

A

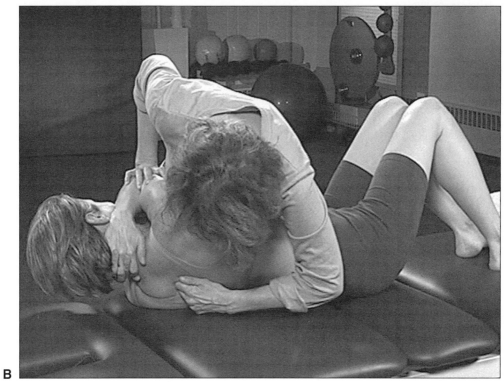

B

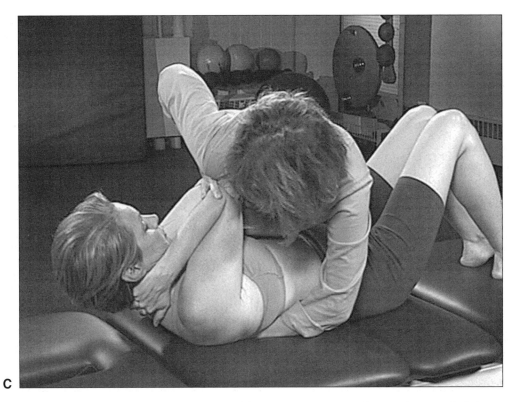

C

FIGURE 12-6. Posterior/superior glide of the more superior vertebra on the more inferior vertebra/manipulation/passive accessory vertebral motion.

POSTERIOR/SUPERIOR GLIDE OF THE MORE SUPERIOR VERTEBRA ON THE MORE INFERIOR VERTEBRA/MANIPULATION/PASSIVE ACCESSORY VERTEBRAL MOTION (Fig. 12-6)

Purpose
- To increase accessory motion in thoracic spine joints
- To increase range of motion at the thoracic spine
- To decrease pain
- To improve periarticular muscle performance

Positioning
1. The patient is supine with the fingers laced together at the base of the neck and the elbows touching.
2. The thoracic spine is placed in midrange in relation to forward/backward bending, side bending, and rotation.
3. The clinician is at the patient's side.
4. A pillow can be used to separate the patient's chest from the clinician.
5. The clinician lifts the patient's contralateral shoulder, rotating the patient toward the clinician, and reaches across the patient's trunk to position the stabilizing hand on the patient's thoracic spine.
6. The stabilizing hand is positioned on the more inferior vertebra such that the hand is closed, the middle phalanx of the index finger is on the patient's transverse process closest to the clinician, the thenar eminence is on the patient's transverse process farthest away from the clinician, and the thumb is along the side of the patient's spinous processes above the motion segment being stabilized (Fig. 12-6B).
7. The clinician repositions the patient in supine position.
8. The clinician locks the more superior vertebrae by forward bending the spine using the patient's arms as a fulcrum to the extent that the motion segment above the one being manipulated is fully flexed, but the motion segment being manipulated has not yet moved.
9. The manipulating hand grips the patient's elbows.

Procedure

1. The stabilizing hand holds the more inferior vertebra in position.
2. The manipulating hand glides the more superior vertebra posteriorly and superiorly by moving the patient's elbows in a posterior and superior direction, directing the force through the long axis of the patient's upper arms. The clinician also should use body weight to assist in directing this force. This technique should be timed to occur as the patient exhales (see Fig. 12-6C).

Particulars

1. The examination procedure for this technique differs from the intervention procedure. To examine for joint mobility, the patient is positioned sitting with arms across the chest. The clinician is facing the side of the patient's trunk with one shoulder positioned in front of the patient's shoulder, the arm reaching across the patient's anterior trunk, and the hand placed on the contralateral shoulder. The clinician palpates the T3-4 motion segment by placing the palpating finger between the T3 and T4 spinous processes, forward bends the patient toward himself or herself until he or she feels motion between T3 and T4, and grades the amount of motion that occurred into forward bending. After grading the motion, the clinician restores slack to the T3-4 motion segment by moving the spine slightly back toward neutral and moves the palpating finger to the T4-5 motion segment. This process is repeated until motion into forward bending at all thoracic vertebral motion segments is graded. It is repeated for backward bending motion (see Fig. 12-6A).

2. The intervention technique should be performed using grade V manipulations.
3. The intervention technique might be especially effective for increasing range of motion into thoracic spine backward bending.
4. The intervention technique might be effective in correcting a thoracic joint forward/backward bending positional fault.

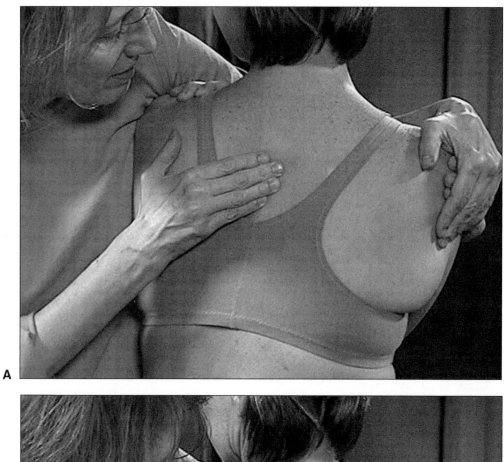

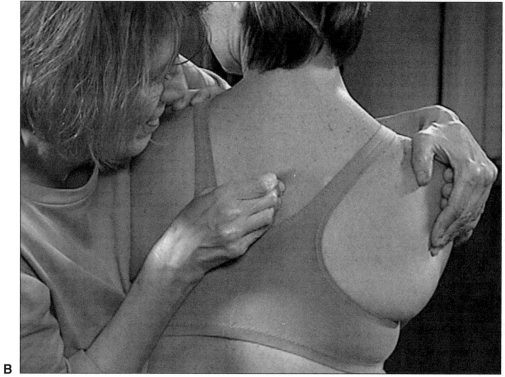

FIGURE 12-7. Rotation glide/passive physiological vertebral motion.

ROTATION GLIDE/PASSIVE PHYSIOLOGICAL VERTEBRAL MOTION (Fig. 12-7)

Purpose

- To increase accessory motion into thoracic vertebral body rotation, and into facet joint distraction on the side toward which the patient is rotating
- To increase range of motion at the thoracic spine
- To decrease pain
- To improve periarticular muscle performance

Positioning

1. The patient is sitting with the arms positioned across the chest.
2. The thoracic spine is placed in midrange in relation to forward/backward bending, side bending, and rotation.
3. The clinician is at the patient's side facing the patient with the clinician's arms across the patient's chest and the clinician's anterior shoulder and hand supporting the patient's shoulders.
4. The clinician locks the more superior vertebrae by rotating the trunk toward the clinician (and to the same side as the direction of intended vertebral body motion) to the extent that the motion segment above the one being mobilized/manipulated is fully rotated, but the motion segment being mobilized/manipulated has not yet moved.
5. The stabilizing hand is positioned with the middle finger on the lateral surface of the more inferior spinous process on the opposite side of the direction of the intended vertebral body motion.

Procedure

1. The clinician applies a grade I traction to the vertebral body by lifting the trunk slightly with the arms of the mobilizing/manipulating hand.
2. The stabilizing hand holds the inferior vertebra in position.
3. The mobilizing/manipulating hand rotates the patient's trunk toward the clinician (see Fig. 12-7B).

Particulars

1. The examination procedure for this technique differs from the intervention procedure. To examine for joint mobility, the patient is positioned sitting with arms across the chest. The clinician is facing the side of the patient's trunk with one shoulder positioned in front of the patient's shoulder, the arm reaching across the patient's anterior trunk, and the hand placed on the contralateral shoulder. The clinician palpates the T3-4 motion segment by placing the palpating finger between the T3 and T4 spinous processes, rotates the patient toward himself or herself until he or she feels motion between T3 and T4, and grades the amount of motion that occurred into rotation. After grading the motion, the clinician restores slack to the T3-4 motion segment by moving the spine slightly back toward neutral and moves the palpating finger to the T4-5 motion segment. This process is repeated until motion into rotation at all thoracic vertebral motion segments is graded. Mobility into left and right rotation is graded (see Fig. 12-7A).
2. The intervention technique might be especially effective for increasing range of motion into thoracic spine rotation in the direction of vertebral body movement.
3. The intervention technique might be effective in correcting a thoracic joint rotation positional fault.

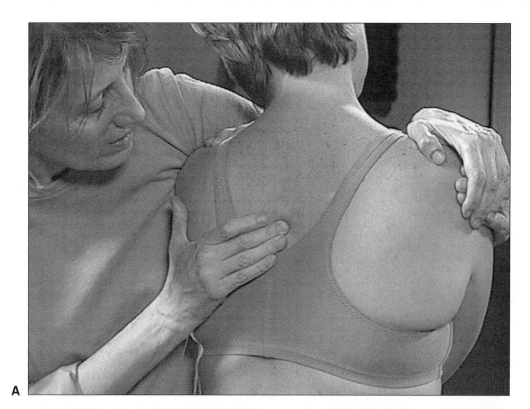

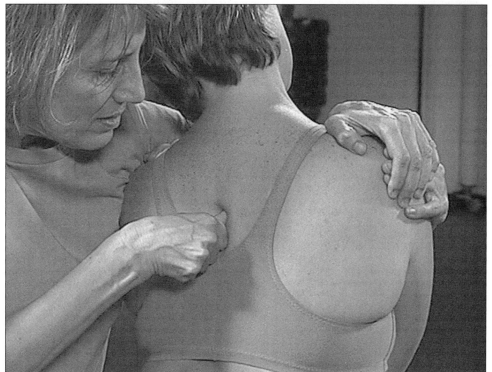

FIGURE 12-8. Side bending glide/passive physiological vertebral motion.

SIDE BENDING GLIDE/PASSIVE PHYSIOLOGICAL VERTEBRAL MOTION (Fig. 12-8)

Purpose

- To increase accessory motion into thoracic joint side bending
- To increase range of motion at the thoracic spine
- To decrease pain
- To improve periarticular muscle performance

Positioning

1. The patient is sitting with the arms positioned across the chest.
2. The thoracic spine is placed in midrange in relation to forward/backward bending, side bending, and rotation.
3. The clinician is at the patient's side facing the patient with the clinician's arm across the patient's chest and the clinician's anterior shoulder and hand supporting the patient's shoulders.
4. The clinician locks the more superior vertebrae by side bending the trunk toward the clinician (and to the same side as the direction of intended vertebral body motion) to the extent that the motion segment above the one being mobilized/manipulated is fully side bent, but the motion segment being mobilized/manipulated has not yet moved.
5. The stabilizing hand is positioned with the thumb or middle finger on either side of the lateral surface of the more inferior spinous process.

Procedure

1. The clinician applies a grade I traction to the vertebral body by lifting the trunk slightly with the arms of the mobilizing hand.
2. The stabilizing hand holds the inferior vertebra in position.
3. The mobilizing/manipulating hand side bends the patient's trunk toward the clinician (see Fig. 12-8B).

Particulars

1. The examination procedure for this technique differs from the intervention procedure. To examine for joint mobility, the patient is positioned sitting with the arms across the chest. The clinician is facing the side of the patient's trunk with one shoulder positioned in front of the patient's shoulder, the arm reaching across the patient's anterior trunk, and the hand placed on the contralateral shoulder. The clinician palpates the T3-4 motion segment by placing the palpating finger between the T3 and T4 spinous processes, side bends the patient toward himself or herself until he or she feels motion between T3 and T4, and grades the amount of motion that occurred into side bending. After grading the motion, the clinician restores slack to the T3-4 motion segment by moving the spine slightly back toward neutral and moves the palpating finger to the T4-5 motion segment. This process is repeated until motion into side bending at all thoracic vertebral motion segments is graded. Mobility into left and right side bending is graded (see Fig. 12-8A).
2. The intervention technique might be especially effective for increasing range of motion into thoracic spine side bending in the direction of vertebral body movement.

RIB JOINTS

Osteokinematic motions:
  Anterior/posterior
  Lateral/medial
  Superior/inferior
  Rotation
Ligaments: Costovertebral joints:
  Capsular ligament
  Radiate ligament
  Intra-articular ligament
Ligaments: Costotransverse joints:
  Capsular ligament
  Costotransverse ligament
Joint orientation:
  Vertebral body: posterior, lateral
  Rib at costovertebral joint: anterior, medial
  Vertebral transverse process: anterior, lateral
  Rib at costotransverse joint: posterior, medial
  Sternum: lateral, inferior
  Rib at costochondral joint: medial, superior
Type of joint:
  Costovertebral joint: synovial
  Costotransverse joint: synovial
  Costochondral joint: synchondrosis
Concave joint surface:
  None, these are plane joints
Resting position:
  Not described by Kaltenborn
Close-packed position:
  Not described by Kaltenborn
Capsular pattern of restriction:
  Not described by Cyriax

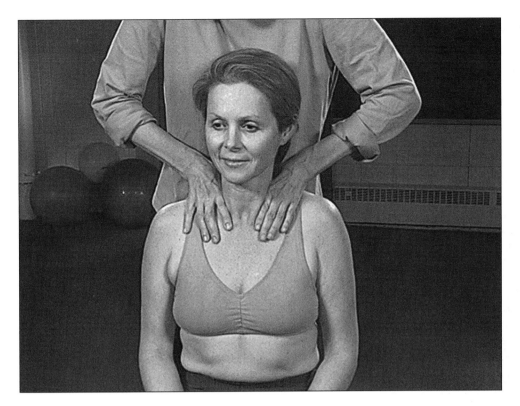

FIGURE 12-9. Inferior glide of the first rib/passive accessory motion.

INFERIOR GLIDE OF THE FIRST RIB/PASSIVE ACCESSORY MOTION (Fig. 12-9)

Purpose

- To examine for first rib joint impairment
- To increase accessory motion in the articulations at the first rib
- To increase range of motion at the first rib
- To decrease pain
- To improve periarticular muscle performance

Positioning

1. The patient is sitting.
2. The trunk is placed in midrange in relation to forward/backward bending, side bending, and rotation.
3. The clinician is behind the patient facing the patient's trunk.
4. The stabilizing hand is positioned on the superior surface of the first rib on the side that is not being mobilized/manipulated.
5. The mobilizing hand is positioned on the superior surface of the first rib on the side being mobilized/manipulated.

Procedure

1. The stabilizing hand holds the rib in position.
2. The mobilizing/manipulating hand glides the rib in an inferior direction as the patient exhales (see Fig. 12-9).

Particulars

1. This technique might be effective in correcting a first rib joint inspiration positional fault or chronic positioning of the first rib into elevation, such as in patients with chronic obstructive pulmonary disease who breathe primarily using the apical musculature. This positional fault might be a contributing factor to the onset of thoracic outlet syndrome.
2. This technique is commonly performed using a grade V manipulation.

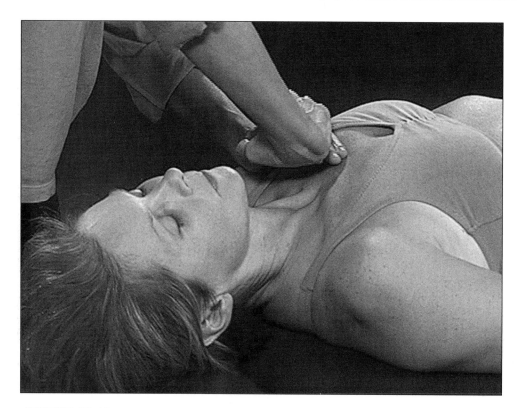

FIGURE 12-10. Expiration glide of ribs two through seven/passive physiological motion.

EXPIRATION GLIDE OF RIBS TWO THROUGH SEVEN/PASSIVE PHYSIOLOGICAL MOTION (Fig. 12-10)

Purpose

- To examine for rib joint impairment
- To increase accessory motion in the articulations at ribs two through seven
- To increase range of motion at ribs two through seven
- To decrease pain
- To improve periarticular muscle performance

Positioning

1. The patient is supine.
2. The trunk is placed in midrange in relation to forward/backward bending, side bending, and rotation.
3. The clinician is at the patient's side facing the patient's trunk.
4. The mobilizing hand is positioned on the anterior or anterolateral surface of the trunk with the medial (ulnar) border of the hand between the rib being mobilized and the one above.
5. The guiding hand is positioned over the mobilizing hand.

Procedure

1. The mobilizing hand guides the rib in a posterior and inferior direction as the patient exhales and resists anterior and superior motion as the patient inhales.
2. The guiding hand controls the position of the mobilizing hand (see Fig. 12-10).

Particulars

1. This is not a grade V manipulation technique.
2. This technique might be especially effective for increasing range of motion into pump-handle expiration at ribs two through seven.
3. This technique might be effective in correcting a rib joint inspiration/expiration positional fault.

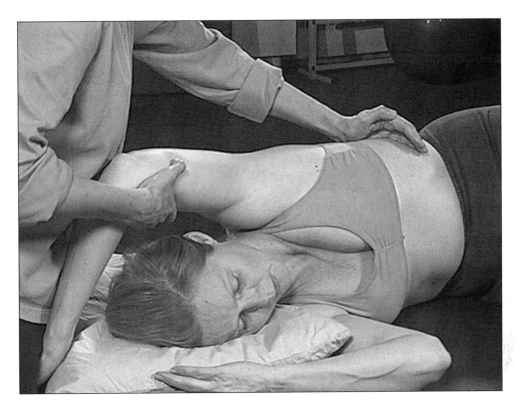

FIGURE 12-11. Expiration glide of ribs 5 through 11/passive physiological motion.

EXPIRATION GLIDE OF RIBS 5 THROUGH 11/PASSIVE PHYSIOLOGICAL MOTION (Fig. 12-11)

Purpose
- To examine for rib joint impairment
- To increase accessory motion in the articulations at ribs 5 through 11
- To increase range of motion at ribs 5 through 11
- To decrease pain
- To improve periarticular muscle performance

Positioning
1. The patient is side lying with the arm positioned over the head.
2. The trunk is placed in midrange in relation to forward/backward bending, side bending, and rotation.
3. The clinician is at the patient's head facing the patient's trunk.
4. The mobilizing hand is positioned on the lateral surface of the trunk with the medial (ulnar) border of the hand between the rib being mobilized and the one above.
5. The guiding hand holds the patient's arm.

Procedure
1. The mobilizing hand guides the rib in a medial and inferior direction as the patient exhales and resists lateral and superior motion as the patient inhales.
2. The guiding hand controls the position of the patient's arm (see Fig. 12-11).

Particulars
1. This is not a grade V manipulation technique.
2. This technique might be especially effective for increasing range of motion into bucket-handle expiration at ribs 5 through 11.
3. This technique might be effective in correcting a rib joint inspiration/expiration positional fault.

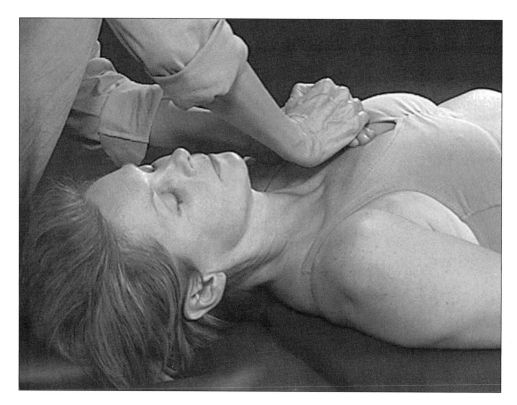

FIGURE 12-12. Inspiration glide of ribs two through seven/passive physiological motion.

INSPIRATION GLIDE OF RIBS TWO THROUGH SEVEN/PASSIVE PHYSIOLOGICAL MOTION (Fig. 12-12)

Purpose
- To examine for rib joint impairment
- To increase accessory motion in the articulations at ribs two through seven
- To increase range of motion at ribs two through seven
- To decrease pain
- To improve periarticular muscle performance

Positioning
1. The patient is supine.
2. The trunk is placed in midrange in relation to forward/backward bending, side bending, and rotation.
3. The clinician is at the patient's side facing the patient's trunk.
4. The mobilizing hand is positioned on the anterior or anterolateral surface of the trunk with the medial (ulnar) border of the hand between the rib being mobilized and the one below.
5. The guiding hand is positioned over the mobilizing hand.

Procedure
1. The mobilizing hand guides the rib in an anterior and superior direction as the patient inhales and resists posterior and inferior motion as the patient exhales.
2. The guiding hand controls the position of the mobilizing hand (see Fig. 12-12).

Particulars
1. This is not a grade V manipulation technique.
2. This technique might be especially effective for increasing range of motion into bucket-handle inspiration at ribs two through seven.
3. This technique might be effective in correcting a rib joint inspiration/expiration positional fault.

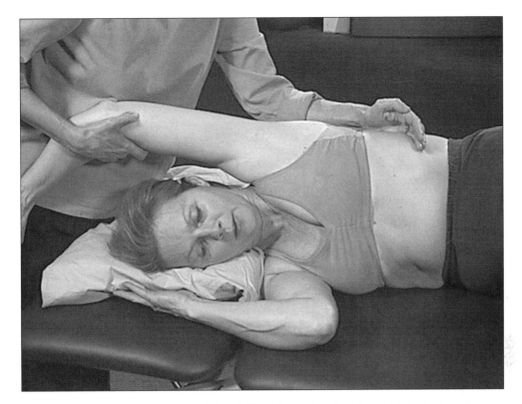

FIGURE 12-13. Inspiration glide of ribs 5 through 11/passive physiological motion.

INSPIRATION GLIDE OF RIBS 5 THROUGH 11/PASSIVE PHYSIOLOGICAL MOTION (Fig. 12-13)

Purpose
- To examine for rib joint impairment
- To increase accessory motion in the articulations at ribs 5 through 11
- To increase range of motion at ribs 5 through 11
- To decrease pain
- To improve periarticular muscle performance

Positioning
1. The patient is side lying with the arm positioned over the head.
2. The trunk is placed in midrange in relation to forward/backward bending, side bending, and rotation.
3. The clinician is at the patient's head facing the patient's trunk.
4. The mobilizing hand is positioned on the lateral surface of the trunk with the medial (ulnar) border of the hand between the rib being mobilized and the one below.
5. The guiding hand holds the patient's arm.

Procedure
1. The mobilizing hand guides the rib in a lateral and superior direction as the patient inhales and resists medial and inferior motion as the patient exhales.
2. The guiding hand controls the position of the patient's arm (see Fig. 12-13).

Particulars
1. This is not a grade V manipulation technique.
2. This technique might be especially effective for increasing range of motion into bucket-handle inspiration at ribs 5 through 11.
3. This technique might be effective in correcting a rib joint inspiration/expiration positional fault.

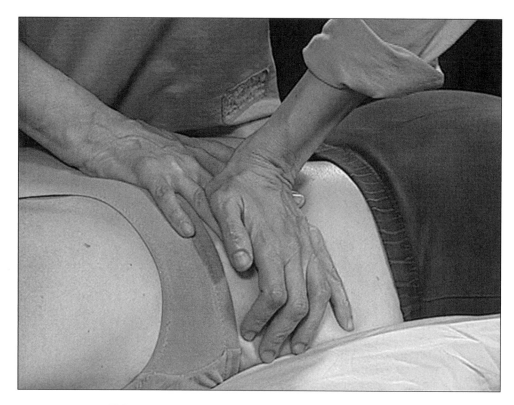

FIGURE 12-14. Anterior glide/passive accessory motion.

ANTERIOR GLIDE/PASSIVE ACCESSORY MOTION (Fig. 12-14)

Purpose

- To examine for rib joint impairment
- To increase accessory motion in the rib articulations
- To increase range of motion at the ribs
- To decrease pain
- To improve periarticular muscle performance

Positioning

1. The patient is prone.
2. The trunk is placed in midrange in relation to forward/backward bending, side bending, and rotation.
3. The clinician is at the patient's side facing the patient's trunk.
4. The mobilizing/manipulating hand is positioned with the palm of the hand over the guiding hand.
5. The guiding hand is positioned with the anterior surface of the middle or index finger on the rib being mobilized/ manipulated.

Procedure

1. The mobilizing/manipulating hand glides the rib anteriorly as the patient exhales.
2. The guiding hand controls the position of the mobilizing/manipulating hand (see Fig. 12-14).

Particulars

1. This technique might be effective in correcting a costovertebral or costotransverse joint positional fault.

REFERENCES

1. Schiller L: Effectiveness of spinal manipulative therapy in the treatment of mechanical thoracic spine pain: a pilot randomized clinical trial. J Manip Physiol Therap 2001;24:394-401.
2. Cyriax J: Textbook of Orthopaedic Medicine, Vol 1: Diagnosis of Soft Tissue Lesions, 8th ed. London, Bailliere Tindall, 1982.

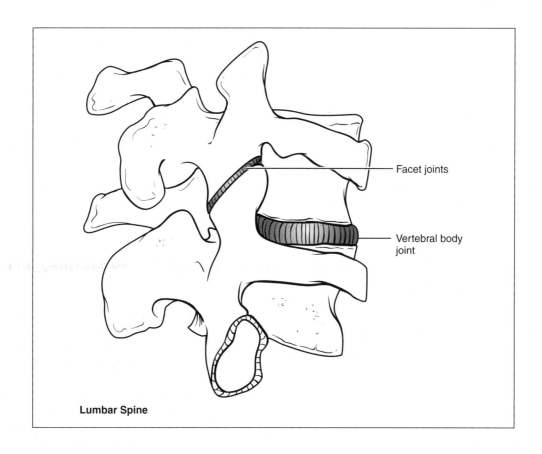

Facet joints

Vertebral body joint

Lumbar Spine

CHAPTER 13

The Lumbar Spine

BASICS

Lumbar Joints

A greater amount of motion exists in the lumbar spine than in the thoracic spine because of the absence of ribs. As in the thoracic and lower cervical joints, the degree and direction of movement in the lumbar spine are dictated by the orientation of the facet joints. The facet joints for the L1 through L4 motion segments are located in the sagittal plane, whereas the L4-5 and L5-S1 facets are aligned closely with the frontal plane. As a result, more forward and backward bending occur in the lower lumbar spine, than in the upper lumbar spine. With forward bending, both facets on the more superior lumbar vertebra glide upward, whereas with backward bending, they glide downward.

RISKS AND BENEFITS OF LUMBAR SPINE MOBILIZATION/MANIPULATION

Risk of serious injury from lumbar spinal manipulation is rare and seems to be limited to cauda equina syndrome. In one review of the literature, the risk of this injury was reported to be one per many millions of manipulations.[1] In the unlikely event that this or any other serious injury occurs, immediate medical attention is necessary to prevent or minimize permanent disability.

SPECIFIC PATHOLOGY AND LUMBAR SPINE MOBILIZATION/MANIPULATION

Mechanical Low Back Pain

Numerous studies have addressed the effect of lumbar mobilization/manipulation on low back pain. Despite the wide interest in this intervention, the methodological quality of many of these studies has been shown to be low.[2]

In a 1994 widely disseminated U.S. Public Health Service–sponsored document that was developed for the purpose of determining optimal treatment for individuals with acute low back pain, the authors made the following recommendations in relation to manipulation:[3]

> "*Manipulation can be helpful for patients with acute low back pain without radiculopathy when used within the first month of symptoms. If symptoms do not improve after one month of treatment, then the treatment should be discontinued and the patient should be reevaluated. If symptoms have been present for more than one month, manipulation is probably safe, but the efficacy of this intervention is unknown. Regardless of acuity, if the patient has radicular signs and symptoms, then there is insufficient evidence to recommend intervention with manipulation.*"

The report's conclusions regarding limiting manipulation interventions to patients without radiculopathy are consistent with a critical review addressing issues related to spinal manipulation that was published concurrently. The investigators specifically advocated performing manipulation techniques exclusively on subjects without radiculopathy.[4] Nevertheless, in a more recent study in which 40 subjects with symptomatic disc herniations were randomly assigned to receive spinal manipulation or chemonucleolysis, subjects who received manipulation experienced a significant reduction in pain and disability at two and six week follow-up. At one-year follow-up, there was no difference between the two groups.[5]

Since the publication of the U.S. Public Health Service document, numerous studies have been performed addressing the effectiveness of mobilization/manipulation for treating patients with nonspecific lower back pain. In an attempt to consolidate the information obtained from these research articles, many critical reviews also have been published. Most reviews have focused on spinal manipulation to the exclusion of mobilization techniques.

In one review, the authors concluded that there was insufficient evidence to support the use of manipulation in the treatment of low back pain. To support this statement, they cited multiple examples of inadequate methodology and conflicting results in the studies they included for review.[6]

In several critical reviews, the authors concluded that manipulation is more effective than placebo and interventions known to be ineffective or harmful in the management of patients with low back pain.[4,7,8] In one other review, the authors reported that there is some evidence supporting the use of spinal manipulation in the clinical setting,[9] whereas in another review, the authors stated that mobilization and manipulation speed recovery and increase range of motion.[10] In a different review, the authors concluded that manipulation is effective in treating acute low back pain and chronic low back pain when accompanied by spinal mobilization.[11] None of these reviews are especially helpful in making clinical decisions because they do not address the relative effectiveness of one viable intervention against that of another and therefore do not permit the reader to judge the efficacy of manipulation in relation to other treatment options.

The conclusions drawn from several additional critical reviews, although more informative, also were lacking in information on the relative effectiveness of spinal manipulation. These researchers concluded that manipulation is similar, but not superior, to other commonly used conservative interventions, such as usual care from a medical practitioner, analgesics, exercise, or back school.[12,13] This was the case regardless of the acuity of injury, whether short-term or long-term effects were being studied, or whether outcomes included pain or function.[12]

The authors of several other reviews contradicted these findings. In one of these reviews, the authors concluded that manipulation is more effective than usual care by a general practitioner, bed rest, analgesics, and massage for patients with chronic low back pain.[7] In another critical review, the stated goal was to investigate the efficacy of chiropractic manipulation. Nevertheless, the articles chosen for review were not limited to those studying chiropractic techniques or performed by chiropractors. The authors concluded that manipulation was more effective than comparative treatments for acute or subacute low back pain uncomplicated by sciatica.[15]

Studies published subsequent to the last of these critical reviews supported these findings that mobilization/manipulation is at least as effective as other interventions commonly used to treat low back pain and suggested that the effects of mobilization/manipulation might be enhanced if combined with exercise. In one of these studies, 49 subjects with chronic low back pain were randomly assigned to receive manipulation, mobilization and stretching, or exercise therapy based on the individual needs of the subject. Outcome measures included pain, disability, and return to work status. The group receiving manipulation, mobilization, and stretching showed significantly greater improvements in all outcome measures immediately after the intervention and at one-year follow-up.[16]

In a separate study, 200 subjects with subacute low back pain were randomly assigned to receive one of four interventions: back school, spinal manipulation, myofascial therapy, or combined manipulation and myofascial therapy. Outcome measures included pain and disability. Although subjects in all the groups improved, there was no difference among the four groups at three-week or six-month follow-up.[17] An explanation for these findings is that studies failed to address the effect of an appropriate combination of treatments that includes spinal mobilization/manipulation.

A much larger study was performed in which care by a general practitioner, exercise, manipulation, and manipulation followed by exercise were compared. A total of 1334 subjects with low back pain were randomly assigned to one of these four groups. The outcome measured was functional disability. The group receiving manipulation and exercise experienced the most improvement. Compared with care by a general practitioner, these subjects achieved a moderate improvement at three months and a small improvement at 12-month follow-up.[18]

Although these latter studies support using mobilization/manipulation for nonspecific low back pain, the evidence is not overwhelming. One reason might be that these researchers have failed to identify subgroups of individuals with low back pain who are most likely to benefit from mobilization/manipulation interventions. In one study, the authors addressed this issue by investigating factors associated with short-term improvement with spinal manipulation. Seventy-one subjects with low back pain without radicular signs or symptoms were treated twice with a spinal manipulation technique described in this book in Chapter 14. Functional outcome was measured using the Oswestry Disability Questionnaire. The following five variables were predictive of a positive outcome after manipulation: (1) duration of symptoms was less than 16 days, (2) at least one hip had more than 35 degrees of medial rotation, (3) one or more lumbar spine levels were hypomobile, (4) there were no symptoms distal to the knee, and (5) Fear Avoidance Behavior Questionnaire work score was less than 19 (indicating low levels of fear avoidance beliefs). The presence of four of these five variables increased the probability of successful outcome after manipulation from 45% to 95%. The investigators suggested that although the manipulation technique used in their study is commonly believed to affect the sacroiliac joint, this manipulation procedure seems to have an effect on the lumbar spine as well.[19]

One concern with this study is the possibility that patients meeting at least some of the criteria determined to be predictive of a positive outcome with manipulation would have improved regardless of the intervention. A follow-up study addressed this methodological concern by evaluating subjects for the five variables determined to predict success with spinal manipulation and randomly assigning these subjects to one of two treatment groups. A total of 131 subjects with low back pain received manipulation with exercise or exercise alone for a four-week period. The manipulation technique was the same technique performed in the original study. Disability and pain were measured at one-week, four-week, and six-month follow-up. Subjects who tested positive for four of the five criteria had a significantly greater probability of success if they received manipulation, with a 92% chance of a successful outcome. Subjects who were not positive on four of the five criteria experienced similar outcomes regardless of intervention.[20] The results of this study provide an explanation for the lack of consistency in the results of prior studies addressing the effectiveness of manipulation because in these other studies there was little attempt to restrict the sample to a homogeneous group. This study also has important implications for determining which patient is most likely to benefit from spinal manipulation.

In summary, the research supports the use of mobilization and manipulation combined with exercise for the treatment of mechanical low back pain. In relation to manipulation, this is especially evident when pain is acute, there is evidence of lumbar spine hypomobility, hip medial rotation range of motion is greater than 35 degrees, pain does not radiate below the knee, and the patient does not exhibit fear avoidance behaviors.

LUMBAR JOINTS

Osteokinematic motions:
  Forward/backward bending
  Side bending
  Rotation
Ligaments:
  Anterior longitudinal ligament
  Posterior longitudinal ligament
  Supraspinous ligament
  Interspinous ligament
  Ligamentum flavum
  Intertransverse ligaments
Joint orientation:
  Inferior facet of superior vertebra through L3-4: anterior, lateral
  Superior facet of inferior vertebra through L3-4: posterior, medial
  Inferior facet of L4-5 and L5-S1: anterior
  Superior facet of L4-5 and L5-S1: posterior
  Superior vertebral body: inferior
  Inferior vertebral body: superior
Type of joint:
  Facets: synovial
  Disc: amphiarthrodial
Concave joint surface:
  None, these are plane joints
Resting position:
  Not described by Kaltenborn
Close-packed position:
  Not described by Kaltenborn
Capsular pattern of restriction:
  Difficult to determine[20]

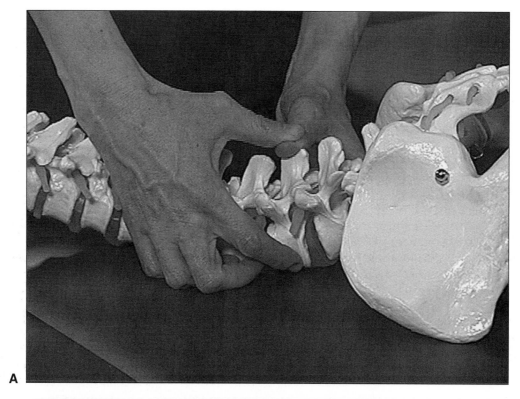

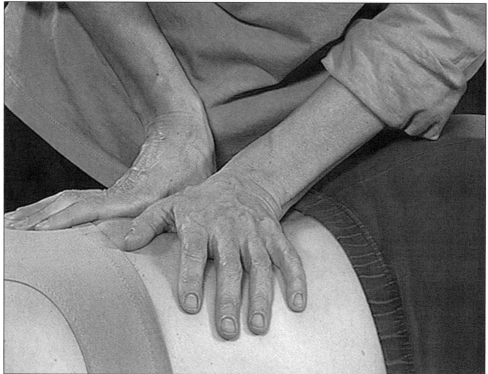

FIGURE 13-1. Anterior glide using the spinous processes/passive accessory vertebral motion.

ANTERIOR GLIDE USING SPINOUS PROCESSES/PASSIVE ACCESSORY VERTEBRAL MOTION (Fig. 13-1)

Purpose

- To examine for lumbar spine joint impairment
- To increase accessory motion into lumbar joint anterior glide
- To increase range of motion at the lumbar spine
- To decrease pain
- To improve periarticular muscle performance

Positioning

1. The patient is prone.
2. The lumbar spine is placed in midrange in relation to forward/backward bending, side bending, and rotation.
3. The clinician is at the patient's side facing the lumbar spine.
4. The mobilizing/manipulating hand is positioned with the heel of the hand or the thumb over the guiding hand.
5. The guiding hand is positioned with the thumb or the middle finger over the spinous process being mobilized/manipulated.

Procedure

1. The mobilizing/manipulating hand glides the spinous process anteriorly as the patient exhales.
2. The guiding hand controls the position of the mobilizing/manipulating hand (see Fig. 13-1).

Particulars

1. This technique also is called *springing*. If it is being performed as an examination technique, the term *spring testing* is used.
2. This technique is commonly performed using a grade V manipulation.
3. This technique has been shown to cause lumbar backward bending at the motion segment below the vertebra being mobilized/manipulated.[21]

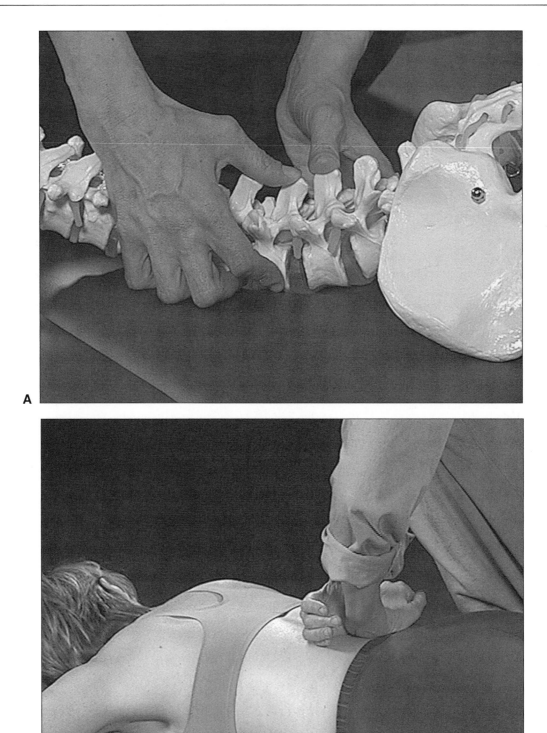

A

B

FIGURE 13-2. Superior glide using the spinous processes/passive accessory vertebral motion: first technique.

SUPERIOR GLIDE USING THE SPINOUS PROCESSES/PASSIVE ACCESSORY VERTEBRAL MOTION: FIRST TECHNIQUE (Fig. 13-2)

Purpose

- To examine for lumbar spine joint impairment
- To increase accessory motion into lumbar joint superior glide
- To increase range of motion at the lumbar spine
- To decrease pain
- To improve periarticular muscle performance

Positioning

1. The patient is prone.
2. The lumbar spine is placed in midrange in relation to forward/backward bending, side bending, and rotation.
3. The clinician is at the patient's side facing the lumbar spine.
4. The stabilizing hand is positioned with the thumb or the medial (ulnar) surface of the pisiform on the spinous process of the more superior vertebra.
5. The mobilizing/manipulating hand is positioned with the thumb or the anterior surface of the pisiform on the most inferior surface of the spinous process of the more inferior vertebra.

Procedure

1. The stabilizing hand holds the vertebra in position.
2. The mobilizing/manipulating hand glides the spinous process superiorly as the patient exhales (see Fig. 13-2).

Particulars

1. This technique might be especially effective for increasing range of motion into lumbar spine backward bending.
2. This technique might be effective in correcting a lumbar joint forward/backward bending positional fault.
3. This technique is commonly performed using a grade V manipulation.

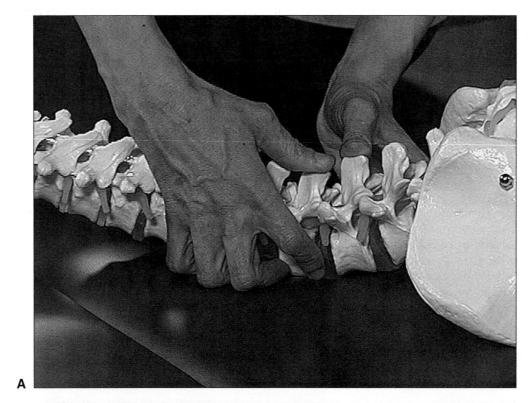

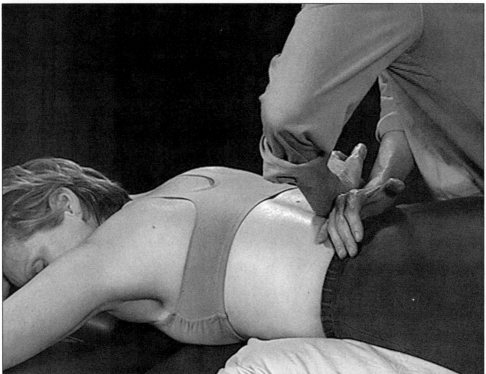

FIGURE 13-3. Superior glide using the spinous processes/passive accessory vertebral motion: second technique.

SUPERIOR GLIDE USING THE SPINOUS PROCESSES/PASSIVE ACCESSORY VERTEBRAL MOTION: SECOND TECHNIQUE (Fig. 13-3)

Purpose

- To examine for lumbar spine joint impairment
- To increase accessory motion into lumbar joint superior glide
- To increase range of motion at the lumbar spine
- To decrease pain
- To improve periarticular muscle performance

Positioning

1. The patient is prone.
2. The lumbar spine is placed in midrange in relation to forward/backward bending, side bending, and rotation.
3. The clinician is at the patient's side facing the lumbar spine.
4. The stabilizing hand is positioned with the thumb or the anterior surface of the pisiform on the spinous process of the more inferior vertebra.
5. The mobilizing/manipulating hand is positioned with the thumb or the medial (ulnar) surface of the pisiform on the most inferior surface of the spinous process of the more superior vertebra.

Procedure

1. The stabilizing hand holds the vertebra in position.
2. The mobilizing/manipulating hand glides the spinous process superiorly as the patient exhales (see Fig. 13-3).

Particulars

1. This technique might be especially effective for increasing range of motion into lumbar spine forward bending.
2. This technique might be effective in correcting a lumbar joint forward/backward bending positional fault.
3. This technique is commonly performed using a grade V manipulation.

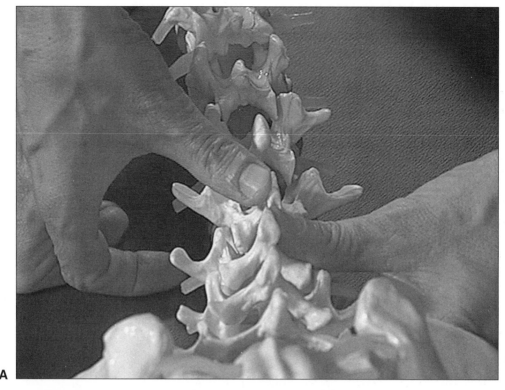

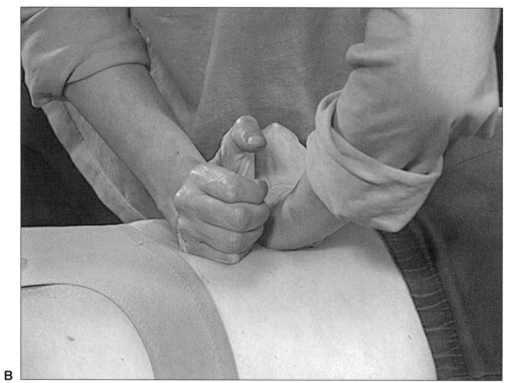

FIGURE 13-4. Lateral glide using the spinous processes/passive accessory vertebral motion.

LATERAL GLIDE USING THE SPINOUS PROCESSES/PASSIVE ACCESSORY VERTEBRAL MOTION (Fig. 13-4)

Purpose

- To examine for lumbar spine joint impairment
- To increase accessory motion into lumbar vertebral body rotation and into facet joint distraction on the side toward which the vertebral body is rotating
- To increase range of motion at the lumbar spine
- To decrease pain
- To improve periarticular muscle performance

Positioning

1. The patient is prone.
2. The lumbar spine is placed in midrange in relation to forward/backward bending, side bending, and rotation.
3. The clinician is at the patient's side facing the lumbar spine.
4. The stabilizing hand is positioned with the thumb or the anterior surface of the pisiform on the lateral surface of the spinous process of the more inferior vertebra.
5. The mobilizing/manipulating hand is positioned with the thumb on the medial (ulnar) surface of the pisiform on the lateral surface of the spinous process of the more superior vertebra opposite the side of the stabilizing hand.

Procedure

1. The stabilizing hand holds the more inferior vertebra in position.
2. The mobilizing/manipulating hand glides the more superior spinous process toward the contralateral side as the patient exhales (see Fig. 13-4).

Particulars

1. This technique might be especially effective for increasing range of motion into lumbar spine rotation in the direction of vertebral body movement (in the direction opposite the movement of the spinous processes).
2. This technique might be effective in correcting a lumbar joint rotation positional fault.
3. This technique is commonly performed using a grade V manipulation.

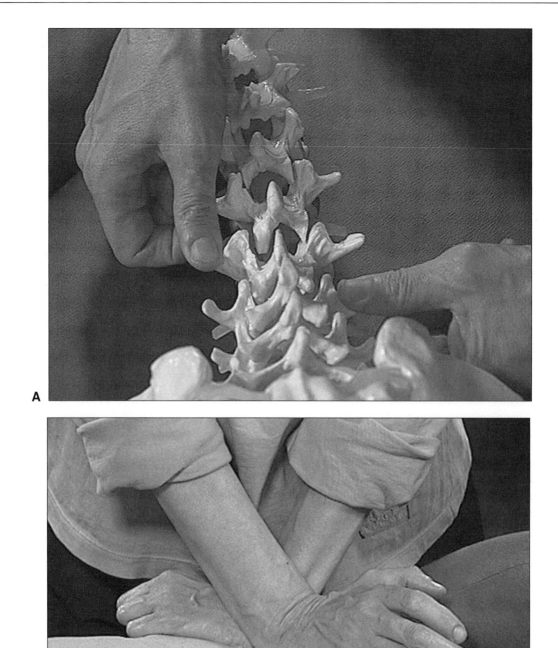

FIGURE 13-5. Anterior glide using the transverse processes/passive accessory vertebral motion.

ANTERIOR GLIDE USING THE TRANSVERSE PROCESSES/PASSIVE ACCESSORY VERTEBRAL MOTION (Fig. 13-5)

Purpose

- To examine for lumbar spine joint impairment
- To increase accessory motion into lumbar vertebral body rotation and into facet joint distraction on the side toward which the vertebral body is rotating
- To increase range of motion at the lumbar spine
- To decrease pain
- To improve periarticular muscle performance

Positioning

1. The patient is prone.
2. The lumbar spine is placed in midrange in relation to forward/backward bending, side bending, and rotation.
3. The clinician is at the patient's side facing the lumbar spine.
4. The stabilizing hand is positioned with the thumb or the anterior surface of the pisiform on the transverse process of the more inferior vertebra.
5. The mobilizing/manipulating hand is positioned with the thumb or the anterior surface of the pisiform on the transverse process of the more superior vertebra opposite the side of the stabilizing hand.

Procedure

1. The stabilizing hand holds the more inferior vertebra in position.
2. The mobilizing/manipulating hand glides the more superior transverse process in an anterior direction as the patient exhales (see Fig. 13-5).

Particulars

1. The L5-S1 motion segment cannot be treated with this technique because the iliac crest obscures the transverse processes.
2. This technique might be especially effective for increasing range of motion into lumbar spine rotation in the direction of vertebral body movement.
3. This technique might be effective in correcting a lumbar joint rotation positional fault.
4. This technique is commonly performed using a grade V manipulation.

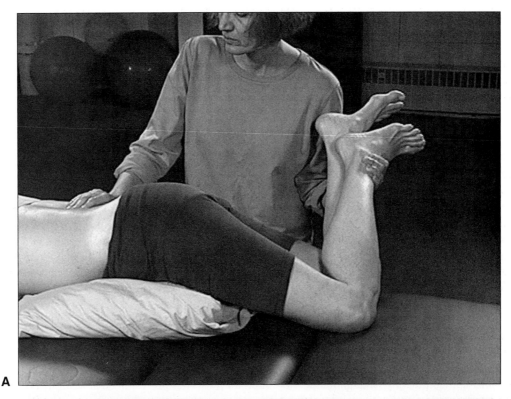

A

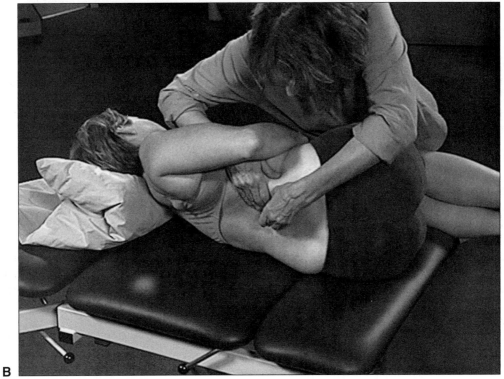

B

FIGURE 13-6. Rotation glide/passive physiological vertebral motion.

ROTATION GLIDE/PASSIVE PHYSIOLOGICAL VERTEBRAL MOTION (Fig. 13-6)

Purpose

- To increase accessory motion into lumbar vertebral body rotation and into facet joint distraction on the side toward which the patient is rotating
- To increase range of motion at the lumbar spine
- To decrease pain
- To improve periarticular muscle performance

Positioning

1. The patient is lying on the side not being treated with the arm resting over the clinician's mobilizing/manipulating arm.
2. The lumbar spine is placed in midrange in relation to forward/backward bending, side bending, and rotation.
3. The clinician is at the side of the treatment table facing the patient's anterior trunk.
4. A pillow can be used to separate the patient's chest from the clinician.
5. The clinician locks the more inferior vertebrae by bringing the patient's knees toward the chest to the extent that the motion segment below the one being mobilized/manipulated is fully flexed, but the motion segment being mobilized/manipulated has not yet moved.
6. The clinician next locks the more superior vertebrae by rotating the upper trunk away from the clinician (and in the direction of the intended vertebral body motion) to the extent that the motion segment above the one being mobilized/manipulated is fully rotated, but the motion segment being mobilized/manipulated has not yet moved.
7. One hand is positioned with the middle finger on the lower lateral surface of the spinous process (the side of the spinous process closest to the treatment table) of the more inferior vertebra and the forearm on the patient's pelvis.
8. The other hand is positioned with the thumb on the upper lateral surface of the spinous process (the side of the spinous process farthest away from the treatment table) of the more superior vertebra and the forearm or elbow anterior and medial to the patient's shoulder.

Procedure

1. The clinician's hand on the more inferior vertebra glides the spinous process upward as the forearm rotates the pelvis forward and the patient exhales.
2. The clinician's hand on the more superior vertebra simultaneously glides the spinous process downward as the forearm rotates the upper trunk backward (see Fig. 13-6B).

Particulars

1. The examination procedure for this technique differs from the intervention procedure. To examine for joint mobility into rotation, the patient is positioned prone with both knees bent to 90 degrees. The clinician is facing the side of the patient's trunk and holds the patient's legs in position at the ankles. The clinician palpates the L5-S1 motion segment by placing the palpating finger between the L5 and S1 spinous processes. With the patient's knees bent, the clinician, moves the patient's ankles toward the clinician, keeping the knees bent rotating the lumbar spine in the same direction in which the ankles are moving. The clinician palpates for motion between L5 and S1 and grades the amount of motion into rotation that occurred. After grading the motion, the clinician restores slack to the L5-S1 motion segment by moving the ankles slightly back toward midline and moves the palpating finger to the L4-5 motion segment. This process is repeated until motion into rotation at all lumbar vertebral motion segments is graded. Mobility into left and right rotation is graded (see Fig. 13-6A).
2. The intervention technique might be especially effective for increasing range of motion into lumbar spine rotation in the direction of vertebral body movement.
3. The intervention technique has been shown to distract the lumbar facet joints.[23]
4. Since this intervention technique also produces distraction of the facet joints, it might also be effective in increasing range of motion into lumbar forward/backward bending and side bending.
5. To examine for joint mobility into forward/backward bending, the patient is positioned side lying with both knees bent. The clinician faces the patient's anterior trunk and holds the patient's legs in position by grasping the ankles and positioning the patient's knees on the clinician's proximal thigh. With the patient's knees bent, the clinician palpates the L5-S1 motion segment by placing the palpating finger between the L5 and S1 spinous processes. The clinician flexes the patient's hips, forward bending the lumbar spine. The clinician palpates for motion between L5 and S1 and grades the amount of motion into flexion that occurred. After grading the motion, the clinician

restores slack to the L5-S1 motion segment by moving the hips slightly into extension and moves the palpating finger to the L4-5 motion segment. This process is repeated until motion into forward bending at all lumbar vertebral motion segments is graded. It is repeated for backward bending. Examination for backward bending motion is best performed with the clinician positioned behind the patient. The examination process for side bending motion is described in the next section, entitled Side Bending Glide/Passive Physiological Vertebral Motion.

6. The intervention technique might be effective in correcting a lumbar joint rotation positional fault.
7. The intervention technique is commonly performed using a grade V manipulation.
8. The clinician can direct most of the mobilizing/manipulating force to the spinous processes if it is important for the motion to be localized to the motion segment being treated, or the clinician can direct most of the mobilizing/manipulating force through the pelvis and trunk if it is not as important for the motion to be localized to the motion segment being treated.
9. Alternatively, if this intervention is appropriate for all the lumbar joints, the clinician can direct the force exclusively through the pelvis and trunk.

SIDE BENDING GLIDE/PASSIVE PHYSIOLOGICAL VERTEBRAL MOTION (Fig. 13-7)

Purpose

- To increase accessory motion into lumbar vertebral body side bending
- To increase range of motion at the lumbar spine
- To decrease pain
- To improve periarticular muscle performance

Positioning

1. The patient is prone.
2. The lumbar spine is placed in midrange in relation to forward/backward bending, side bending, and rotation.
3. The clinician is at the side of the treatment table facing the patient's thigh.
4. The clinician locks the more inferior vertebrae by abducting the hip to the extent that the motion segment below the one being mobilized/manipulated is fully side bent, but the motion segment being mobilized/manipulated has not yet moved.
5. The stabilizing hand is positioned with the thumb or middle finger on either side of the lateral surface of the more superior spinous process.
6. The mobilizing/manipulating hand is positioned on the medial surface of the distal thigh with the clinician's arm and trunk supporting the patient's lower leg.

Procedure

1. The stabilizing hand holds the vertebra in position.
2. The mobilizing/manipulating hand brings the leg into more abduction (see Fig. 13-7B).

Particulars

1. The examination procedure for this technique differs from the intervention procedure. The patient is positioned side lying facing the clinician with both knees bent. The clinician faces the patient's anterior trunk and holds the patient's legs in position by grasping the ankles and positioning the patient's knees on the clinician's proximal thigh. With the patient's knees bent, the clinician palpates the L5-S1 motion segment by placing the palpating finger between the L5 and S1 spinous processes. The clinician flexes the patient's hips, forward bending the lumbar spine. The clinician palpates for motion between L5 and S1 and grades the amount of motion into side bending that occurred. After grading the motion, the clinician restores slack to the L5-S1 motion segment by moving the hips slightly into extension. The clinician lifts the patient's ankles upward, side bending the lumbar spine in the same direction as the direction in which the legs are moving. After grading the motion, the clinician restores slack to the L5-S1 motion segment by moving the ankles back into the original position and moving the hips slightly into extension. The clinician moves the palpating finger to the L4-5 motion segment. This process is repeated until motion into side bending at all lumbar vertebral motion segments is graded. Mobility into left and right side bending is graded (see Fig. 13-7A).
2. The intervention technique should be performed only if movement at the motion segments below the one being mobilized/manipulated can be eliminated or if movement at these segments would not have any adverse effects.
3. The intervention technique might be especially effective for increasing range of motion into lumbar spine side bending in the direction of vertebral body movement.

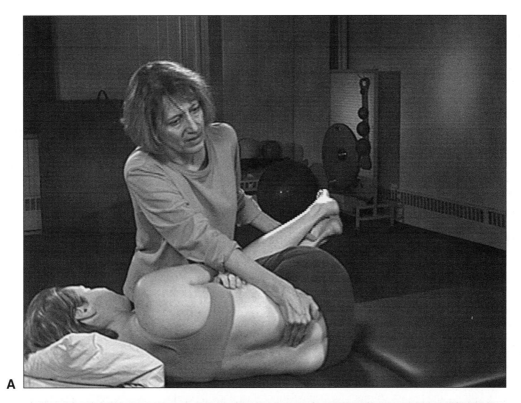

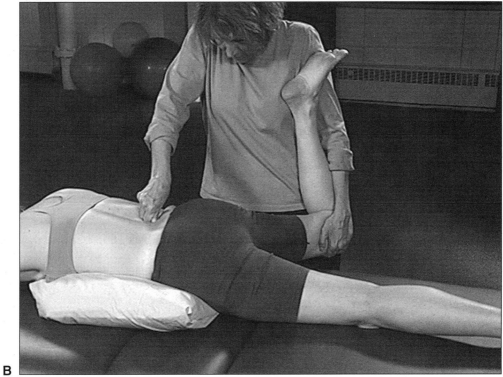

FIGURE 13-7. Side bending glide/passive physiological vertebral motion.

REFERENCES

1. Assendelft WJJ, Bouter LM, Knipschild PG: Complications of spinal manipulation: a comprehensive review of the literature. J Fam Pract 1996;42:475-480.
2. Koes BW, Bouter LM, van der Heijden JMG: Methodological quality of randomized clinical trials on treatment efficacy in low back pain. Spine 1995;20:228-235.
3. Bigos S, Bowyer O, Braen G, et al: Acute Low Back Problems in Adults. ACHPR Publication No. 95-0642. Rockville, Md, Agency for Health Care Policy and Research, Public Health Service, U.S. Department of Health and Human Services, 1994.
4. Shekelle PG: Spine update: spinal manipulation. Spine 1994;19:858-861.
5. Burton AK, Tillotson KM, Cleary J: Single-blind randomized controlled trial of chemonucleolysis and manipulation in the treatment of symptomatic lumbar disc herniation. Eur Spine J 2000; 9:202-207.
6. Koes BW, Assendelft WJJ, van der Heijden JMG, et al: Spinal manipulation for low back pain: an updated systematic review of randomized clinical trials. Spine 1996;21:2860-2873.
7. van Tulder MW, Koes BW, Bouter LM: Conservative treatment of acute and chronic nonspecific low back pain: a systematic review of randomized controlled trials of the most common interventions. Spine 1997;22:2128-2156.
8. Fiechtner JJ, Brodeur RR: Manual and manipulation techniques for rheumatic disease. Rheum Dis Clin North Am 2000;26:83-96.
9. Haigh R, Clarke AK: Effectiveness of rehabilitation for spinal pain. Clin Rehabil 1999;13(suppl):63-81.
10. Twomey L, Taylor J: Spine update: exercise and spinal manipulation in the treatment of low back pain. Spine 1995;20:615-619.
11. Bromfort G: Spinal manipulation: current state of research and its indications. Neurol Clin North Am 1999;17:91-111.
12. Assendelft WJJ, Morton SC, Yu EI, et al: Spinal manipulative therapy for low back pain: a meta-analysis of effectiveness relative to other therapies. Ann Intern Med 2003;138:871-881.
13. Cherkin DC, Sherman KJ, Deyo RA, et al: A review of the evidence for the effectiveness, safety and cost of acupuncture, massage therapy, and spinal manipulation for back pain. Ann Intern Med 2003;138:898-906.
14. Mohseni-Bandpei MA, Stephenson R, Richardson B, et al. Spinal manipulation in the treatment of low back pain; a review of the literature with particular emphasis on randomized controlled clinical trials. Phys Ther Reviews 1998;3:185-194.
15. Coulter ID: Efficacy and risks of chiropractic manipulation: what does the evidence suggest? Integr Med 1998;1:61-66.
16. Aure OF, Hoel Nilsen J, Vasseljen O: Manual therapy and exercise therapy in patients with chronic low back pain: a randomized, controlled trial with 1-year follow-up. Spine 2003;28:525-531.
17. Hsieh C-YJ, Adams AH, Tobis J, et al: Effectiveness of four conservative treatments for subacute low back pain: a randomized clinical trial. Spine 2002;27:1142-1148.
18. UK BEAM Team Trial: UK Back Pain Exercise and Manipulation (BEAM) randomized trial: effectiveness of physical treatments for back pain in primary care. BMJ 2004;329:1377-1380.
19. Flynn T, Fritz J, Whitman J, et al: A clinical prediction rule for classifying patients with low back pain who demonstrate short-term improvement with spinal manipulation. Spine 2002;27:2835-2843.
20. Childs JD, Fritz JM, Flynn TW, et al: A clinical prediction rule to identify patients with low back pain most likely to benefit from spinal manipulation: a validation study. Ann Intern Med 2004;141:920-928.
21. Cyriax J: Textbook of Orthopaedic Medicine, Vol 1: Diagnosis of Soft Tissue Lesions, 8th ed. London, Bailliere Tindall, 1982.
22. Kulig K, Landel R, Powers C: Assessment of lumbar spine kinematics using dynamic MRI: a proposed mechanism of sagittal plane motion induced by manual posterior-to-anterior mobilization. J Orthop Sports Phys Ther 2004;34:57-61.
23. Cramer GD, Gregerson DM, Knudsen JT, et al: The effects of side-posture positioning and spinal adjusting on the lumbar Z joints: a randomized controlled trial with sixty-four subjects. Spine 2002;27:2459-2466.

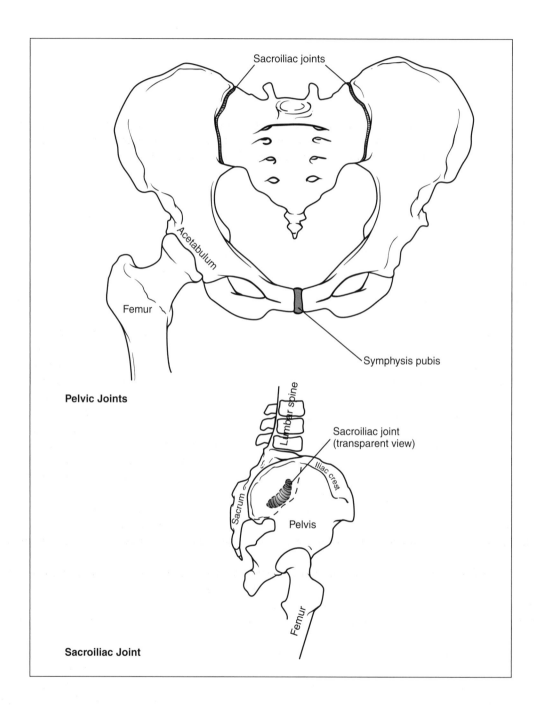

Sacroiliac joints

Acetabulum

Femur

Symphysis pubis

Pelvic Joints

Lumbar spine

Sacroiliac joint
(transparent view)

Iliac crest

Sacrum

Pelvis

Femur

Sacroiliac Joint

CHAPTER 14

Pelvic Joints

BASICS

The pelvis consists of three joints: two sacroiliac joints and one pubic joint. Since these joints are configured in the formation of a ring, impairment at one joint could easily cause impairment at one or more of the other pelvic joints. Movement at these three joints is minimal and does not depend on muscular control.

Sacroiliac Joints

Motion at the sacroiliac joints is greater in women and decreases with age in both sexes. The decrease in motion occurs from progressive roughening of the iliac articular surfaces.

Despite the fact that pelvic joint motion has been investigated in numerous studies, there is little consensus regarding the specifics of movement at this joint. The most commonly used joint mobilization/manipulation techniques address the movements of posterior and anterior rotation of the ilium on the sacrum. The direction of rotation (posterior or anterior) is defined by the movement of the iliac crests. These two motions are classified as specific types of *iliosacral joint motion,* even though the joint itself is referred to as the sacroiliac joint. Conversely, movement of the sacrum on the ilium is called *sacroiliac joint motion*. The most commonly referenced sacroiliac joint motion mobilization/manipulation techniques address the motions of flexion (also called *nutation*) and extension (also called *counternutation*) of the sacrum on the iliac articulations. Sacral flexion and extension are determined by the direction of motion of the superior surface of the sacrum in relation to the sacral inferior surface. Sacral flexion occurs when the superior surface of the sacrum moves in an anterior direction and extension occurs when the superior surface moves in a posterior direction. Most sources agree that posterior rotation of the ilium entails the same joint movement as sacral flexion, and anterior rotation of the ilium entails the same joint movement as sacral extension. These two movements, iliosacral posterior/anterior rotation and sacroiliac flexion/extension, are differentiated from one another by the number of joints moving. If the motion occurs at one sacroiliac joint, or is asymmetrical, the motion is described as iliac posterior or anterior rotation (iliosacral joint motion) and is accompanied by motion at the symphysis pubis. If simultaneous and symmetrical motion occurs at both sacroiliac joints, the motion is described as sacral flexion or extension (sacroiliac joint motion).

Motion at the sacroiliac joint is affected by movement at adjacent joints. For example, it is likely that increasing the lumbar lordosis causes sacroiliac joint flexion, whereas unilateral hip flexion causes iliosacral joint posterior rotation.

The etiology and prevalence of sacroiliac joint impairment have been studied widely, with little consensus. One problem with studies of sacroiliac joint impairment is the insufficient reliability and validity of tests commonly used to identify and isolate sacroiliac joint impairment from other low back pain conditions, possibly because these tests rely heavily on palpation of minute asymmetries of the position and motion of pelvic and lower extremity bony landmarks.

Nevertheless, many clinicians believe that sacroiliac joint impairment is often a result of joint hypermobility, resulting in a positional fault. When a positional fault is identified, the recommended treatment is a mobilization/manipulation technique performed in the direction opposite the direction of the positional fault. The most commonly described positional fault occurs when one ilium rotates in a posterior or anterior direction on the sacrum. Numerous other positional faults of the ilium and the sacrum have been described in the literature, but they are not as frequently acknowledged as sources of sacroiliac joint impairment as positional faults involving anterior and posterior rotations.

This approach to evaluating and treating sacroiliac joint pain has been challenged by some researchers, who argue that the tests designed to identify the presence and direction of a sacroiliac joint positional fault have not been shown to be reliable. The validity of this approach also has been called into question by studies in which there were no demonstrable changes in the position of the ilium on the sacrum after manipulation. In one of these studies, positional changes were measured by stereophotogrammetric analysis,[1] whereas in another study, measurements were taken using a slide pointer.[2]

These conclusions were not supported by results of a different study, in which changes in alignment were evident after manipulation, when measured using calipers. In this study, subjects were included only if they had positive results for at least three of four specific tests of sacroiliac joint impairment.[3] Although the result of this latter study provides some validation for the use of manipulation for the treatment of sacroiliac joint impairment, the study results do not provide insight into determining the appropriate direction of the mobilization/manipulation force.

As a result of these issues, some clinicians have proposed that sacroiliac joint impairment be identified by the presence of a positive result on several sacroiliac joint tests and treated with a nonspecific manipulation procedure. Since the identification of sacroiliac joint impairment has been shown to improve when several examination procedures designed to evaluate for sacroiliac joint impairment are positive, this approach addresses the issue of correct identification of a sacroiliac joint condition. Furthermore, it does not require that the clinician correctly identify the direction of the positional fault. This approach to the evaluation and treatment of sacroiliac joint impairments has been shown to be effective in several studies, and are described below.

Symphysis Pubis

Sacroiliac joint movement is believed to produce motion at the symphysis pubis. This motion is most often described as a gliding movement in a superior/inferior direction, although pivoting of the two articular surfaces also has been hypothesized.

SPECIFIC PATHOLOGY AND SACROILIAC JOINT MOBILIZATION/ MANIPULATION

Sacroiliac Joint Pain

Several investigators have studied the effect of a manipulation procedure that is commonly used to treat patients with sacroiliac joint impairment. Subjects were included in these studies if they had low back pain that was classified into a treatment-oriented category that the investigators called *extension/mobilization*. Classification into this category was determined by responses to lumbar movement and sacroiliac joint tests. Specifically, subjects must have experienced pain that either decreased or centralized with movement into extension, and must have had a positive response to three of four sacroiliac joint tests: the standing forward bending test, supine-long-sitting test, prone knee bend test, and asymmetrical anterior and posterior superior iliac crest height in the sitting position. In the first study, subjects were randomly assigned to receive extension exercises and manipulation or flexion exercises. Subjects receiving extension and manipulation responded with a significantly greater decrease in pain and increase in function than subjects receiving flexion exercises.[4] To determine whether these results occurred from the manipulation or the exercise program, a second study was performed. Subjects were randomly assigned to receive either manipulation with flexion and extension exercises or specific exercises into extension. Subjects receiving manipulation and exercises into flexion and extension responded with a greater decrease in pain and increase in function than subjects receiving specific extension exercises.[5] Evidently, manipulation and exercise is more effective in treating pain and functional limitations than exercise alone in this subcategory of patients.

Hip Pain

In a study of 20 runners with reports of hip pain and evidence of sacroiliac joint impairment, subjects were randomly assigned to receive inferior glide mobilization to the hip or manipulation to the sacroiliac joint. At follow-up, subjects receiving the sacroiliac joint manipulation had significantly less pain than the group receiving hip mobilization.[6]

SACROILIAC JOINTS

Osteokinematic motions:
    Ilium: anterior/posterior rotation
    Sacrum: extension/flexion

Ligaments:
    Posterior sacroiliac ligaments (transverse, oblique, longitudinal)
    Anterior sacroiliac ligament
    Iliolumbar ligament
    Sacrospinous ligament
    Sacrotuberous ligament
Joint orientation:
    Sacrum: lateral, posterior
    Ilia: medial, anterior
Type of joint:
    Part synovial, part syndesmotic
Concave joint surface:
    None, this is a plane joint
Resting position:
    Not described by Kaltenborn
Close-packed position:
    Not described by Kaltenborn
Capsular pattern of restriction:
    Pain when the joints are stressed[7]

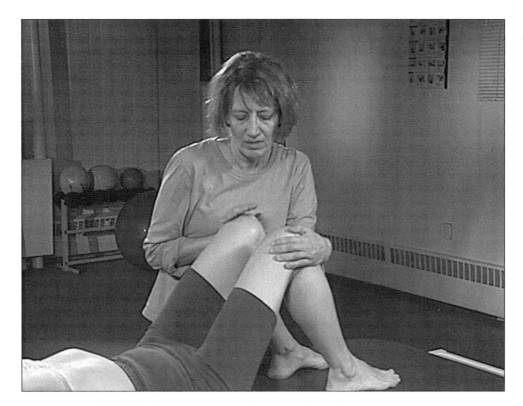

FIGURE 14-1. Distraction of the sacroiliac joint/muscle energy.

DISTRACTION OF THE SACROILIAC JOINT/MUSCLE ENERGY (Fig. 14-1)

Purpose

- To increase accessory motion into sacroiliac joint distraction
- To increase range of motion at the sacroiliac joint
- To decrease pain
- To improve periarticular muscle performance

Positioning

1. The patient is supine with the knees bent, feet flat on the treatment table, and hips abducted.
2. The spine and pelvis are placed in midrange in relation to forward/backward bending, side bending, and rotation.
3. The clinician is at the patient's side facing the pelvis.
4. Both hands are positioned such that each hand is on the lateral surface of each of the patient's knees.

Procedure

1. The clinician instructs the patient to perform an isometric contraction of the abductors by resisting a force provided by the clinician into hip adduction, thus distracting the iliac joint surfaces away from the sacrum as the abductors contract and pull on their attachments to the iliac crest.
2. This contraction is held for approximately 5 seconds.
3. The clinician brings the hips into more adduction.
4. This procedure can be repeated several times (see Fig. 14-1).

Particulars

1. The determination of the appropriateness of this technique involves evaluating the results of several tests of sacroiliac joint impairment.
2. This technique might be effective in correcting an iliosacral joint positional fault.

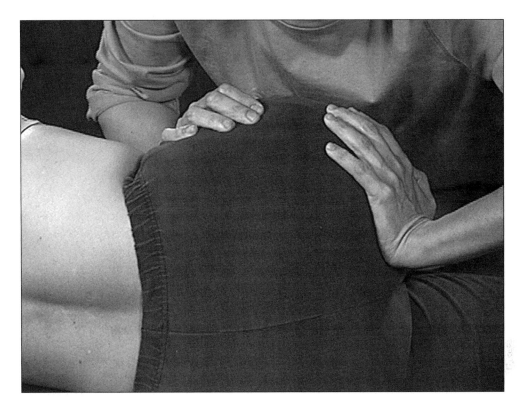

FIGURE 14-2. Posterior glide of the iliac crest/passive accessory vertebral motion.

POSTERIOR GLIDE OF THE ILIAC CREST/PASSIVE ACCESSORY VERTEBRAL MOTION (Fig. 14-2)

Purpose

- To examine for iliosacral joint impairment
- To increase accessory motion in the sacroiliac joint
- To increase range of motion at the sacroiliac joint
- To decrease pain
- To improve periarticular muscle performance

Positioning

1. The patient is lying on the unaffected side, with the hip on the side to be mobilized/manipulated in flexion and the contralateral hip in extension.
2. The sacroiliac joint is approximating the restricted range into posterior rotation.
3. The clinician is at the patient's side facing the anterior pelvis.
4. The mobilizing/manipulating hand is on the patient's anterior superior iliac spine and the anterior surface of the iliac crest.
5. The guiding hand is on the patient's ischium.

Procedure

1. The clinician applies a grade I traction to the joint by lifting the pelvis slightly with the arms of the mobilizing/manipulating and guiding hands.
2. The mobilizing/manipulating hand glides the anterior superior iliac spine and the anterior surface of the iliac crest in a posterior direction.
3. The guiding hand guides the ischium anteriorly (see Fig. 14-2).

Particulars

1. This technique might be effective in correcting an iliosacral joint anterior rotation positional fault.

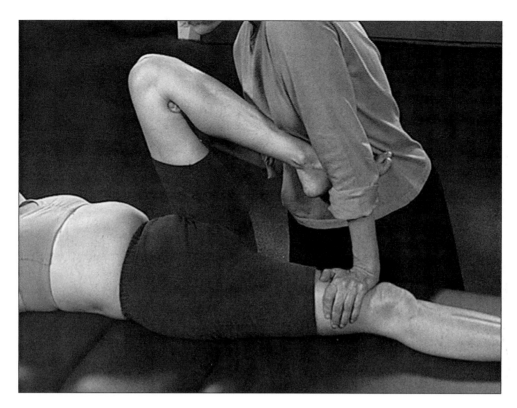

FIGURE 14-3. Posterior glide/muscle energy.

POSTERIOR GLIDE/MUSCLE ENERGY (Fig. 14-3)

Purpose

- To increase accessory motion in the sacroiliac joint
- To increase range of motion at the sacroiliac joint
- To decrease pain
- To improve periarticular muscle performance

Positioning

1. The patient is supine, with the side to be mobilized positioned with the hip flexed to the end of the available range and the unaffected side positioned with the hip extended.
2. The unaffected side can be positioned with the knee flexed off the edge of the treatment table.
3. The sacroiliac joint is approximating the restricted range into posterior rotation.
4. The clinician is at the patient's knee facing the pelvis.
5. The stabilizing hand is positioned on the anterior surface of the distal thigh on the unaffected side.
6. The mobilizing hand is positioned on the posterior surface of the distal thigh on the affected side with the clinician's trunk reinforcing the hand position.

Procedure

1. The clinician instructs the patient to perform an isometric contraction of the gluteus maximus by resisting a force provided by the clinician into hip flexion, thus gliding the pelvis into posterior rotation as the gluteus maximus contracts and pulls on its attachment to the posterior surface of the ilium.
2. This contraction is held for approximately 5 seconds.
3. The clinician next brings the hip into more flexion until an increase in resistance is met.
4. This procedure can be repeated several times (see Fig. 14-3).

Particulars

1. The patient can be taught to perform this technique as part of a home program.
2. The determination of the appropriateness of this technique involves evaluating the results of several tests of sacroiliac joint impairment.
3. This technique might be effective in correcting an iliosacral joint anterior rotation positional fault.

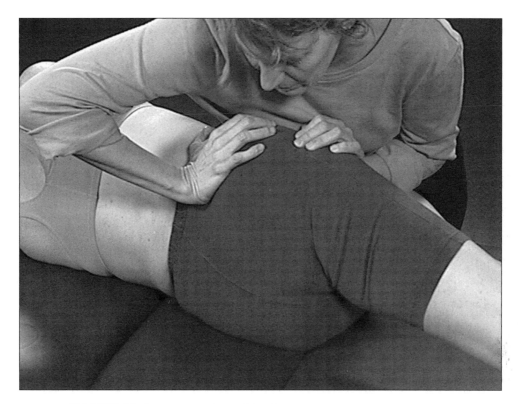

FIGURE 14-4. Anterior glide of the iliac crest/passive accessory motion.

ANTERIOR GLIDE OF THE ILIAC CREST/PASSIVE ACCESSORY MOTION (Fig. 14-4)

Purpose

- To examine for iliosacral joint impairment
- To increase accessory motion in the sacroiliac joint
- To increase range of motion at the sacroiliac joint
- To decrease pain
- To improve periarticular muscle performance

Positioning

1. The patient is lying on the unaffected side, with the hip on the side to be mobilized/manipulated in extension and the contralateral hip in flexion.
2. The sacroiliac joint is approximating the restricted range into anterior rotation.
3. The clinician is at the patient's side facing the anterior pelvis.
4. The mobilizing/manipulating hand is positioned over the posterior surface of the iliac crest.
5. The guiding hand is on the anterior and lateral surface of the pelvis distal to the anterior superior iliac spine.

Procedure

1. The clinician applies a grade I traction to the joint by lifting the pelvis slightly with the arms of the mobilizing/ manipulating and guiding hands.
2. The mobilizing/manipulating hand glides the iliac crest anteriorly.
3. The guiding hand guides the anterior and lateral surface of the pelvis posteriorly (see Fig. 14-4).

Particulars

1. This technique might be effective in correcting an iliosacral joint posterior rotation positional fault.

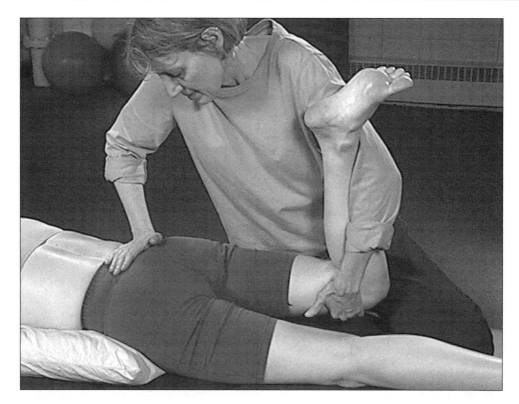

FIGURE 14-5. Anterior glide/muscle energy.

ANTERIOR GLIDE/MUSCLE ENERGY (Fig. 14-5)

Purpose

- To increase accessory motion in the sacroiliac joint
- To increase range of motion at the sacroiliac joint
- To decrease pain
- To improve periarticular muscle performance

Positioning

1. The patient is prone, with the side to be mobilized positioned with the hip extended and the knee flexed. The unaffected side can be positioned with the hip flexed off the edge of the treatment table.
2. The sacroiliac joint is approximating the restricted range into anterior rotation.
3. The clinician is at the patient's knee facing the pelvis.
4. The mobilizing hand is positioned over the posterior surface of the iliac crest.
5. The guiding hand is on the anterior surface of the distal thigh with the clinician's arm or trunk supporting the patient's lower leg.

Procedure

1. The clinician lifts the thigh off of the treatment table and instructs the patient to perform an isometric contraction of the rectus femoris by resisting a force provided by the clinician into hip extension and knee flexion, thus gliding the pelvis into anterior rotation as the rectus femoris contracts and pulls on its attachment to the anterior inferior iliac spine.
2. This contraction is held for approximately 5 seconds.
3. The clinician next brings the hip into more extension and the knee into more flexion until an increase in resistance is met.
4. This procedure can be repeated several times (see Fig. 14-5).

Particulars

1. The determination of the appropriateness of this technique involves evaluating the results of several tests of sacroiliac joint impairment.
2. This technique might be effective in correcting an iliosacral joint posterior rotation positional fault.

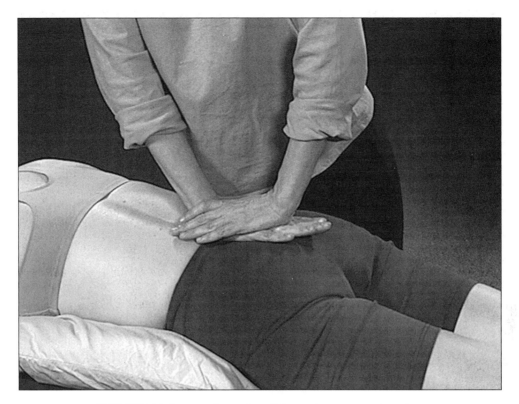

FIGURE 14-6. Sacral anterior glide/passive accessory motion.

SACRAL ANTERIOR GLIDE/PASSIVE ACCESSORY MOTION (Fig. 14-6)

Purpose

- To examine for sacroiliac joint impairment
- To increase accessory motion in the sacroiliac joint
- To increase range of motion at the sacroiliac joint
- To decrease pain
- To improve periarticular muscle performance

Positioning

1. The patient is prone.
2. The spine and pelvis are placed in midrange in relation to forward/backward bending, side bending, and rotation.
3. The clinician is at the patient's side facing the pelvis.
4. The heel of the mobilizing/manipulating hand is positioned over the superior surface of the sacrum.
5. The guiding hand is positioned over the mobilizing/manipulating hand.

Procedure

1. The mobilizing/manipulating hand glides the superior surface of the sacrum anteriorly, directing the sacrum into flexion (nutation).
2. The guiding hand controls the position of the mobilizing/manipulating hand (see Fig. 14-6).

Particulars

1. This technique might be effective in correcting a sacroiliac joint positional fault.

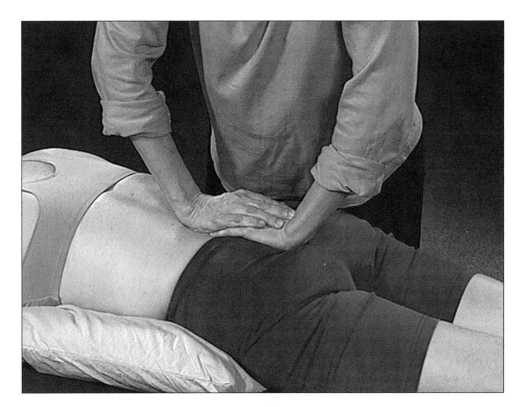

FIGURE 14-7. Sacral posterior glide/passive accessory motion.

SACRAL POSTERIOR GLIDE/PASSIVE ACCESSORY MOTION (Fig. 14-7)

Purpose
- To examine for sacroiliac joint impairment
- To increase accessory motion in the sacroiliac joint
- To increase range of motion at the sacroiliac joint
- To decrease pain
- To improve periarticular muscle performance

Positioning
1. The patient is prone.
2. The spine and pelvis are placed in midrange in relation to forward/backward bending, side bending, and rotation.
3. The clinician is at the patient's side facing the pelvis.
4. The heel of the mobilizing/manipulating hand is positioned over the inferior surface of the sacrum.
5. The guiding hand is positioned over the mobilizing/manipulating hand.

Procedure
1. The mobilizing/manipulating hand glides the inferior surface of the sacrum anteriorly, directing the sacrum into extension (counternutation).
2. The guiding hand controls the position of the mobilizing/manipulating hand (see Fig. 14-7).

Particulars
1. This technique might be effective in correcting a sacroiliac joint positional fault.

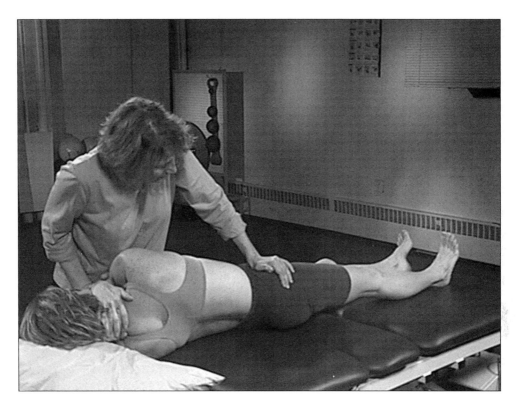

FIGURE 14-8. Rotation glide/manipulation/passive physiological vertebral motion.

ROTATION GLIDE/MANIPULATION/PASSIVE PHYSIOLOGICAL VERTEBRAL MOTION (Fig. 14-8)

Purpose
- To decrease pain in the sacroiliac and lumbar regions
- To improve periarticular muscle performance

Positioning
1. The patient is supine with the fingers laced together at the base of the neck and the elbows touching.
2. The spine and pelvis are placed in midrange in relation to forward/backward bending, side bending, and rotation.
3. The clinician is at the patient's asymptomatic side facing the pelvis.
4. The clinician side bends the patient away from the clinician and then rotates the patient's upper trunk toward the clinician, using the patient's folded arms as a fulcrum.
5. The stabilizing hand holds the patient's arms in position on the treatment table, maintaining the upper trunk in rotation.
6. The manipulating hand is positioned over the anterior superior iliac spine.

Procedure
1. The stabilizing hand holds the upper trunk in position.
2. The manipulating hand thrusts the anterior superior iliac spine in a posterior, lateral, and inferior direction (see Fig. 14-8).

Particulars
1. The determination of the appropriateness of this technique involves evaluating the results of several tests of sacroiliac joint impairment.
2. This technique should be performed using grade V manipulations.

3. This technique has been shown to be effective with a treatment-based classification subgroup of patients defined as *extension/manipulation*.[4,5]

4. This technique has been shown to be effective with patients with nonradicular low back pain[8,9] (see Chapter 13).

5. This technique might be effective in correcting an iliosacral joint rotation positional fault.

SYMPHYSIS PUBIS

Osteokinematic motion:
    None
Ligament:
    Arcuate ligament
Joint orientation:
    Both pubic bones: medial
Type of joint:
    Syndesmotic
Concave joint surface:
    None, this is a plane joint
Resting position:
    Not described by Kaltenborn
Close-packed position:
    Not described by Kaltenborn
Capsular pattern of restriction:
    Pain when the joints are stressed[7]

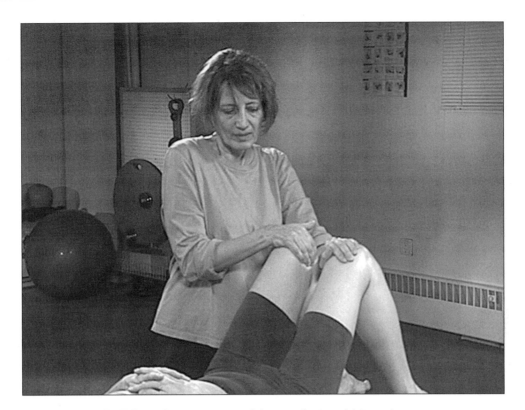

FIGURE 14-9. Distraction of the symphysis pubis/muscle energy.

DISTRACTION OF THE SYMPHYSIS PUBIS/MUSCLE ENERGY (Fig. 14-9)

Purpose

- To increase accessory motion into symphysis pubis joint distraction
- To increase range of motion at the symphysis pubis
- To decrease pain
- To improve periarticular muscle performance

Positioning

1. The patient is supine with the knees bent, feet flat on the treatment table, and hips adducted.
2. The spine and pelvis are placed in midrange in relation to forward/backward bending, side bending, and rotation.
3. The clinician is at the patient's side facing the pelvis.
4. Both hands are positioned such that each hand is on the medial surface of each of the patient's knees.

Procedure

1. The clinician instructs the patient to perform an isometric contraction of the adductors by resisting a force provided by the clinician into hip abduction, thus distracting the symphysis pubis joint surfaces away from one another as the adductors contract and pull on their attachments to the pubic rami.
2. This contraction is held for approximately 5 seconds.
3. The clinician brings the hips into more abduction until an increase in resistance is met.
4. This procedure can be repeated several times (see Fig. 14-9).

Particulars

1. The determination of the appropriateness of this technique involves evaluating the results of palpation and spring testing of the pubis symphysis.
2. This technique might be effective in correcting a symphysis pubis positional fault.

REFERENCES

1. Tullberg T, Blomberg S, Branth B, et al: Manipulation does not alter the position of the sacroiliac joint: a roentgen stereophotogrammetric analysis. Spine 1998;23:1124-1128.
2. Smith RL, Sebastian BA, Gajdosik RL: Effect of sacroiliac joint mobilization on the standing position of the pelvis in healthy men. J Orthop Sports Phys Ther 1988;10:77-84.
3. Cibulka MT, Delitto A, Koldehoff RM: Changes in innominate tilt after manipulation of the sacroiliac joint in patients with low back pain: an experimental study. Phys Ther 1988;68:1359-1363.
4. Delitto A, Cibulka MT, Erhard RE, et al: Evidence for an extension/mobilization category in acute low back pain: a prescriptive validity pilot study. Phys Ther 1993;73:216-228.
5. Erhard R, Delitto A, Cibulka MT: Relative effectiveness of an extension program and a combined program of manipulation and flexion and extension exercises in patients with acute low back syndrome. Phys Ther 1994;74:1093-1100.
6. Cibulka MT, Delitto A: A comparison of two different methods to treat hip pain in runners. J Orthop Sports Phys Ther 1993;17:172-176.
7. Cyriax J: Textbook of Orthopaedic Medicine, Vol 1: Diagnosis of Soft Tissue Lesions, 8th ed. London, Bailliere Tindall, 1982.
8. Flynn T, Fritz J, Whitman J, et al: A clinical prediction rule for classifying patients with low back pain who demonstrate short-term improvement with spinal manipulation. Spine 2002;27:2835-2843.
9. Childs JD, Fritz JM, Flynn TW, et al: A clinical prediction rule to identify patients with low back pain most likely to benefit from spinal manipulation: a validation study. Ann Intern Med 2004;141:920-928.

Index

Note: Page numbers followed by f indicate figures; those followed by t indicate tables.

344

Rotation glide—*cont'd*
of lumbar joints, 310f, 311–312
of sacroiliac joint, 327–328, 327f
of thoracic joints, 284f, 285

S

Sacral anterior glide, 325, 325f
Sacral extension, 317
Sacral flexion, 317
Sacral posterior glide, 326, 326f
Sacroiliac joints, 316f, 317–328
anterior glide/muscle energy for, 324, 324f
capsular pattern of restriction of, 319
distraction/muscle energy for, 320, 320f
extension/mobilization of, 318
iliac crest of
anterior glide/passive accessory motion of,
323, 323f
posterior glide/passive accessory motion of,
321, 321f
impairment of, 10, 317–318
and hip pain, 318
ligaments of, 319
motion at, 317
orientation of, 319
osteokinematic motions of, 318
pain in, 317–318
positional faults of, 317
posterior glide/muscle energy for, 322, 322f
rotation glide/manipulation/passive
physiological vertebral motion of, 327–328,
327f
sacral anterior glide/passive accessory motion
of, 325, 325f
sacral posterior glide/passive accessory motion
of, 326, 326f
Scapulothoracic joint, 37, 50–57
concave surface of, 50
distraction of, 51, 51f
inferior glide of, 54f, 55
lateral glide of, 57, 57f
medial glide of, 56, 56f
orientation of, 50
osteokinematic motions of, 50
superior glide of, 52f, 53
Sellar joints, 23, 25f
Shoulder joint(s), 36–66, 36f
acromioclavicular, 36f, 37, 63–66
anterior glide of, 65, 65f
posterior glide of, 64, 64f
superior glide of acromion on clavicle of, 66,
66f
adhesive capsulitis of, 38
glenohumeral, 36f, 37, 38–49
anterior glide of, 46f, 47, 48f, 49
decreased range of motion of, 38

Shoulder joint(s)—*cont'd*
distraction of, 40f, 41
inferior glide of, 42f, 43
posterior glide of, 44f, 45
impingement syndrome of, 38
nonspecific pain in, 38
scapulothoracic, 37, 50–57
distraction of, 51, 51f
inferior glide of, 54f, 55
lateral glide of, 57, 57f
medial glide of, 56, 56f
superior glide of, 52f, 53
specific pathology of, 37–38
sternoclavicular, 36f, 37, 58–62
anterior glide of clavicle on sternum of, 62,
62f
inferior glide of, 60, 60f
posterior glide of, 61, 61f
superior glide of, 59, 59f
Side bending glide
of lower cervical joints, 262f, 263
with passive physiological vertebral motion,
262f, 263
of lumbar joints, 312, 313f
of thoracic joints, 286f, 287
Side glide, of lower cervical joints, with passive
accessory vertebral motion, 258f, 259
Somatic dysfunction, 3
Spinal joint(s), 225–228
appendicular *vs.*, 225
coupled motion in, 227–228
disc herniation of, reduction of, 11–12
evaluation *vs.* intervention for, 227
joint locking for, 226–227
motion of, 225
passive accessory *vs.* passive physiologic, 226
precautions and contraindications to
mobilization/manipulation of, 13–14,
225–226
range of motion of, 8
springing of, 227
terminology for, 225
Spinning, 22, 22f
Spinous processes
cervical
anterior glide/passive accessory vertebral
motion using, 248f, 249
anterior/superior glide/passive accessory
vertebral motion using, 250f, 251, 252f, 253
lateral glide/passive accessory vertebral
motion using, 254f, 255
lumbar
anterior glide using, 300f, 301
lateral glide using, 306f, 307
superior glide using, 302f, 303, 304f, 305
thoracic, 267